Aggregatibacter actinomycetemcomitans: A D-3 (Dysbiosis, Damage, Disease) Periodontal Pathobiont

Aggregatibacter actinomycetemcomitans: A D-3 (Dysbiosis, Damage, Disease) Periodontal Pathobiont

Guest Editor

Daniel H. Fine

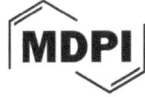

Basel • Beijing • Wuhan • Barcelona • Belgrade • Novi Sad • Cluj • Manchester

Guest Editor
Daniel H. Fine
Department of Oral Biology
School of Dental Medicine
Rutgers, The State University
of New Jersey
Newark, NJ
USA

Editorial Office
MDPI AG
Grosspeteranlage 5
4052 Basel, Switzerland

This is a reprint of the Special Issue, published open access by the journal *Pathogens* (ISSN 2076-0817), freely accessible at: https://www.mdpi.com/journal/pathogens/special_issues/CYI2W1LM71.

For citation purposes, cite each article independently as indicated on the article page online and as indicated below:

Lastname, A.A.; Lastname, B.B. Article Title. *Journal Name* **Year**, *Volume Number*, Page Range.

ISBN 978-3-7258-3063-3 (Hbk)
ISBN 978-3-7258-3064-0 (PDF)
https://doi.org/10.3390/books978-3-7258-3064-0

Contents

About the Editor

Daniel H. Fine

Daniel H. Fine, DMD is Professor & Chair of the Department of Oral Biology in Rutgers School of Dental Medicine (RSDM) & Senior Associate Dean in The School of Graduate Studies at Rutgers University. Dr. Fine attained a Doctor of Dental Medicine in 1965 from the University of Pennsylvania, a certificate in Periodontology and Oral Medicine from New York University in 1967. He began his career at the University of Pittsburgh as an Instructor in Periodontology and a Research Associate in the Department of Microbiology. Dr. Fine joined Columbia School of Dental and Oral Surgery in 1970 as a Post-Doctoral student in the Department of Pathology and Cell Biology at Columbia University College of Physicians and Surgeons (PNS). He became a tenured faculty in the School of Dentistry in 1977 and Professor in 1987. Dr. Fine's was a (1) Visiting Scientist (Guy's Hospital, London from 1979–1980), (2) NIH Senior Research Fellow PNS 1988–1990, and (3) a Visiting Scientist in 2006 at the American Museum of Natural History in Molecular/Microbial Evolution & Genomics. Dr. Fine's research focuses on genetic regulation of bacterial virulence and pathogenicity. His studies converge on Localized Aggressive Periodontitis (now Stage III Grade C periodontitis) and *Aggregatibacter actinomycetemcomitans*. He has published close to 200 scientific articles, had over 70 funded grants from the National Institutes of Health and industry and has been invited speaker at Universities nationally & internationally.

Preface

The preface to this Special Issue includes a summary of each of the 12 articles contained within the Special Issue that puts each contribution into a logical framework and acknowledges each author's gracious contribution. The over-arching goal of the Special Issue is to illustrate how studies of Localized Aggressive Periodontitis (LAgP) and its association with *Aggregatibacter actinomycetemcomitans* have moved the field forward and contributed to progress in infectious disease research in general.

The aim of this Special Issue is to present microbial factors related to the dysbiosis, damage, and "disease" associated with *A. actinomycetemcomitans*, a microbe resulting in a unique form of inflammatory periodontal disease that occurs predominantly in children and adolescents of African descent. A World Workshop Consensus Conference (WWCC) held in 2017 eliminated "Localized Aggressive Periodontitis" (LAgP) as a distinct disease and lumped it into a category called Stage III/Grade C Periodontitis. This new classification ignores the age-related occurrence and familial distribution that characterizes LAgP. The WWCC decision made by a mere majority of participants provided the motivation to delve into (1) the way in which consensus conferences are typically conducted, (2) how this conference deviated from consensus conference standards, and (3) the impact the WWCC decisions have had and will continue to have on research and scholarship as a result of the deviations from standards used by other branches of the health sciences.

After reviewing broadly accepted criteria developed for other comparable consensus conferences, it became clear that the WWCC decision was ill-advised. Publications 6 years prior to the WWCC new classification were compared to publications from the 6 years following the conference decision. Web-based searches in pertinent databases using mesh terms LAgP, Aggressive Periodontitis, Periodontitis, and Stage III/Grade C Periodontitis were conducted. A significant decrease in publications for "Aggressive Periodontitis" and LAgP were seen in the 6 years following the WWCC re-classification whereas a considerable increase in publications with the more general term "Periodontitis" were seen over this same time span (Fine et al., 2024). Few publications explored the well-defined disease previously called LAgP. Thus the WWC conference failed (1) to discuss the standards of agreement required for consensus prior to the conference, and (2) to present the "dissenting point of view" in the published document. This Special Issue of *Pathogens* was designed to encourage our community to maintain a classification for this unique disease. The significant association of *A. actinomycetemcomitans* and its relationship to the initiation and progression of LAgP are emphasized in this Special Issue. Furthermore, two overlapping audiences of the health profession are addressed: (1) those involved in academic and scholarly pursuits, tasked with organizing consensus conferences, and (2) those involved in providing clinical care to patients who wish to equip themselves with a comprehensive understanding as to how summary decisions can guide current and future ways of dealing with the diagnosis, prevention, and treatment of a disease.

Contribution 1 is an overall editorial (Fine, 2024), while contributions 2–4 are more clinical in nature and point to the importance of recognition of the distinction between the newly named Stage III, Grade C periodontitis that melds several forms of periodontal diseases as opposed to separating LAgP and other forms of more slowly progressive periodontal disease that occur in adults (Fine et al., 2024, Miguel and Shaddox, 2024, Ryder et. al., 2024). Each of these contributions describe how this unique form of disease in children and adolescents should be viewed.

In Contribution 2 (Fine et al., 2024), the focus is on the pressing need to re-instate the classification of this unique disease as a distinct entity since its recent elimination in a World Workshop Consensus Conference (WWCC). This paper challenges the WWCC decision to remove Localized Aggressive Periodontitis (LAgP) as a disease classification in spite of its unique clinical and microbiological features that separate it from adult forms of periodontitis. The paper describes how the new Staging and Grading system advocated by the WWCC minimizes the importance of specific diagnostic assessments of disease and lumps all forms of periodontitis into Stages and Grades. This paper attributes the failure to make distinctions between LAgP and other forms of periodontal disease is due to the use of inaccurate/overlapping case definitions used in the recent WWCC doctrine. The paper proposes that the new definition of disease has already, and will continue to, have a dramatic impact on research and scholarly activity as well as treatment choices. The paper proposes a need to re-think this WWCC shift in classification based on considerations such as (1) the age of onset, (2) the rapidity of tissue destruction, (3) the localized nature of the disease, and (4) the familial patterns of inheritance which are unique to this disease (formerly called LAgP). It appears as if these distinctive factors have been overlooked by the WWCC. The paper then assesses the influence of this new classification on progress in this field of research by considering articles published using PubMed, Scopus, and The World Wide Web that examine publications 6 years prior to the WWCC re-classification as compared to publications 6 years following this change. In addition to these considerations, the strength of the association of *A. actinomycetemcomitans* in conjunction with a unique microbial consortium that includes *Filifactor alocis* and other oral micro-organisms is also presented as a rationale for re-instating LAgP as a distinct disease entity. Features of *A. actinomycetemcomitans* are evaluated using the Bradford Hill criteria, that document how this oral microbe can adapt to various environments, influence its biofilm neighbors, and move through the blood and lymphatics that attest to its relevance in oral and non-oral diseases. With this line of reasoning presented, the paper suggests that the use of inaccurate/overlapping case definitions should be abandoned and more accurate definitions re-instated. In addition, the paper proposes that clinicians weigh treatment success as the time from treatment to relapse of infection to more accurately gauge (1) reversal or continuance of local disease and (2) reduction in the possibility for spread of these highly adaptable microbes to sites distant from the oral cavity. As such, the paper proposes that existing measurements of overall reduction in periodontal tissue destruction include "extended-time to return of disease", or relapse as a worthy treatment goal *. At this moment, since several longitudinal studies have identified a distinctive microbial consortium that includes *A. actinomycetemcomitans* that precede this disease, these characteristics could be tested, along with potential biomarkers, as potential diagnostic tools in efforts to distinguish this unique disease from generalized adult periodontitis. * (Note that on page 24 (Fine et al., 2024) case B describes a 20 mm reduction which should be a .20 mm reduction).

Contribution 3 provides support for the uniqueness of the disease now classified as Stage III Grade C periodontitis (Miguel and Shaddox, 2024). A review of several studies illustrate that the Localized Grade C disease may not be restricted to the permanent dentition. In fact, the diagnosis of this aggressive, rapidly progressing form of periodontitis may be detected early in primary and mixed dentitions in patients with permanent Grade C/Molar/Incisor Periodontitis (C-MIP disease). The paper also presents data showing that periodontal treatment in the primary dentition can lead to a favorable clinical response that can lead to a healthy permanent dentition. Moreover, the paper provides data showing that early *A. actinomycetemcomitans* colonization plays an important role in C-MIP development (RR = 7.3), increasing the risk of bone loss either with JP2 (OR = 14.3) or non-JP2 genotypes (OR = 3.4) of the species. In these instances, *A. actinomycetemcomitans*' high prevalence is observed in both primary and permanent dentitions (85% and 71%, respectively).

Along with *A. actinomycetemcomitans*, *F. alocis* and *P. gingivalis*, *T. denticola*, and *T. forsythia* seem to also play a significant role in this disease. Furthermore, the paper points out that the subgingival biofilm in periodontally healthy children retained these periodontopathogens even after biofilm maintenance was performed in the adult parents, suggesting a possible contribution of microbial risk derived early-on from family members. It can also be surmised that familial aggregation of this disease implies a genetic predisposition, which is also suggested by a hyperinflammatory response to bacterial LPS in healthy siblings. Biomarkers for bone loss, cytokines, and chemokines associated with disease may also be found in clinically healthy siblings of affected parents. Since periodontitis is typically seen in adults and rarely seen in children and adolescents, this important paper highlights the critical relevance of early diagnosis especially in this aggressive form of disease. In many diseases, age is considered to be an important characteristic of disease susceptibility. This paper uniquely illustrates how early age is an important feature of this form of aggressive periodontitis and describes genetic, biologic, and microbiological evidence of disease in children and adolescents. Furthermore, as is the case with juvenile diabetes, an age-associated disease, diagnosis and therapy can be improved if age is factored into the diagnostic criteria in Grade C/MIP. In summary, this paper provides strong support for the need to restore a definitive classification so that early diagnosis and appropriate therapies can be used to better define cases for continuing research and successful treatment.

Contribution 4 describes the geography of the oral microbiome on a global (macro) level and local (micro) level, and in so doing, the authors address *A. actinomycetemcomitans* and its ethnic, racial, and familial distribution in Localized Aggressive Periodontitis, a rapidly progressive disease, as well as its intraoral distribution at first molar and incisor sites (Ryder et al., 2024). They also discuss other pathobionts and their positioning in the plaque biofilm and how this positioning can affect disease. In this review, the authors remind readers that this pathobiont and its more pathogenic clone, the JP2 clone, a "b" serotype that expresses excessive levels of leukotoxin, originated in Mediterranean Africa and moved from Western Africa to the Americas due in part to the patterns of the slave trade. Furthermore, this paper reports on studies showing that the microbe can be transferred from mother to child, contributing to data suggesting that the disease occurs in young children. An interesting description of plaque biofilm formation on a local geographical level is also described in this paper that presents both a philosophical and biological characterization of disease. Moreover, the paper describes local geography in plaque and points to the importance of considering geographical proximity, chemical communication among microbes, as well as biological interactions for both the benefit and detriment of biofilm members.

Contributions 5 and 6 focus on *A. actinomycetemcomitans* and point to the importance of growth phase, media, and strain variation in the assessment of in vitro virulence traits and their impact on disease.

In Contribution 5, the authors present information about how *A. actinomycetemcomitans* strain D7S-1 (wild-type rough colony) and D7SS (isogenic smooth variant of D7S-1) react to nutrient deficiencies (Tjokro et al., 2024). The assumption in this study is that laboratory conditions that study strains in enriched media mis-represent "natural/challenging" growth conditions that occur in vivo. To this end, the authors tested the growth of a clinical strain, D7S-1, and an isogenic laboratory strain, D7SS, in nutrient-deficient (ND) and nutrient-limited (NL) media as compared to a nutrient-enriched (NE) laboratory medium and then studied the effects of these growth conditions on the viability of these strains. Viability is evaluated by culturing, and cell morphology as assessed by both Transmission and Scanning Electron Microscopy. As expected, bacteria in NE exhibit typical growth phases, ending in the death phase. In contrast, *A. actinomycetemcomitans* strains grown in

NL and ND media, following the stationary phase, display a dormancy-like phenotype with minimal growth but prolonged viability up to 15 days. These studies open the door to examining genes related to this dormancy phenotype, which may be similar to the phenotype of *A. actinomycetemcomitans* in vivo.

In Contribution 6, Kalfas and colleagues (2024) examine leukotoxin (LtxA) production by different strains of *A. actinomycetemcomitans* under different growth conditions, finding that LtxA that attacks leukocytes, causing the release of Il-1, while LtxA's reaction with macrophages can provoke the release of the NLRP3 inflammasome resulting in LtxA-induced death. The focus of this study is on various strains (Y-4, b serotype non-JP2; SUNYab&75, serotype a; NCTC 9710, serotype c; and HK 1519, serotype b/JP2), growth conditions (PYG vs. BM broth), and growth phases (late logarithmic and stationary phase) leading to LtxA production. Both cells with LtxA attached and cell-free LtxA were examined. The JP2 strain showed the greatest level of LtxA production, which was not affected by growth phase in the cell free state but did show greater levels of LtxA in stationary phase in both PYG and BM media. The Y4 strain showed slightly higher levels of LtxA in BM in the stationary phase but was always lower than the HK1519 strain. In LtxA that was cell attached the levels of LtxA in HK 1519 growth was higher in the stationary phase, while Y 4 showed lower growth when compared to the JP2 strain. PMN lysis was assessed via release of lactate dehydrogenase. The *cagE* gene has the potential for elevated LtxA, and perhaps since Y4 lacks the *cagE* gene and HK1519 has this gene, the authors postulate that it is possible that this gene deletion accounts for the difference in LtxA levels seen between these two strains. However, more evidence is needed.

Contributions 7 and 8 are related to *A. actinomycetemcomitans* and its association with systemic diseases. Contribution 6 describes emaA, an autotransporter protein that adheres to injured heart valves and can act as a contributor to infectious endocarditis, while Contribution 7 describes a study of *A. actinomycetemcomitans* and its association with Rheumatoid Arthritis.

In Contribution 7, Mintz et al. (2024) investigate the role of a proteinaceous surface structure of *A. actinomycetemcomitans* in infective endocarditis. The relationship between oral bacteria and infective endocarditis, a disease of the endocardial surface of the heart, is well established. Binding of bacteria to underlying matrix proteins or platelets activate circulating platelets which leads to fibrin deposition. The subsequent formation of an infective mass or vegetation, composed of bacteria and coagulation byproducts, disrupts blood flow through the heart. Infective endocarditis is typically associated with Gram-positive organisms. However, a minority of cases are associated with Gram-negative bacteria. *A. actinomycetemcomitans*, a Gram-negative bacterium, has been implicated in the causation of this disease. This association occurs despite the low prevalence of *A. actinomycetemcomitans* in the adult population, implying a more frequent level of *A. actinomycetemcomitans* than expected in adult patients diagnosed with infective endocarditis. A gene, extracellular matrix protein adhesin A (*emaA*) encoding a 200,000 MW protein was identified by a loss of function transposon mutagenesis screen. This gene product mediates the binding of *A. actinomycetemcomitans* to specific types of collagen, an abundant protein found in the extracellular matrix of most tissues. Furthermore, EmaA binds to native collagen and induces disease in a well-established rabbit endocarditis model. The individual protein monomers are synthesized and targeted to the membrane by an extraordinarily long signal sequence and are transported across the inner membrane. The carboxyl termini of three protein monomers form a pore in the outer membrane through which the passenger domains are transported for presentation on the outer surface of the bacterium. Based on sequence and structural homology, EmaA is assigned to the class of type V secreted proteins, which form non-fimbrial oligomeric, coil–coil adhesins, and includes YadA of Yersiniae species as a prototypic member. In this chapter, the authors (Mintz et al., 2024) summarize a series of elegant studies investigating the known biochemical, molecular, and structural aspects of this protein including collagen binding and biofilm formation, and how this adhesin contributes to the pathogenicity of this organism.

Contribution 8 was designed to determine whether the presence of antibody to *A. actinomycetemcomitans* in saliva or serum could be associated with an increased prevalence of Rheumatoid Arthritis (Svard et al., 2024) This study provides another way of considering evidence of the association of *A. actinomycetemcomitans* with Rheumatoid Arthritis (RA) as presented by Konig et al., (2016) and where data suggest that *A. actinomycetemcomitans*, in particular, was distinct from other periodontal pathogens in triggering the dysregulation of citrullinating enzymes in neutrophils resembling autoantibody activity in joint fluid obtained from RA patients. That paper (Konig et al., 2016) showed that *A. actinomycetemcomitans* species induced hypercitrullination in host neutrophils that mimics autoantigen citrullination in the RA joint and that antibodies to LtxA are enhanced in RA patients as compared to healthy controls (ref). It was difficult to discern in that paper whether the decision to examine patients with *A. actinomycetemcomitans* was somewhat biased in that the authors claimed that *A. actinomycetemcomitans* or products derived from it were tied to RA as opposed to reactions from other oral bacteria. Results derived from gingival crevice fluid from patients with disease had reactions derived from LtxA from *A. actinomycetemcomitans*, and in particular, these fluids induced hypercitrullination similar to that seen in RA joints. Furthermore, it should be pointed out that the patients studied by these authors were older than those typically seen to carry *A. actinomycetemcomitans*, and although they showed levels of reactions to LtxA and serum antibody to LtxA, their in vitro studies were related to PMN degradation and netosis by LtxA. A second paper (Gomez-Banuelos et al., 2020) did not show an association with IgG antibody to LtxA and RA in any stage of RA disease; therefore, the authors suggested a time of transition from asymptomatic to RA disease status. They showed the existence of some relationship of IgM to LtxA, suggested as pre-symptomatic for RA. Svard and co-authors (2024) approached this question in a different manner by examining a group of RA patients regardless of their *A. actinomycetemcomitans* status and determined what percent of RA patients had serum or saliva antibody to *A. actinomycetemcomitans* among these subjects. The authors very clearly pointed to the limitations of their study, since the RA patients assessed showed a very low level of *A. actinomycetemcomitans* in both saliva and serum as compared to healthy controls. So, unlike the Konig et al. paper (2016), in the Svard et al. paper, subjects with LtxA producing *A. actinomycetemcomitans* were minimal, not dominant, and not related to the disease (RA). For the purposes of this Special Issue, however, the Svard et al., (2024) paper provides a good reference to the fact that *A. actinomycetemcomitans*, as has been reported previously, occurs in low levels in otherwise periodontally healthy patients or patients who are not defined as LAgP subjects. This data contrasts to the array of data that show that *A. actinomycetemcomitans* is uniformly present as a necessary member of the consortia found in patients who are younger and diagnosed with LAgP.

Contributions 9 and 10 focus on two prominently important virulence factors, cytolethal distending toxin and complement resistance factors possessed by *A. actinomycetemcomitans* that have an effect on the early stages of periodontal disease. These factors affect the epithelial cell lifestyle, which can result in microbial invasion, as well as ApiA, a trimeric autotransporter protein related to autoaggregation, epithelial cell binding, and complement resistance.

In Contribution 9, it is proposed that *A. actinomycetemcomitans* cytolethal distending toxin (Cdt) acts as a perilous accessory pathogenic trait that can be responsible for translocation of *A. actinomycetemcomitans* from the gingival space through the gingival epithelium into the underlying connective tissue (Shenker et al., 2024). This penetration enables substances to progress further via blood vessels and lymphatics to distant organs. The authors describe how Cdt an *A. actinomycetemcomitans* exotoxin, composed of three proteins subunits, Cdt A, B and C, can cause epithelial senescence and also affects lymphocytes, macrophages, and mast cells. Three unique properties are described for Cdt, as follows: (1) exploitation of cholesterol as a pervasive cell receptor; (2) engagement with the host cell protein, cellugyrin, via a combination of Cdt B and C that affects cell entry and trafficking; and (3) blockade of the PI-3K signaling pathway. Cdt-induced gingival epithelial senescence involves the acquisition of a new phenotype characterized by sustained cell cycle (G2/M) arrest and accumulation of senescence-associated beta galactosidase (SA-beta-gal), lipofuscin, and cytokines, the latter collectively known as the senescence-associated secretory phenotype (SASP). The authors propose that Cdt-induced gingival epithelia senescence leads to altered epithelial barrier integrity and, in turn, alterations in the subgingival microflora.

In Contribution 10, a paper is presented that studies ApiA, a multi-functional trimeric autotransporter protein that is produced by *A. actinomycetemcomitans* (Jacob et al., 2024). While ApiA in *A. actinomycetemcomitans* was first described in the early 2000s, little new information has emerged that specifically defines its importance in complement resistance. In this paper, Jacob and colleagues (2024) have chosen to focus their attention on surface-related ApiA complement functionality, which includes autoaggregation and epithelial cell binding. Gene regions within *apiA* that correspond to autoaggregation, epithelial cell binding, and complement resistance are described in an *Escherichia coli* host. The paper focuses on the relationship of ApiA to the alternative pathway of complement resistance which was first described 20 years ago by Asakawa et al. (2003) but the specific region of this gene responsible for serum resistance was not well defined and has been elusive. This study was designed to define the gene regions related to epithelial cell attachment and autoaggregation, with a special emphasis on the alternative complement pathway and Factor H binding. Factor H originated as a host protein that protects human cells from complement induced cell pore formation and death. Over the years, bacterial cells have evolved a mechanism of hijacking Factor H to protect themselves from complement sensitivity. This paper has identified a 12 mer derived from ApiA that binds Factor H and thus resists both complement sensitivity and cell death. When examined in *A. actinomycetemcomitans*, *apiA* expression is tied to the regulation of several prominent *A. actinomycetemcomitans* adaptability genes that include *oxyR*, *katA*, *ompA1*, and *ompA2*. This work opens the door to a better understanding of the role of complement resistance in the early stages of periodontal inflammation.

Contributions 11 and 12 illustrate how understanding of microbial factors can lead to transformative therapeutic approaches far removed from typical dental diseases. These approaches include inventions derived from exploration of *A. actinomycetemcomitans* virulence factors that have been applied to staphylococcal infections and cancer-related lymphomas.

In Contribution 11, the focus is on dispersin B, a broad-spectrum anti-biofilm glycoside hydrolase derived from *A. actinomycetemcomitans* (Kaplan et al., 2024). Biofilms form from densely packed microbial communities that attach to surfaces and shield the inner core of microbes from otherwise hazardous biocide interactions. Dispersin B, a biofilm-degrading enzyme, disassembles the biofilm polysaccharide poly-β(1–6)-*N*-acetylglucosamine (PNAG), thereby freeing cells in the inner core of the biofilm and permitting these cells to migrate to vulnerable sites distant from the original biofilm. This paper proposes that dispersin B is therefore more useful in preventing biofilm development as opposed to the treatment of existing biofilms. For commercialization, a dispersin B has been formulated in a gel to be placed on the skin and has been studied in a pig wound-healing model. Clinical trials for chronic wounds and acne vulgaris are expected to begin in 2025. Dispersin B could be used as a topical agent for treatment of surgical wound sites, burns, diabetic foot ulcers, as well as eye infections.

In contribution 12 Kachlany and Vega present a paper that describes the therapeutic applications of leukotoxin derived from *A. actinomycetemcomitans*. This toxin will kill white blood cells (WBCs) and subvert the host immune system. The toxin, leukotoxin A (LtxA) interacts with lymphocyte function associated antigen -1 (LFA-1), a beta-2 integrin that is formed as a dimer from CD11a and CD18 and is expressed exclusively on the surface of WBCs and is the receptor of LtxA. The LtxA protein activates numerous cell death pathways making it an exceptional therapeutic candidate for hematologic and autoimmune/inflammatory diseases. LFA-1 has 3 unique configurations, low, intermediate and high affinity binding. This variety of affinity is a major reason that LtxA can be used therapeutically. In the low affinity state, the normal state, CD11a and CD18 are hidden and unavailable and thus not affected by LtxA. In the high affinity state, the diseased state, CD11a and CD18 are fully accessible and thus can make contact between LFA-1 and LtxA results in rapid death of WBCs, critical cells for immune protection. Neutrophils and monocytes show the highest level of LFA-1 followed by T-cells and B-cells. The paper describes how LtxA, with the proposed commercial name of Leukothera has been been used for treatments as diverse as leukemia, Lymphoma, psoriasis, allergic asthma, inflammatory bowel disease and Chron's disease.

Papers by Kaplan et al., (2024) and Kachlany and Vega (2024) illustrate how in-depth study of bacterial-induced diseases such as Localized Aggressive Periodontitis can show broad application to other infections and conditions supporting the premise that "to name a disease and to study it" can lead to a deep understanding of strategies by which bacteria participate in the ecological forces that promote disease. This in turn can provide a deeper understanding of disease, its treatment, and prevention. Discoveries such as these have not only helped explain biofilm formation by *A. actinomycetemcomitans*, its lifestyle, and its association with periodontitis but may ultimately have a major impact on diagnosis and therapeutic interventions that can go far beyond initial expectations and thus affect other seemingly unrelated diseases and conditions.

Daniel H. Fine
Guest Editor

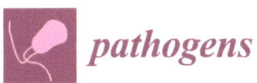 *pathogens*

Editorial

New Classification of Periodontal Diseases, the Obstacles Created and Opportunities for Growth

Daniel H. Fine

Department of Oral Biology, Rutgers School of Dental Medicine, 110 Bergen, Newark, NJ 07103, USA; finedh@sdm.rutgers.edu

Citation: Fine, D.H. New Classification of Periodontal Diseases, the Obstacles Created and Opportunities for Growth. *Pathogens* **2024**, *13*, 1098. https://doi.org/10.3390/pathogens13121098

Received: 9 December 2024
Accepted: 10 December 2024
Published: 12 December 2024

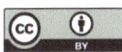
1. Gaps in the Knowledge, Opening a Forum for Discussion and Future Directions

The purpose of this Editorial is to expose the gaps in the knowledge created by a decision by the World Workshop Consensus Conference (WWCC), held in 2017, which was focused on the re-classification of periodontal diseases [1]. This newly developed classification system has had a negative impact on our ability to understand a specific form of periodontal disease [2]. This Special Issue of Pathogens focuses on the newly developed classification system and how it affects our ability to understand a specific form of periodontal disease, Localized Aggressive Periodontitis (LAgP), and the microorganism *Aggregatibacter actinomycetemcomitans*, which is intimately involved in disease initiation and progression [2]. As a result of the conclusions of the 2017 conference, research related to LAgP and *Aggregatibacter actinomycetemcomitans* has been minimized, as have the unique features of (1) LAgP, the "disease" (2) the key essential microbe related to this disease, and (3) replicated research that supports the uniqueness of both the microbe and the disease have been squelched [3,4]. This Special Issue also illustrates how important studies of *Aggregatibacter actinomycetemcomitans* in well-defined cases of LAgP have led to scientific discoveries that have extended far beyond this field of research, into areas as diverse as staphylococcal infections and lymphomas [5,6]. The editorial below will discuss (1) the developments that led to this current state of affairs, (2) the outsized influence this conference has had on this field of study, (3) the failures of this particular consensus conference, and (4) the way in which future failures can be overcome by well-designed consensus conferences.

A review of recent history will provide a better understanding of how these "new" definitions evolved and the effect these "new" definitions have had on this field of study. In the specialty of periodontology, over the last 60 years or more, there have been repeated efforts to review the current literature and update information regarding disease classification [7]. Global workshops have occurred, typically every 7 to 10 years, which were designed to review diagnosis, treatment, and prevention, with the goal of presenting the most current data that could function as a guide for practitioners, academicians, and researchers [7,8]. The direction over the past thirty to forty years has been focused on efforts to separate diseases based on their unique presentation [9]. However, the most recent workshop has taken a distinctly conservative and restrictive approach to periodontal disease and more or less minimized the value of disease classifications that distinguished between aggressive/rapidly progressive forms of disease, disease that is refractory to standard treatment, and diseases that are slowly progressive [1,10,11]. This strategy goes against the fundamental approach in the health profession that led to personalized/precision medicine, which is designed to emphasize subtle differences in diseases with an eye toward providing a more precise guide to treatment and prevention [12]. Interestingly, the relationship between periodontal disease and its effect on systemic diseases such as diabetes [13] and coronary heart disease, as well as their effects on periodontal disease, have been retained [1,11,14]. While data related to cohorts of bacteria and their relationship with the local host response and forms of periodontitis have been accumulating, this aspect has been minimized. In many cases, scientific truths take time to be accepted; however, in some cases, misguided objections to factual data can outweigh proven truths. What seems obvious to some is an anathema to others [15,16].

Research is intended to uncover scientific principles based on facts through a process of repeated testing and replication intended to support or refute the original hypothesis. However, research is conducted by humans, all of whom have foibles that can introduce prejudices and biases that can undermine the intentions and findings of the original research. The recognition that specific forms of the most common dental diseases, caries, and periodontitis are dependent on a complex imbalance in the local ecology, with overriding genetic and sociological component is logical [17,18]. The data supporting these linkages are convincing but still have missing fragments. Putting these pieces together takes time and is a common goal in several other branches of biological research; however, throwing the baby out with the bathwater is also common and an ill-conceived approach [19]. It appears as if profound experimental proof changes some opinions; however, landmark experiments occur infrequently and are usually dependent on a small group of insightful/influential researchers [20]. Max Planck developed a principle that suggests that "new scientific truth does not occur by convincing opponents but results from the death of its opponents" [15]. Simply put, scientific progress, as per Planck, occurs one funeral at a time [16]. While the direction of oral biology has been moving forward, we are facing the feeling that some of our major decisionmakers are unwilling or unable to accept the concept of personalized/precision medicine. Proof of the relevance of the specificity and importance of an accurate diagnosis can be seen in another branch of our specialty, the area of pediatric dentistry, where the diagnosis of subtypes of caries has had a major impact on the prevalence of caries in children [2]. The diagnosis of occlusal as opposed to proximal caries resulted in the use of occlusal sealants, reducing the prevalence of occlusal decay [21]. In the case of the diagnosis of early childhood caries (ECC), dietary restrictions resulted in a reduction in ECC [22]. In the most recent World Workshop on Periodontal Diseases, the "consensus" reached by a group of individuals gathered at this world workshop in 2017 reversed scientific progress. This may be explained by the death of major advocates of the microbiology and immunology of periodontal diseases, allowing the doubters to emerge as the more influential and powerful group [23,24].

One example of this cycle of discovery and lack of support took place in 1848, when Dr. Ignaz Ignaz Semmelweis, a Hungarian physician/obstetrician, observed and reported that puerperal fever at the time of birth resulted from poor antiseptic practices by the physicians who were in charge of delivery [25]. He noted that the midwives in the surgical ward he attended washed their hands prior to the delivery of pregnant mothers, whereas the physicians who had just come from teaching anatomy entered the operatory without washing their hands prior to delivery. This omission, he postulated, resulted in the much higher death rate in the babies delivered by physicians as compared to deliveries attended to by midwives [26]. He then conducted a simple set of experiments, which compared delivery after hand-washing with a chlorine rinse to delivery after no hand-washing and showed conclusively that puerperal fever was significantly reduced if those delivering the babies washed their hands thoroughly prior to delivery. His presentations to societies throughout Europe fell on deaf ears and were only accepted after Dr. Joseph Lister repeated these experiments by demanding hand-washing and spraying phenolic acid in the delivery rooms he supervised [27]. These studies were first presented in 1865 and were published in 1867. However, in 1865, Semmelweis was committed to a mental institution and died never knowing that his basic experiment was finally accepted by his medical colleagues.

This editorial and the upcoming book were designed to provide an open forum for discussion among researchers and clinicians who are opposed to the position taken at the last consensus conference. Vigorous discussion has not been encouraged, nor has there been any significant discussion related to this new classification [28]. This failure in communication needs to be corrected and is especially unacceptable in a complex scientific endeavor. As a result, an active field of research has been affected, and this failure will continue to hamper research and clinical care in a specific form of periodontitis that occurs in children and adolescents of African descent [2]. We used this Special Issue to focus on LAgP, but other forms of periodontitis need to be considered as well. The rationale for the emphasis on LAgP is that tooth loss occurs at an early age and the severity of the disease can possibly compromise the overall health of the individuals affected.

The book will describe the outsized influence the WWCC decision has had on this field of research, resulting from the failure (1) to follow best practices for consensus conferences, (2) to show an open-minded appreciation of longitudinal studies that have been replicated and support key elements demonstrating differences in this silent and orphan, or rare, "disease" as compared to other forms of periodontitis, and (3) to separate disease categories into well-defined groupings and to differentiate the subtle and unique differences between divergent forms of periodontal disease [28].

The second part of this Editorial will present a brief background of oral microbiology and how it fits into the overall scheme of microbiological discoveries that currently relate to periodontitis. The final piece of the editorial will present a very brief overview of the organization of the articles contained within the Special Issue.

2. A Brief Overview of the Long History of Oral Microbiology and Periodontal Disease

Oral microbiology has been intimately connected to general microbiology since its inception. For those unfamiliar with the history of microbiology and oral disease, a brief review focusing on the connection between oral microbes in the oral cavity and microbiologically induced diseases in general is provided. Antonie van Leeuwenhoek (1632–1723), originally a haberdasher from the Dutch Republic who later became a lens-maker and self-taught biologist, notably documented the microbes (he termed them "animalcules") that he visualized in his simple microscope [29,30]. Generally regarded as the "Father of Microbiology", Van Leeuwenhoek started examining pond water, saliva, and almost everything he could find, extensively documenting the size and shape of the things he magnified with his primitive microscope. His diagrams and descriptions of the images he visualized were published for the benefit of his scientific peers. In his words, "I...took the material...from the gums above my front teeth...I found a few living animalcules." He hand-drew pictures of creatures including cocci, spirochetes, and fusiform bacteria. In another one of his observations, he said "I took in my mouth some very strong wine-Vinegar, and closing my teeth, I gargled and rinsed them very well... but there were an innumerable quantity of animalcules yet remaining... I took a very little wine-Vinegar and mixt it with the water...[i.e., in vitro] whereupon the Animals dyed presently.... From hence...I conclude, that the Vinegar with which I washt my Teeth, kill'd only those Animals which were on the outside... but did not pass thro the whole substance of it...the scurf" [this "scurf" is what we now refer to as a biofilm] [29,30].

Two hundred years later, Louis Pasteur (1822–1895) and Robert Koch (1843–1910) founded the fields of immunology and microbiology [31,32]. Fortunately for the emerging field of dentistry, Willoughby Miller (1853–1907), a dentist trained at the Philadelphia Dental College, traveled to Germany in 1879, stayed there for many years, and studied classical methods of microbiology in the laboratory of Koch starting in the 1890s [33]. There, he proposed that the fermentation of carbohydrates occurs in the presence of oral bacteria, resulting in the formation of acid and destruction of enamel [34]. He also proposed the "focal theory of infection", stating that oral microbes play a role in diseases at sites distant from the oral cavity [34]. This theory was not substantiated. Miller's career choice was influenced by his father-in-law, Dr. Alexander Abbott (1860–1935), director of the "Laboratory of Hygiene", located next door to the Dental College, who authored the first textbooks of microbiology in the USA, called *The Hygiene of Transmissible Diseases* and Principles of Bacteriology [33]. Furthermore, Dr. David Bergey (1860–1937), a member of Abbott's department and the creator of Bergey's Manual of Determinative Bacteriology, was another key contributor to bacteriology in the USA [33]. A young student from England, Theodor Rosebury (1904–1976), enrolled at the University of Pennsylvania Dental School, attained his dental degree in 1928, and then was offered a fellowship at Columbia University, where he immersed himself in microbiology and began to study caries and periodontal disease from a microbiological perspective [35]. Although microbiology was a field in its embryonic stages, numerous publications related to oral microbiology and disease were starting to appear. Those further interested in this history can peruse a 1918 article by Kritchevsky and Seguin [36], a 1918 paper by Turner and Drew [37], and a 1929 report by Beckwith et al. [38]. These publications likely stimulated Rosebury in his pursuit of a career in microbiology. Over the years, Rosebury and colleagues pioneered vaccine development for caries, and developed the methodologies used to study anaerobic microorganisms [35]. Famous for his work on the anaerobic chamber and anaerobic microbiology, during WWII he was appointed the Director of Germ Warfare at Fort Detrick, Maryland [35]. Rosebury notably was a mentor of JB MacDonald (1918–2014), the first director of the Forsyth Institute (appointed in 1956), who assembled a team of researchers that included Dr Sigmund Socransky (1934–2011) and Dr. Ronald Gibbons (1932–1996), among others [35]. This very brief and limited historical review omits many researchers who made important contributions to field, such as Hemmens and Harrison (1942; [39]), Fish (1937; [40]), Box (1947; [41]), Waerhaug and Steen (1952; [42]), and Shultz Haudt et al. (1954; [43]). Toward the end of the 1950s, the question as to whether infectious diseases are caused by a single microbe such as *Bacteroides melaninogenicus* (proposed by JB MacDonald and the Forsyth group [44] or by a consortium of microbes (proposed by Rosebury and colleagues [45] was disputed by microbiologist of that era; this was a forerunner of the hypotheses that provided possible explanations regarding the causes of periodontal diseases (Loesche, 1976; [46]. This controversy more than likely stimulated Walter Loesche (1935–2012), a graduate student at MIT/Forsyth/Harvard, to propose "The Specific Plaque Hypothesis (SPH) and Non-Specific Plaque Hypotheses (NSPH)", as discussed below (Loesche, 1976; [46]). The difficulties in growing anaerobic subgingival bacteria stimulated Socransky and his colleagues (1991; 1998; [47,48]), Wade et al. (1997; [49]) Floyd Dewhirst and Bruce Paster [50,51], who were among the forerunners of the development of methods used to enumerate the uncultivable microbes that lead to qPCR.

Over the years, several hypotheses have been presented by microbiologists, intended to guide researchers in their studies and to establish proofs of the relationships between microbes and infectious diseases. Notable among these were original concepts proposed by Friedrich Gustav Henle (1809–1885), which were later modified by Koch, who, in 1890, proposed his "postulates", which required several steps of proof to conclude that a specific microbe causes a disease. First, these postulates proposed that the microbe of interest must be found in the disease but not seen in healthy subjects. Then, the microbe must be isolated from the diseased person and grown in pure culture. Second, once isolated in pure culture, this microbe should be placed into a healthy animal and a similar pattern of disease should emerge. Finally, the organism should be re-isolated from the experimentally induced diseased animal [31,32]. These postulates were modified many times. The postulates were especially difficult to prove when the diseases were viral in nature, or when "causative" microbes could not be isolated in pure culture. Nonetheless, these postulates provided a framework for exploration. Other obstacles occurred when the "focal theory of infection" was proposed. With reference to oral infections, this theory proposed that commensal microbes from the oral cavity that were not necessarily pathogenic in nature were suspected of causing diseases distant from the oral cavity [52]. More recently, the "Bradford Hill Criteria", proposed in 1965, included nine proofs that ideally must be met in order to conclude that the proposed microbe is causative of the disease in question [53]. While more comprehensive than Koch's postulates, the criteria do not emphasize the importance of host susceptibility. These criteria are discussed in more detail in this Special Issue/Book [2]. With respect to dental diseases, several important hypotheses have been proposed in efforts to understand the etiology of these diseases, which include the following: (1) The Specific Plaque Hypothesis (SPH), the Non-Specific Plaque Hypothesis (NSPH) [46], the Ecological Plaque Hypothesis (EPH) ([Marsh 1994; [54]), and the Keystone Plaque Hypothesis (KPH; Hajishengalis et al., 2012 [55]).

These hypotheses propose alternative conceptual explanations of disease initiation in efforts to guide treatment and prompt further study. The SPH suggests that a particular microbe or group of microbes are responsible for a particular form of dental disease, which can be treated by reducing the particular microbe(s) with either antibiotics or antiseptics. The NSPH suggests that the accumulation of a quantity of plaque leads to disease, which can be managed by reducing the volume of plaque or its metabolic components. The EPH states that microbial ecology is influenced by the nutrients supplied to the plaque environment, either through external factors such as (1) sugars in the case of caries, or (2) microbiologically induced growth factors, and/or (3) through the host and/or microbial factors produced in response to environmental shifts. These factors can be attributed to the results that progressing disease has on microbial succession or host response elements (Marsh, 1994 [53]). Thus, in one example, the excessive consumption of carbohydrates will cause a plummet in dental plaque pH, which will increase the likelihood of the overgrowth of acidogenic (acid-producing) microbes living within that biofilm/plaque matrix. In another example, heme and menadione, derived from red blood cells emanating from microbial-induced inflammation in gingival tissues, can provide an ecological advantage to *Porphyromonas gingivalis* through promoting its continued growth and survival thanks to the nutritional factors derived from inflamed tissue. The KPH proposes that particular low-abundance microbes such as *P. gingivalis* can act as a "Keystone" microbe that modulates the host immune system to protect itself and other members of the subgingival microflora. This host modulation can support and encourage the growth of other less adaptable microbes that are biogeographically close to the co-inhabiting *P. gingivalis* microbes and that provide a cover for these less adaptable microbes in a hostile subgingival environment (Hajishengalis et al., [55]).

Our research group used the phrase "social influencer" to capture the idea that microbes like *Aggregatibacter actinomycetemcomitans* and *P. gingivalis*, even at low numbers, can have an outsized influence on the surrounding microbes by encouraging their growth and survival [2]. We propose that the "one" can influence the "many" by suppressing the host immune system at the local level. While each of these hypotheses has contributed to our understanding of disease in the oral cavity, each has focused on the bacteria and minimized the importance of alternative ways to assess damage to the host's periodontal tissues. As a result, we now favor "The Damage/Response Framework" presented by Casadevall and Pirofski [56]. The features of this framework that differentiate it from other microbe- or host-centric hypotheses are that (1) contributions from both the host and the microbe are required to cause virulence (a microbe-centric term), (2) the ultimate outcome of the interaction of the microbe and host is determined through the damage to the host, thus incorporating the role of the host into the concepts of virulence and pathogenicity (a more host-centric term), and (3) the concept that host damage is tied to interactions between the host and microbes that vary with time. Time-related disease can be best illustrated by two viral diseases, chicken pox [57] and polio [58]. In chicken pox, the disease appears under control but flares up in some older individuals and is manifested as shingles due to the re-emergence of the Herpes Zoster virus. In polio even though the virus is undetected, symptoms can emerge in elderly individuals due to host damage that occurred decades ago.

In the mid-1960s, dental academics' and practitioners' interest in the relationship between microbiology and periodontal disease was re-invigorated by the work of Keyes and Fitzgerald (1962; [59]) and Loe and colleagues (1965; [60]). However, in the year 1976, the impetus to create tools and hypotheses designed to explore the relationship between microbiology and dental disease occurred in a more systematic manner. First, two independent investigators discovered that Localized Juvenile Periodontitis (later called, LAgP) was associated with a Gram-negative capnophilic cocco-bacillus, which was named *Actinobacillus actinomycetemcomitans* at the time [61,62]. These discoveries coincided with the introduction of the Specific Plaque Hypothesis developed by Walter Loesche (1976; [46]).

As shown in Figure 1, modified from Casadevall and Pirofski [56], we propose that periodontal disease, especially localized aggressive periodontitis, is most compatible with the damage/response framework. In this case, we propose that either a weakened local host response or an over-exuberant local host response will encourage disease at the local site.

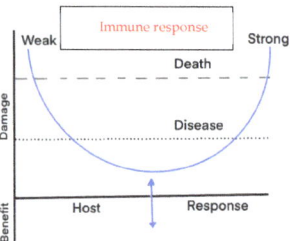

Figure 1. Damage/response framework. The more extreme the host response is (weaker or stronger) the worse the outcome.

3. Overview of the Special Issue

The Special Issue is divided into three portions: (1) a clinical overview of the disease and the data that show its unique features; (2) the microorganism, *Aggregatibacter actinomycetemcomitans*, which is not sufficient but necessary for the disease to occur through altering the ecology enough to overwhelm the host; (3) discoveries centered around *Aggregatibacter actinomycetemcomitans* that developed as a result of intense molecular studies of this microbe. These intensive molecular investigations resulted in therapies being developed for diseases as wide-ranging as psoriasis, lymphomas, and staph infections, as well as other polymicrobial diseases, and are described in the final two papers.

Conflicts of Interest: The author declares no conflict of interest.

References

1. Papapanou, P.N.; Sanz, M.; Buduneli, N.; Dietrich, T.; Feres, M.; Fine, D.H.; Flemmig, T.F.; Garcia, R.; Giannobile, W.V.; Graziani, F.; et al. Periodontitis: Consensus report of workgroup 2 of the 2017 World Workshop on the Classification of Periodontal and Peri-Implant Diseases and Conditions. *J. Periodontol.* **2018**, *89* (Suppl. 1), S173–S182. [CrossRef] [PubMed]
2. Fine, D.H.; Schreiner, H.; Diehl, S.R. A Rose by Any Other Name: The Long Intricate History of Localized Aggressive Periodontitis. *Pathogens* **2024**, *13*, 849. [CrossRef] [PubMed]
3. Hoglund Aberg, C.; Kwamin, F.; Claesson, R.; Dahlen, G.; Johansson, A.; Haubek, D. Progression of attachment loss is strongly associated with presence of the JP2 genotype of Aggregatibacter actinomycetemcomitans: A prospective cohort study of a young adolescent population. *J. Clin. Periodontol.* **2014**, *41*, 232–241. [CrossRef] [PubMed]
4. Razooqi, Z.; Tjellstrom, I.; Hoglund Aberg, C.; Kwamin, F.; Claesson, R.; Haubek, D.; Johansson, A.; Oscarsson, J. Association of Filifactor alocis and its RTX toxin gene ftxA with periodontal attachment loss, and in synergy with Aggregatibacter actinomycetemcomitans. *Front. Cell. Infect. Microbiol.* **2024**, *14*, 1376358. [CrossRef]
5. Kaplan, J.B.; Sukhishvili, S.A.; Sailer, M.; Kridin, K.; Ramasubbu, N. Aggregatibacter actinomycetemcomitans Dispersin B: The Quintessential Antibiofilm Enzyme. *Pathogens* **2024**, *13*, 668. [CrossRef]
6. Kachlany, S.C.; Vega, B.A. Therapeutic Applications of Aggregatibacter actinomycetemcomitans Leukotoxin. *Pathogens* **2024**, *13*, 354. [CrossRef]
7. Armitage, G.C. Learned and unlearned concepts in periodontal diagnostics: A 50-year perspective. *Periodontology 2000* **2013**, *62*, 20–36. [CrossRef]
8. Armitage, G.C. A brief history of periodontics in the United States of America: Pioneers and thought-leaders of the past, and current challenges. *Periodontology 2000* **2020**, *82*, 12–25. [CrossRef]
9. Armitage, G.C. Comparison of the microbiological features of chronic and aggressive periodontitis. *Periodontology 2000* **2010**, *53*, 70–88. [CrossRef]
10. Armitage, G.C. Periodontal diseases: Diagnosis. *Ann. Periodontol.* **1996**, *1*, 37–215. [CrossRef]
11. Caton, J.G.; Armitage, G.; Berglundh, T.; Chapple, I.L.C.; Jepsen, S.; Kornman, K.S.; Mealey, B.L.; Papapanou, P.N.; Sanz, M.; Tonetti, M.S. A new classification scheme for periodontal and peri-implant diseases and conditions—Introduction and key changes from the 1999 classification. *J. Clin. Periodontol.* **2018**, *45* (Suppl. 20), S1–S8. [CrossRef] [PubMed]
12. Snyderman, R. Personalized health care: From theory to practice. *Biotechnol. J.* **2012**, *7*, 973–979. [CrossRef] [PubMed]
13. Sanz, M.; Ceriello, A.; Buysschaert, M.; Chapple, I.; Demmer, R.T.; Graziani, F.; Herrera, D.; Jepsen, S.; Lione, L.; Madianos, P.; et al. Scientific evidence on the links between periodontal diseases and diabetes: Consensus report and guidelines of the

joint workshop on periodontal diseases and diabetes by the International Diabetes Federation and the European Federation of Periodontology. *J. Clin. Periodontol.* **2018**, *45*, 138–149. [CrossRef] [PubMed]

14. Sanz, M.; Del Castillo, A.M.; Jepsen, S.; Gonzalez-Juanatey, J.R.; D'Aiuto, F.; Bouchard, P.; Chapple, I.; Dietrich, T.; Gotsman, I.; Graziani, F.; et al. Periodontitis and Cardiovascular Diseases. Consensus Report. *Glob. Heart* **2020**, *15*, 1. [CrossRef]

15. Hull, D.L.; Tessner, P.D.; Diamond, A.M. Planck's Principle. *Science* **1978**, *202*, 717–723. [CrossRef]

16. Azoulay, P.; Fons-Rosen, C.; Zivin, J.S.G. Does Science Advance One Funeral at a Time? *Am. Econ. Rev.* **2019**, *109*, 2889–2920. [CrossRef]

17. Hajishengallis, G.; Lamont, R.J. Beyond the red complex and into more complexity: The polymicrobial synergy and dysbiosis (PSD) model of periodontal disease etiology. *Mol. Oral. Microbiol.* **2012**, *27*, 409–419. [CrossRef]

18. Hajishengallis, G.; Liang, S.; Payne, M.A.; Hashim, A.; Jotwani, R.; Eskan, M.A.; McIntosh, M.L.; Alsam, A.; Kirkwood, K.L.; Lambris, J.D.; et al. Low-abundance biofilm species orchestrates inflammatory periodontal disease through the commensal microbiota and complement. *Cell Host Microbe* **2011**, *10*, 497–506. [CrossRef]

19. Mukherjee, S. *The Emperor of All Maladies: A Biography of Cancer*; Scribner: New York, NY, USA, 2010.

20. Porta, M. One hundred years ago: The dawning of the insulin era. *Acta Diabetol* **2021**, *58*, 1–4. [CrossRef]

21. Sheykholeslam, Z.; Buonocore, M.G. Bonding of resins to phosphoric acid-etched enamel surfaces of permanent and deciduous teeth. *J. Dent. Res.* **1972**, *51*, 1572–1576. [CrossRef]

22. Folayan, M.N.O.; Amalia, R.; Kemoli, A.; Sun, I.G.; Duangthip, D.; Abodunrin, O.; Virtanen, J.I.; Masumo, R.M.; Vukovic, A.; Al-Batayneh, O.B.; et al. Can the sustainable development goal 9 support an untreated early childhood caries elimination agenda? *BMC Oral. Health* **2024**, *24*, 776. [CrossRef] [PubMed]

23. Giannobile, W.V.; Tonetti, M.S. Sigmund S. Socransky, D.D.S., 1934–2011. *J. Clin. Periodontol.* **2012**, *39*, 415–416. [CrossRef] [PubMed]

24. Teles, R.P.; Teles, F.R.; Loesche, W.J.; Listgarten, M.; Fine, D.; Lindhe, J.; Malament, K.; Haffajee, A.D. Rediscovering Sig Socransky, the genius and his legacy. *J. Dent. Res.* **2012**, *91*, 433–439. [CrossRef] [PubMed]

25. Stang, A.; Standl, F.; Poole, C. A twenty-first century perspective on concepts of modern epidemiology in Ignaz Philipp Semmelweis' work on puerperal sepsis. *Eur. J. Epidemiol.* **2022**, *37*, 437–445. [CrossRef]

26. Poczai, P.; Karvalics, L.Z. The little-known history of cleanliness and the forgotten pioneers of handwashing. *Front. Public Health* **2022**, *10*, 979464. [CrossRef]

27. Thurston, A.J. Of blood, inflammation and gunshot wounds: The history of the control of sepsis. *Aust. N. Z. J. Surg.* **2000**, *70*, 855–861. [CrossRef]

28. Fine, D.H.; Armitage, G.C.; Genco, R.J.; Griffen, A.L.; Diehl, S.R. Unique etiologic, demographic, and pathologic characteristics of localized aggressive periodontitis support classification as a distinct subcategory of periodontitis. *J. Am. Dent. Assoc.* **2019**, *150*, 922–931. [CrossRef]

29. Fred, E.B. Antony van Leeuwenhoek: On the Three-hundredth Anniversary of his Birth. *J. Bacteriol.* **1933**, *25*, 2–18. [CrossRef]

30. Robertson, L.A. Antoni van Leeuwenhoek 1723–2023: A review to commemorate Van Leeuwenhoek's death, 300 years ago: For submission to Antonie van Leeuwenhoek journal of microbiology. *Antonie Van Leeuwenhoek* **2023**, *116*, 919–935. [CrossRef]

31. Fredricks, D.N.; Relman, D.A. Sequence-based identification of microbial pathogens: A reconsideration of Koch's postulates. *Clin. Microbiol. Rev.* **1996**, *9*, 18–33. [CrossRef]

32. Schwartz, M. Dr. Jekyll and Mr. Hyde: A short history of anthrax. *Mol. Asp. Med.* **2009**, *30*, 347–355. [CrossRef] [PubMed]

33. Rosan, B.; Hammond, B.F. A Philadelphia story--featuring Ned Williams: Microbiology at the University of Pennsylvania School of Dental Medicine. *J. Dent. Res.* **2000**, *79*, 1451–1457. [CrossRef] [PubMed]

34. Miller, W.D. *The Micro-Organisms of the Human Mouth*; S. Karger: Basel, Switzerland, 1890; p. 364.

35. Fine, D.H. Dr. Theodor Rosebury: Grandfather of Modern Oral Microbiology. *J. Dent. Res.* **2006**, *85*, 990–995. [CrossRef] [PubMed]

36. Kritchevsky, B.; Seguin, P. The Pathogenesis and Treatment of Pyorrhea Alveolaris. *Dent. Cosmos* **1918**, *60*, 781–784.

37. Turner, J.G.; Drew, A.H. An Experimental Inquiry into the Bacteriology of Pyorrhoea. *Proc. R. Soc. Med.* **1919**, *12*, 104–118. [CrossRef]

38. Beckwith, T.; Williams, A.; Rose, E. The role of bacteria in pyorrhea. *Med. J. Record* **1929**, *129*, 333–336.

39. Hemmens, E.; Harrison, R. Studies of the Anaerobic Bacterial Flora of Suppurative Periodontitis. *J. Infect. Dis.* **1942**, *70*, 131–146. [CrossRef]

40. Fish, E.W. Local and Remote Sequelae of Infection in the Parodontal Sulcus: (Section of Odontology). *Proc. R. Soc. Med.* **1937**, *30*, 1149–1165.

41. Box, H.K. New aspects of periodontal research. *J. Can. Dent. Assoc.* **1947**, *13*, 3–10.

42. Waerhaug, J.; Steen, E. The presence or absence of bacteria in gingival pockets and the reaction in healthy pockets to certain pure cultures; a bacteriological and histological investigation. *Odontol. Tidskr.* **1952**, *60*, 1–24.

43. Schultz-Haudt, S.; Bruce, M.A.; Bibby, B.G. Bacterial factors in nonspecific gingivitis. *J. Dent. Res.* **1954**, *33*, 454–458. [CrossRef] [PubMed]

44. Gibbons, R.J.; Macdonald, J.B. Hemin and vitamin K compounds as required factors for the cultivation of certain strains of Bacteroides melaninogenicus. *J. Bacteriol.* **1960**, *80*, 164–170. [CrossRef] [PubMed]

45. Rosebury, T.; Clark, A.R.; Macdonald, J.B.; O'Connell, D.C. Studies of fusospirochetal infection. III. Further studies of a guinea pig passage strain of fusospirochetal infection, including the infectivity of sterile exudate filtrates, of mixed cultures through ten transfers, and of recombined pure cultures. *J. Infect. Dis.* **1950**, *87*, 234–248. [CrossRef] [PubMed]
46. Loesche, W.J. Chemotherapy of dental plaque infections. *Oral. Sci. Rev.* **1976**, *9*, 65–107.
47. Socransky, S.S.; Haffajee, A.D.; Smith, C.; Dibart, S. Relation of counts of microbial species to clinical status at the sampled site. *J. Clin. Periodontol.* **1991**, *18*, 766–775. [CrossRef]
48. Socransky, S.S.; Haffajee, A.D.; Cugini, M.A.; Smith, C.; Kent, R.L., Jr. Microbial complexes in subgingival plaque. *J. Clin. Periodontol.* **1998**, *25*, 134–144. [CrossRef]
49. Wade, D.N.; Kerns, D.G. Acute necrotizing ulcerative gingivitis-periodontitis: A literature review. *Mil. Med.* **1998**, *163*, 337–342. [CrossRef]
50. Paster, B.J.; Boches, S.K.; Galvin, J.L.; Ericson, R.E.; Lau, C.N.; Levanos, V.A.; Sahasrabudhe, A.; Dewhirst, F.E. Bacterial diversity in human subgingival plaque. *J. Bacteriol.* **2001**, *183*, 3770–3783. [CrossRef]
51. Dewhirst, F.E.; Chen, T.; Izard, J.; Paster, B.J.; Tanner, A.C.; Yu, W.H.; Lakshmanan, A.; Wade, W.G. The human oral microbiome. *J. Bacteriol.* **2010**, *192*, 5002–5017. [CrossRef]
52. Burket, L.W.; Burns, C.G. Bacteremias following dental extraction. *J. Dent. Res.* **1937**, *16*, 521–530. [CrossRef]
53. Hill, A.B. The Environment and Disease: Association or Causation? *Proc. R. Soc. Med.* **1965**, *58*, 295–300. [CrossRef] [PubMed]
54. Marsh, P.D. Microbial ecology of dental plaque and its significance in health and disease. *Adv. Dent. Res.* **1994**, *8*, 263–271. [CrossRef] [PubMed]
55. Hajishengallis, G.; Darveau, R.P.; Curtis, M.A. The keystone-pathogen hypothesis. *Nat. Rev. Microbiol.* **2012**, *10*, 717–725. [CrossRef]
56. Casadevall, A.; Pirofski, L.A. Host-pathogen interactions: Redefining the basic concepts of virulence and pathogenicity. *Infect. Immun.* **1999**, *67*, 3703–3713. [CrossRef]
57. Garnett, G.P.; Grenfell, B.T. The epidemiology of varicella-zoster virus infections: A mathematical model. *Epidemiol. Infect.* **1992**, *108*, 495–511. [CrossRef]
58. Wandell, P.; Borg, K.; Li, X.; Carlsson, A.C.; Sundquist, J.; Sundquist, K. The risk of post-polio syndrome among immigrant groups in Sweden. *Sci. Rep.* **2023**, *13*, 6044. [CrossRef]
59. Keyes, P.H.; Fitzgerald, R.J. Dental caries in the Syrian hamster. IX. *Arch. Oral. Biol.* **1962**, *7*, 267–277. [CrossRef]
60. Loe, H.; Theilade, E.; Jensen, S.B. Experimental Gingivitis in Man. *J. Periodontol.* **1965**, *36*, 177–187. [CrossRef]
61. Slots, J. The predominant cultivable organisms in juvenile periodontitis. *Scand. J. Dent. Res.* **1976**, *84*, 1–10. [CrossRef]
62. Newman, M.G.; Socransky, S.S.; Savitt, E.D.; Propas, D.A.; Crawford, A. Studies of the microbiology of periodontosis. *J. Periodontol.* **1976**, *47*, 373–379. [CrossRef]

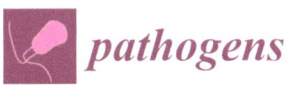 *pathogens*

Review

A Rose by Any Other Name: The Long Intricate History of Localized Aggressive Periodontitis

Daniel H. Fine *, Helen Schreiner and Scott R. Diehl

Department of Oral Biology, Rutgers School of Dental Medicine, 110 Bergen Street, Newark, NJ 07101, USA; hschrein@sdm.rutgers.edu (H.S.); diehlsd@sdm.rutgers.edu (S.R.D.)
* Correspondence: finedh@sdm.rutgers.edu; Tel.: +1-973-985-6181

Abstract: This review addresses the recent World Workshop Consensus Conference (WWCC) decision to eliminate Localized Aggressive Periodontitis (LAgP) in young adults as a distinct form of periodontitis. A "Consensus" implies widespread, if not unanimous, agreement among participants. However, a significant number of attendees were opposed to the elimination of the LAgP classification. The substantial evidence supporting a unique diagnosis for LAgP includes the (1) incisor/molar pattern of disease, (2) young age of onset, (3) rapid progression of attachment and bone loss, (4) familial aggregation across multiple generations, and (5) defined consortium of microbiological risk factors including *Aggregatibacter actinomycetemcomitans*. Distinctive clinical signs and symptoms of LAgP are presented, and the microbial subgingival consortia that precede the onset of signs and symptoms are described. Using Bradford–Hill guidelines to assess causation, well-defined longitudinal studies support the unique microbial consortia, including *A. actinomycetemcomitans* as causative for LAgP. To determine the effects of the WWCC elimination of LAgP on research, we searched three publication databases and discovered a clear decrease in the number of new publications addressing LAgP since the new WWCC classification. The negative effects of the WWCC guidelines on both diagnosis and treatment success are presented. For example, due to the localized nature of LAgP, the practice of averaging mean pocket depth reduction or attachment gain across all teeth masks major changes in disease recovery at high-risk tooth sites. Reinstating LAgP as a distinct disease entity is proposed, and an alternative or additional way of measuring treatment success is recommended based on an assessment of the extension of the time to relapse of subgingival re-infection. The consequences of the translocation of oral microbes to distant anatomical sites due to ignoring relapse frequency are also discussed. Additional questions and future directions are also presented.

Keywords: aggressive periodontitis; *Aggregatibacter actinomycetemcomitans*; treatment success; consensus conferences; microbiome consortia; damage/response framework

Citation: Fine, D.H.; Schreiner, H.; Diehl, S.R. A Rose by Any Other Name: The Long Intricate History of Localized Aggressive Periodontitis. *Pathogens* **2024**, *13*, 849. https://doi.org/10.3390/pathogens13100849

Academic Editors: Jens Kreth and Anders Johansson

Received: 30 July 2024
Revised: 20 September 2024
Accepted: 27 September 2024
Published: 29 September 2024

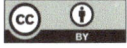

1. Introduction: Importance of Recognizing Subtypes of Periodontitis for Scientific Discovery

The primary purpose of this hybrid review is to present evidence that Localized Aggressive Periodontitis (LAgP; recently reclassified as Stage III Grade C Periodontitis) is a unique disease that deserves its own classification as a distinct form of periodontitis. The aim of this review is to describe the features that make this disease distinctive on a clinical and microbiological level. A more complete understanding of the roles of genetics and host responsiveness in young individuals requires additional research (described in Miguel and Shaddox (This Special Issue). Additional efforts to gain this important information may be thwarted if LAgP is abandoned as a distinct entity. This review will be structured into sections that support the role of *A. actinomycetemcomitans* in this unique disease. The manuscript is somewhat unconventional and consists of a hybrid paper that contains literature review material, opinions based on evidence, and examples of LAgP related to tooth loss and assessment of treatment success or failure. The paper stresses the clinical and microbiological aspects of LAgP, especially in vulnerable populations. The review presents these unique features in distinctive sub-headings as follows: (1) Overall Introduction, (2) Influence of the World Workshop Consensus Conference (WWCC) on Disease Classification, (3) Benefits of Precise Disease Classification, (4) Brief History of Landmark Experiments that Support Microbiological Associations with Dental Diseases, (5) The Damage/Response Framework, (6) Examples of Distinct Characteristics of LAgP, and (7) Conclusions and Future Directions.

The paper presents information that challenges the decision made by the WWCC to eliminate LAgP as a unique disease entity [1,2]. Many ways of classifying different forms of periodontal disease have been proposed, but the recent Stage III Grade C classification no longer recognizes the disease previously known as Localized Aggressive Periodontitis (LAgP), Periodontosis, Localized Juvenile Periodontitis, and Early Onset Periodontitis [1,3]. The Staging and Grading method of classification adopted by the leadership of the WWCC is a scheme that has been used extensively by cancer researchers and clinicians for purposes of creating a consistent system for prognosis and treatment [4]. However, the classification of the disease by staging and grading was never intended to serve as a substitute for a robust framework for disease diagnosis [5]. As noted above, throughout the extensive history of efforts to characterize LAgP, many name changes have evolved, but several features unique to this disease have remained constant, including (1) the early age of onset of disease, (2) the disease is localized, at least initially affecting incisors and first molars, and (3) the rapid rate of severe bone loss compared to forms of periodontitis presenting in adults [3,6]. It has also been obvious that, unlike adult periodontitis, LAgP frequently exhibits strong familial aggregation with transmission across multiple generations [7]. LAgP also exhibits a far higher prevalence of 2.05% in African Americans aged 14–17 compared to only 0.14% in persons of European ancestry in the United States, a nearly 15-fold difference in frequency [8].

The revised classification of LAgP as Stage III Grade C ignores the distinct clinical, microbiological, and genetic differences in this aggressive form of periodontitis as compared to adult forms of the disease [9]. Historical revisions of nomenclature that reflect shifting opinions are valid, but in this case, the WWCC change fails to reflect the most current scientific knowledge, especially with respect to clinical and microbiological features [10]. One goal of this review is to illustrate the negative effects that this "new" classification is already having on research aimed at understanding the etiology and progression of LAgP and the impacts that this "classification" has on clinical diagnosis and treatment. This paper will focus on (1) the unique clinical presentation of LAgP, (2) the unique microbiological risk factors associated with LAgP, and (3) historical and clinical examples that show why LAgP should continue to be recognized as a unique disease entity.

2. Influence of Consensus Conference and Key Microbiological Influences on Disease Classification

(A) WWCC impact on Disease Classification.

Dental biology does not exist in a vacuum. The WWCC focus on histopathological differences as the ultimate discriminator for periodontal disease classification is narrow. Histopathological discrimination is unlikely until biopsy material related to active disease has been collected [11]. In time, it is likely that both histopathological and genetic differences between periodontitis in older adults and LAgP in children and young adults will be uncovered [12]. However, at this moment, it is inappropriate to ignore the major clinical signs and symptoms that are unique to LAgP [13]. As for genetics, thus far, etiology based on a single gene of major effect causing LAgP appears unlikely, aside from rare syndromic forms such as those caused by mutations in the cathepsin C gene [14]. Instead, it is more probable that an ensemble of genes of small to moderate effect, combined with environmental risk factors, play a prominent role in susceptibility to the disorder [12,15]. The WWCC argument that cases of LAgP are too rare to warrant recognition as a unique diagnosis is inconsistent with standard practice in medicine where orphan diseases (affecting less than 200,000 individuals in the U.S.) routinely receive specific diagnoses [16]. The 2.05% prevalence among the 11+ million African American adolescents in the United States alone would mean that approximately 225,000 individuals are likely to be affected by LAgP. Moreover, necrotizing diseases are also very uncommon, but despite their limited numbers, these diseases were still recognized with a unique diagnosis by the WWCC [17,18]. The suggestion that the determinations of the WWCC are unalterable is invalid because changes in the WWC classification have occurred previously [19].

Necrotizing diseases such as Acute Necrotizing (AN) Gingivitis and AN Periodontitis provide good examples as to how disease categorization can be implemented by the WWCC based on new information despite their low prevalence. Further, AN diseases illustrate how "impairment of the host immune system" can create a dysbiotic state. In the examples of necrotizing diseases, histopathological differences are extolled [17]. We propose that patients with LAgP fit into the same category, also having an impaired host immune system but in this case at the local level, as demonstrated by polymorphonuclear leukocyte dysfunction that in itself supports the concept that this is a specific category of disease [20]. In spite of these inconsistencies, the WWCC authors failed to create a separate case definition for LAgP as a distinctive disease entity [1]. There is no recognition of the uniqueness of LAgP in the WWCC decision despite the fact that many expert reports in the literature, including the foundation paper on LAgP written for the WWCC, clearly point to specific signs and symptoms, especially in patients of African descent who have excessive bone loss at an early age [11,21]. In fact, the decision to eliminate LAgP as a disease entity, despite its characteristically unique clinical features that separate it from other forms of periodontitis, lacked the widespread agreement among the Workshop participants normally required for a decision to be characterized as a "consensus" [22].

(B)   Support for Maintaining LAgP as a Disease entity.

We have used this section to provide support for maintaining LAgP as a distinct disease entity, offering a rationale for this support that is more accessible to both clinicians and researchers.

Over the years, disease diagnoses have been debated among the "lumpers" and "splitters". These terms originated in evolutionary biology but could be used in any form of biology [22]. Most simply put, "lumpers" tend to join things together, while 'splitters' separate things so that they can be examined individually in greater detail. In the words of Siddhartha Mukherjee, author of the bestselling book *"The Emperor of All Maladies"* [23], there is great value in differentiating cancer types for diagnosis and therapy. In his words, "How can you treat something you can't name?". As one example, Dr. Mukherjee points out that targeted immunotherapy is successful because definitions of disease highlighting different types of cancers can be affected by specific targeted treatments [23]. This reasoning can also be applied to LAgP. Staging and Grading, first introduced in the 1940s and 1950s by Dr. Pierre Denoix, was never intended as a diagnostic strategy [24].

Personalized/Precision Medicine was promulgated by the insightful work of Dr. Ralph Snyderman (former member of the immunology section of the National Institute of Dental and Craniofacial Research and Dean of Duke University Medical School) [25]. Personalized Medicine makes great efforts to define diseases precisely as opposed to lumping different forms of a disease into a single group [21].

i. Age as a consideration for case determination. A close look at the new WWCC definition of LAgP (now called Stage III Grade C Periodontitis) reveals that there is no distinction within this framework that discriminates between a young adolescent with the disease and older patients presenting with a similar pattern of disease [13]. It appears as if the extensive data on cases of Localized Aggressive Periodontitis in adolescents or children who show extreme levels of disease were overlooked for reasons not enumerated [26].

There is no dispute that subgingival bacteria initiate a host damage response in both LAgP and other forms of periodontitis [27]. However, it appears as if factors such as age of onset, ethnicity, and rate of disease progression are ignored in the recent Consensus document [18]. The Consensus summary states that differences in the pathobiology of aggressive and chronic forms of periodontitis are not significant enough to establish distinct disease entities [1]. Of curiosity, age as a factor for periodontitis is reported by one of the foundation papers, but here, age assessment begins with individuals 30 and above [28]. The paper concludes that ..."empirical evidence-driven definitions of CAL (Clinical Attachment Level) thresholds signifying disproportionate severity of periodontitis by age are feasible [28] and that ..."age is a significant determinant of the clinical presentation of periodontitis..." and "... individuals with fewer remaining teeth have higher mean CAL and PD measures" [28]. The age determinant is especially true for LAgP, but the age range for an LAgP disease classification is not considered in the paper. The focus of those of us who study LAgP has usually been on individuals aged 20 and younger, but this age group was not recognized [29].

ii. Rate of bone loss as a consideration for disease classification. The most prominent illustration of differences in the rate of disease progression occurs when comparing LAgP to Adult Periodontitis (AP). The rate of disease progression is a difficult parameter to measure unless longitudinal studies are performed [30,31]. A simple examination of specific site disease progression can be determined when LAgP and adult periodontitis patients are compared and age is introduced as a parameter. There is no denying that 6 to 8 mm of bone loss is rarely seen in a short period of 2–3 years in any other forms of periodontitis aside from LAgP [11,32]. However, even in LAgP, this very significant fact (rate of bone loss) is hidden when mean clinical attachment levels (CAL) are averaged over all teeth with up to 168 sites [30] (see Section 6 B).

iii. Etiology as a consideration for disease classification. The hazardous, often challenging, shifting, and, at times, impaired oral environment (e.g., irradiated salivary glands, dry mouth, circadian rhythms) has resulted in a highly adaptable oral microbiome [33]. As the main entryway into the body, bacteria first reaching the oral cavity face enormous environmental obstacles and a multitude of surfaces for colonization [34]. The more we explore, the more we realize that oral bacteria are not only involved in dental disease but that these highly adaptable bacteria can and have been shown to escape their initial oral habitat and move to remote sites to exacerbate diseases at sites distant from the oral cavity [35,36]. While we first thought of specific bacteria as the etiological agents of dental diseases, our thinking based on well-designed longitudinal clinical studies has changed our focus to reflect the fact that the consortia of oral bacteria are most likely the provocateurs [29,37]. These consortia operate as a well-organized dysbiotic community and challenge the host's ability to defend itself [38,39].

(C)   Influence of WWCC decision on LAgP publications.

The WWCC's decision to ignore LAgP as a unique diagnosis has had an outsized influence on diagnosis, treatment, prevention, and scholarship in the areas of microbiology, immunology, and pathobiology of periodontal disease. It was our expectation that the elimination of LAgP as a disease would lead to less research, more limited treatment options, and risk further divorcing our field's biological initiatives from that of modern medicine. To explore our concern that the new classification has already had an impact on research and clinical scholarship, we performed a database search using mesh terms that included Periodontitis, Aggressive Periodontitis, Localized Aggressive Periodontitis, and Stage III Grade C Periodontitis. We limited the time span of the search to 12 years (6 years prior to the change in terminology, from 2012 to 2017, and 6 years following the classification change from 2018 to 2023). We used these terms to search PubMed, Web of Science, and Scopus databases. Data derived from these searches were used to compare the number of papers published within these time frames in each of the categories specified (Table 1). The results show an overall increase in papers with "Periodontitis" in their title and/or abstract six years following the WWCC but a 33% decrease in those with "Aggressive Periodontitis". It is abundantly clear that the elimination of LAgP as a case definition has had a major negative impact on the number of publications focusing on patients who previously were classified as LAgP (see Table 1).

Table 1. Numbers of publications by periodontitis disease categories 2012–2023.

Disease Category	Pub Med Years		Web of Science Years		Scopus Years	
	2012–2017	2018–2023	2012–2017	2018–2023	2012–2017	2018–2023
Periodontitis	6492	6287	10,181	16,420	13,000	18,926
Aggressive Periodontitis	884	534	1053	817	1030	679
Localized Aggressive Periodontitis	179	114	134	102	118	80
* Stage III Grade C Periodontitis		* 148		* 138		* 135

Comparisons between 6 years prior and 6 years following category changes are seen below as percentages disclosed by each search engine. Periodontitis changes varied from −3% to +38%. Aggressive Periodontitis changes varied from −22% to −40%. Localized Aggressive Periodontitis changes varied from −24% to −36%. * Stage III Grade C includes all forms of Aggressive Periodontitis and does not discriminate between adolescents and adults who have the disease; thus, the number of publications is at a minimum of 60% less when compared to LAgP; in addition, 20% of these publications define the new classification and did not present clinical data.

3. Benefits of Precise Disease Definitions

In the section below, we describe two examples of how well-defined disease definitions lead to accurate diagnosis and improved treatment outcomes. One example relates to dental disease, and one relates to diseases that are sexually transmitted. First, Pediatric Dentistry has deemed it appropriate and beneficial to go with the "splitters" approach and name diseases that have similar outcomes but have distinctive characteristics that can be recognized by clinicians and can be treated in ways that benefit patients [40]. For example, the biological processes of caries, despite their various locations in the mouth, are very similar, and all varieties are related to acid-producing, aciduric microbes that affiliate themselves with tooth surfaces and demineralize the surface and subsurface to create a carious lesion [41]. Nevertheless, for Pediatric dentists, the caries process has been recognized as having distinct subtypes: (1) occlusal caries, (2) proximal caries, and (3) root caries [42]. Moreover, early childhood caries (ECC) has been recognized as a distinct clinical entity [43]. These well-defined diagnoses have led to specific treatments such as (1) sealants used to obliterate occlusal pits and fissures [44], (2) fluoride varnishes for proximal decay [45], and (3) dietary counseling for prevention of ECC [46]. These treatments have resulted in changes in caries prevalence that benefit dental and overall health [47]. Unfortunately, our field's new WWCC guidelines fail to make similar distinctions for a major subtype of periodontitis, and it is our premise that these guidelines are going to have a negative impact on the treatment and prevention of this unique disease.

Sexually transmitted diseases (STDs) provide a second example where sub-division has had a prominent effect on disease diagnosis treatment success [48]. Naming the specificity of these diseases has led to successful outcomes. For instance, Syphilis is initiated by *Treponema pallidum*, Gonorrhea is due to *Neisseria gonorrhoeae*, and Chlamydia is due to infection by *Chlamydia trachomatis*. Hepatitis B, Herpes Simplex virus (HSV), Human Papillomavirus (HPV), and AIDS initiated by HIV are infections due to specific viruses [49]. In contrast, some diseases can be initiated by a variety of infectious agents and promote morbidity and mortality resulting from disparate confounding factors. For example, Kaposi's sarcoma can be caused by (1) Herpes virus (HHV-8), (2) AIDS-related HIV, (3) iatrogenic transplant associations, (4) advanced age, most common in Eastern Europeans, Middle Eastern, and Mediterranean men, and (5) endemic Kaposi's sarcoma, occurring in young people in Africa [50]. These distinctions in diseases and the resulting tissue damage point to distinct therapies since they are complex and are best described by the Damage Response Framework introduced by Casadevall and Pirofski [51,52]. These authors described how HIV, the primary infectious agent in AIDS, typically is not the cause of mortality or morbidity [51,52]. The disease and irreversible tissue and organ damage were due to the immunocompromised host being unable to counteract damage inflicted by otherwise harmless microorganisms [53–55]. The lead WWCC authors' effort to compartmentalize Periodontal Diseases and Conditions fails to distinguish between diagnosis, treatment, and prognosis. On the positive side, their decisions may have improved opportunities for reimbursement by third-party payers, but that outcome remains to be seen.

4. Brief History of Landmark Experiments That Support Microbiological Associations with Dental Diseases

(A) Seminal Discoveries of Microbes and Dental Diseases.

Infectious diseases, by definition, have a microbial etiology, and thus, specific infectious agents are used to define the disease of interest. The recognition of microbiological aspects of dental disease began in full force in the earliest days of microbiology, when it first became an accepted field of biology. W.D. Miller, one of the first graduates of the Pennsylvania Dental College (graduating in 1879), went to Berlin to study in the laboratory of Robert Koch. Miller developed the chemo-parasitic theory of caries, suggesting that oral bacteria fermented sugars and produced acids that demineralized enamel [56]. He also developed the focal theory of infection, which suggested that bacteria or products of bacteria can travel to sites distant from the oral cavity and play a role in the development of various diseases that can affect the brain, lungs, and stomach. Sometime thereafter, Kritchevsky and Seguin [57], two French microbiologists, focused on periodontal disease and its treatment. They also believed that oral disease could be implicated in systemic diseases. Over time, the focal theory of infection was abandoned because treatments such as full mouth extraction designed to eliminate oral infection had no impact on the systemic diseases that these oral microbes were proposed to cause. Immunological research in the same era examined the role of oral microbes on immune responsiveness. Notable among them were papers by Beckwith and colleagues, who showed in dramatic fashion how oral bacterial plaque provoked a severe full-body immunological/inflammatory response [58].

However, the emphasis on microbiology and immunology did not receive substantial attention from the dental and research community until two dramatic experiments made a profound and lasting impact. In retrospect, these advances were not without their flaws, and thus, these landmark experiments need to be put into context based on our current understanding of disease [42].

The series of rigorous experiments by Paul Keyes and colleagues clearly showed that caries could be passed from mother to child when he compared the caries experiences of Golden Hamsters to Albino Hamsters [59]. Keyes was interested in dietary influences on the caries process but accidentally stumbled on the fact that Golden Hamsters were highly susceptible to carious dental lesions while Albino Hamsters were carie-free. By shifting newly born Albino pups into cages with Golden Hamster Dames, he found that these pups, delivered by cesarian section in a germ-free chamber, would now show caries because they were suckled by caries-exposed Dames. In contrast, Albino Dames, who suckled Golden Hamster pups, also delivered by cesarian section, showed no caries. It was found that penicillin could impede the carious process, and finally, it was shown that the agent provocateur was a Gram-positive coccus (later identified as Streptococcus). These experiments showed that caries were caused by oral microbes in animals fed carbohydrates and that the microbes could be passed from mother to child. These experiments were dramatic and demonstrated the importance of acid production and demineralization, but it is important to point out that the experiments were conducted in the absence of a fully developed microbiome. As a result, dysbiosis and homeostatic imbalance were not studied (Figure 1).

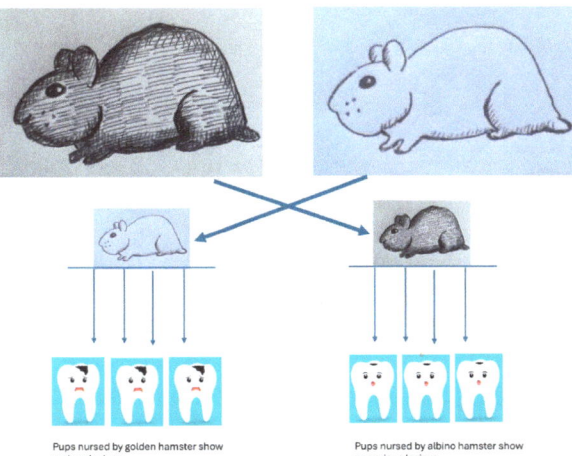

Figure 1. Illustration of the Golden and Albino Hamster experiments showing transmission from mother to child. Golden Hamster Dame (caries positive) is on the left, and Albino Hamster Dame (caries negative) is on the right side. Hamster pups are delivered in a sterile chamber by cesarian section under sterile conditions, and then albino pups are put in the cage of the Golden Hamster pups to be suckled by the Albino Dame (bottom right side of illustration) while the albino pups are suckled by the Golden Hamster Dame (bottom left side of the illustration). As shown, the Golden pups have no caries now (**bottom right**), while the albino pups have caries (**bottom left**).

The second seminal experiment was initiated and developed by Harald Löe and colleagues in Denmark [60]. The battleground was the junctional epithelium, the epithelial barrier that formed a boundary between the subgingival pocket area and the gingival and periodontal complex [61]. This complex boundary tissue contained all the elements that could thwart the inward progress and extension of supragingival bacteria to the subgingival space and provoke the ingress of destructive bacterial elements such as toxins, enzymes, antigens, lipoproteins, polysaccharides, and teichoic acids, etc. It was proposed that these substances could weaken the barrier and lead to the ingress of noxious elements, which could result in overall aberrant host responsiveness, tissue alteration, and disease at the local tissue site [62,63]. These experiments opened the door to our recognition that microbes formed on teeth in an ordered, deliberate manner. Exploration of this model showed that over time, the shift from a clean tooth surface to one colonized sequentially by microbial pioneers, followed by a complex mass of bacteria over time, moved from above to below the gum line. This progression from an aerobic to an anaerobic microbiome led to tissue inflammation (Figure 2). These studies showed that resumption of toothbrushing and other oral hygiene methods after abstention for a three-week period caused the removal of microbial masses and a return to gingival health and implied that the supragingival microflora was needed to supply nutrients to subgingival colonizers. This simple, elegant model permitted our colleagues to investigate plaque biofilm development and the associated effect of microbial dysbiosis on tissue inflammation. Sophisticated microbiological and histopathological studies provided a new and vital understanding of how microbes interacted and how they may have affected the underlying epithelial and connective tissue response [64,65]. However, these experiments also illustrated how host inflammation provided a feedback loop for nutritional supplementation that might have accounted for microbial expansion [66]. It was also shown that not all subjects responded in the same way and to the same extent relative to the microbiological challenge and that within the same mouth, different sites responded differently [67,68]. While now appreciated to be much more complicated than previously thought, these experiments resulted in more questions than answers and stimulated new areas of research that have moved well beyond dentistry. The whole field of coaggregation initiated by Paul Kolenbrander and colleagues was derived from these primitive but elegant experiments [69,70].

Zero time   7 days

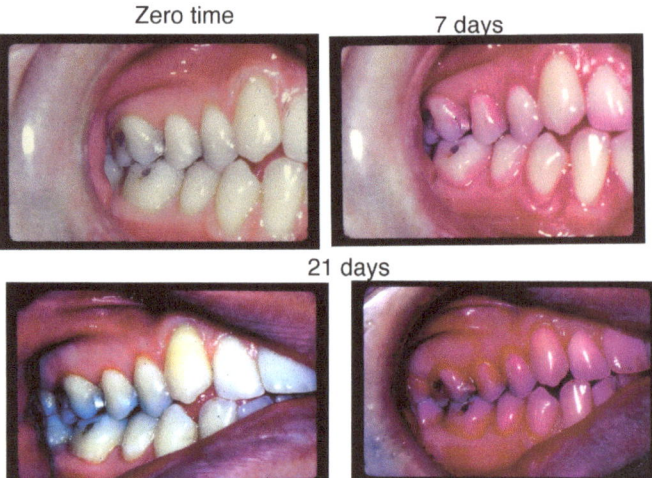

21 days

Figure 2. Illustration of the experimental gingivitis model. **Panel Upper Left:** illustration of pre-experimental gingival health of a student prior to abstaining from oral hygiene. **Panel Lower Left:** Gingival indices indicate punctate areas of redness around marginal ginigivae, especially in the upper premolar and molar areas 21 days after abstaining, while incisors show minimal inflammation. **Panel Upper Right:** Plaque disclosure seven days following abstaining from oral hygiene using erythrocin staining. Note minimal levels of plaque around the gingival margin of the teeth. **Panel Lower Right:** Plaque disclosure 21 days after abstaining from oral hygiene. Note the increased intensity of erythrocin staining, which illustrates increased plaque thickness, and how upper anterior teeth show less staining, i.e., less plaque accumulation.

These understandings re-awakened interest in the movement of bacteria from oral to distant sites [63]. Local destruction was thought to result from the direct result of bacterial by-products such as enzymes, toxins, etc., or from an overactive host response initially designed to stem the tide in favor of healing [71]. However, many believed that an excessive host response could also be responsible for local tissue destruction and/or disease. The experimental gingivitis model of Harald Löe and colleagues provided a close examination of the chronological association of oral bacteria in supragingival plaque and the coordinated dysregulation of the host response to accumulating bacteria [72] (Figure 2). In the figure above, a dental student abstained from all oral hygiene for a 3-week period, and both gingival and plaque indices were recorded at 7, 14, and 21 days after abstention. In addition, after this 21-day period, the student brushed and flossed their teeth, and the plaque and its resulting gingivitis returned to pre-abstention levels. The figure above illustrates the dramatic changes resulting from abstinence from oral hygiene (Figure 2).

(B)   Microbiology / *A. actinomycetemcomitans* and LAgP.

In an effort to abbreviate the long history of aggressive periodontitis in adolescents, it is worth mentioning the significance of the original recognition of what was first called periodontosis by Dr. Bernhard Gottlieb in Vienna in 1923 [10]. In the "modern era", Dr. Paul Baer (1971) presented a prescient, more detailed clinical description of this entity, then called Localized Juvenile Periodontitis (LJP) [6]. His description depicted rapid bone loss in younger individuals and was founded on a minimum of the following five clinical features: (1) the age of onset, (2) a family history, (3) the lack of relationship between local factors and deep pockets, (4) the rapid rate of progression, and (5) the effect on primary teeth. In the over five decades since this publication, the name of this disease and the disease itself have often been debated [1,3,73]. Unfortunately, since Baer's descriptive and thorough paper, many twists and turns have resulted in great confusion that has and will continue to seriously impede efforts to understand the microbiology, pathology, clinical definition, and treatment of this silent (often painless symptomatology) and uncommon condition.

In 1976, *Actinobacillus actinomycetemcomitans* (*Aa*; now *Aggregatibacter*) was shown to be associated with what was then called Localized Juvenile Periodontitis (LJP) [74,75]. This discovery coincided with an effort to demonstrate that specific microbial entities were responsible for specific forms of periodontal disease and led to the birth of the Specific Plaque Hypothesis (SPH) as its counter-part the Non-Specific Plaque Hypothesis (NSPH) [76,77]. *Aa*, a Gram-negative capnophilic microbe, was discovered in 1912 by Klinger [78] in a disease called Actinomycosis (lumpy jaw disease). Interestingly, *Aa* was not presented as the sole actor in this disease, and *Aa* was shown to have acted in concert with *Actinomyces israelii*; hence, the species name "actinomycetemcomitans" or in common with *Actinomyces* [78]. The SPH stimulated a significant body of research that explored specific microbes and their relationship to specific clinically recognizable forms of disease [79]. They were significant hypotheses for their time and stimulated a voluminous literature that examined the biological features of several microbes associated with both caries and periodontitis [80–82]. This intellectually challenging approach added significant scientific information to microbial features related to these diseases that were here-to-fore unexplored [83]. The understanding of dental diseases, as well as the biology and pathogenicity of several microorganisms associated with distinct forms of dental disease studied, benefited from these broad hypotheses. These microbes included but were not limited to *Streptococcus mutans* and its relationship to caries [41], *Actinobacillus* (now *Aggregatibacter*) *actinomycetemcomitans* and its relationship to LJP [74,75], *Bacteroides melaninogenicus* (now *Porphyromonas gingivalis*) [81,84] and its relationship to adult periodontitis, and *Actinomyces viscosus* and its relationship to root caries [85,86]. In retrospect, this appears to be a naïve approach, but nevertheless, it stimulated a plethora of research that led to a better understanding of glucans and dextrans in the case of *S. mutans* [87], leukotoxin and cytolethal distending toxin in the case of *Aa* [88], gingipains [89], hemolysins [90], and collagenases in the case of *P. gingivalis*, etc. [91]. The choice between the SPH and the NSPH was replaced by the Ecological Plaque Hypothesis [92], which, though modified over the years, has highlighted how dental diseases are influenced by ecological interactions and how ecological interactions can influence and modify dental diseases.

(C) Bradford–Hill Guidelines for Determining Causation: Association of *A. actinomycetemcomitans* in a Microbial Consortium with LAgP.

Of all dental diseases, LAgP is the closest to fulfilling the Bradford–Hill Guidelines for the association of provocative agents and disease [93]. LAgP, if defined in the most stringent manner, focusing on (1) adolescents with bone loss in the molar or incisor region and (2) young individuals typically of African descent, satisfies six of the nine aspects of the Bradford–Hill criteria. These associations are required to show (1) temporality, or exposure to the agent prior to disease; (2) strength of association, or the level of association of the microbe as determined statistically; (3) a biological gradient or dose-related response of a biologically-active substance as related to tissue damage, thus, the higher the exposure, the greater the disease; (4) consistency or reproducibility of critical experiments by others; (5) plausibility of the association of the agent with its pathological consequences such as tissue damage caused by the microbe; (6) alteration of the disease, or experimental evidence that intervention alters the provoking agent (either the bacteria, bacterial complex, or virulence agents) and the disease (See Table 2).

The associations presented in items 1 to 6 in the table below are based on a longitudinal model designed to study the transition from health to disease and demonstrate that a specified consortium of microbes, in addition to *Aa*, is required for the disease to occur (*Aa* is necessary but not sufficient) [29]. It is possible that the consortia can be expanded to include other microbes, but the original observation and the replication of the consortia by others who conducted longitudinal studies in well-defined adolescent patients of African descent have shown that *Aa* is a critical member in the disease process (see Table 2). We suggest that

Aa is a social influencer that, despite its low level, has an outsized influence on microbial community geography and behavioral interactions. The most likely rationale is that *Aa* impairs local immune responsiveness by production of leukotoxin, cytolethal distending toxin, and upregulation of complement resistance to allow for its survival as well as the survival of less adaptable subgingival microbes. Models and clinical studies suggest that the consortia consist of *Aa* and *Filifactor alocis*, among other subgingival microbes [29,94]. It appears as if *F. alocis* invades the biofilm at the later stages of subgingival biofilm formation but then provokes an aggressive and damaging host response by continuing to alter the local immune responsiveness with the production of its own form of leukotoxin. It appears as if both *Aa* and *F. alocis* relationships with disease could be strain related [95]. Other studies have found somewhat different consortia associated with periodontitis in older patients [96]. There is a great deal of evidence that points to bacteria as initiators of cell-mediated tissue loss in periodontitis [80,81,97]. Linking this to typical environmental factors of suspicion is still in its infancy. In contrast, studies of carious lesions are clearly dependent on environmental factors, such as carbohydrate consumption, that stimulate the growth and survival of acid-producing–acid-loving microbes [41,83]. It is still too early to conclude, but highly likely, that nutritional elements derived from the host and bacterial community co-inhabitants are important in microbial biogeography in LAgP, but these factors require more in-depth study, another reason to maintain recognition of the condition as a distinct clinical diagnosis.

Table 2. Causation of disease by microbial consortia assessed by Bradford–Hill criteria.

Hill Criteria	Example	Feasibility Yes/No?	Impact of Study and Reference
1. Temporal relationship	Exposure to agent precedes outcome	Yes	Longitudinal; healthy controls; age approp *Aa*; [98,99] Longitudinal; health controls age approp *Aa* + consort; [29,100]
2. Strength of Association	Size of association determined statistically	Yes	Show stats *Aa*; [98] Show stats *Aa* + consort; [29,100]
3. Dose-Response	^exposure > ^response	Yes	Measure consort vs. *Aa* alone; [29,100]
4. Consistency	Experiments reproduced	Yes	Show consort X-sect; [101,102] Show consort longitude; [29,100]
5. Plausibility	Assoc agrees with pathobiological explanations	Yes	Cdt has impact; [103] Ltx has impact; [95] Consortia passed from mother with disease to Child: local debridement improves inflammation, but consort remains; [104]. Consort metabolomics; [94]
6. Experimental evidence	Disease altered By intervention	Yes	Tetracycline admin reduces disease; [105] Tetracycline eliminates *Aa* and reduces disease; [106] Amox/Metra reduces disease, no antibiotic, no improvement; [107]
7. Alternative explanation	Rule out other explanations	? Open ? Open	[29,98,100]
8. Specificity	Cause produces effect	Yes	Flp and no disease; [108] Ltx and more bone loss; [109] Pga B is modified, and disease is reduced; [110]
9. Coherence	Theory consistent with Existing knowledge	Yes	Ltx and infections; [111] Cdt and infections; [112] Metabolomics and consortia; [94]

To support these associations in the Bradford–Hill guidelines, we required a minimum of three independent longitudinal studies that test for categories 1 through 6. For positive proof, at least two to three longitudinal studies were required to show a microbial consortia or virulence complex that was implicated in the disease prior to detection of disease. Due to the dearth of longitudinal studies performed using the appropriate populations, we proposed that one of the three studies showing that the presence of *Aa* alone could, at this moment, satisfy categories 1 through 6. Guidelines 7 to 9 were also assessed. Guideline 7 evaluates specificity and requires that the study demonstrates that a cause can produce an effect. Guideline 8 evaluates experimental alteration, which requires demonstrating that the disease can be altered by an intervention that reduces the overall damage response. Guideline 9 discusses coherence, which requires that the theory presented is in keeping with existing knowledge. Guidelines 7 to 9 have been limited to *Aa* and its effects because studies with the consortia in these categories have not yet been reported. While newer approaches to data integration have been used to expand the interpretation of the Bradford–Hill guidelines, they remain an important way to associate infectious agents with the etiology of disease.

5. Damage/Response Framework and LAgP

(A) Overview.

During the early period of microbiological studies, there was also an appropriate and important emphasis placed on the host immunological response [113]. At this time, the disease process was thought of as a war between "bad" bacteria and the host's responsiveness to those bacteria [114]. Notable experiments and descriptions by Page and Schroeder [64], work by Taubman et al. [115], Genco and Sanz [116], Taichman and colleagues [117,118], and Lehner and colleagues [113] emphasized stages in the inflammatory process that highlighted the prominence of specific cells such as polymorphonuclear leukocytes (PMNs), monocytes, macrophages, and plasma cells. The importance of each of these cell types in the process of tissue damage was carefully described, and particular emphasis was placed on plasma cells and their ability to destroy bone via osteoclastic activity. In parallel to this work, hemolysins, collagenases, and a host of destructive microbial factors derived from *B. melaninogenicus*, as well as a leukotoxin derived from *Aa*, were uncovered. The apparent emphasis and conflicts between microbiologists and immunologists became perceptible in many forms of infectious diseases [114]. More recently, periodontal research has shown that shifting levels of cytokines and chemokines act as signaling molecules that encourage cellular activity [68]. The emergence of the Damage/Response Framework shifted the emphasis away from a competition between microbes and the host to the intimate interaction between the microbe and its host in relation to disease progression [51] (Figure 3).

The oral cavity provides an ideal place to study host/microbial interactions [119,120]. First and foremost, the oral cavity is the entry point for most external substances. Material derived from the mouth is easily accessible for longitudinal analysis. Analysis of the interaction of cellular and acellular material can be collected and normalized for quantitative assessment. Oral collections can be performed painlessly, without aggressive/invasive/destructive methodologies, and with little to no interference with bodily function [119]. Finally, host influences, as well as external influences such as diet, radiation, circadian rhythms, drug effects, stress, aging, trauma healing, etc., can be documented in vivo [121,122].

The landmark experiments by Keyes and Löe provided the impetus for studies of microbial colonization of teeth and oral soft tissue from birth to senescence, which proved to be thorough and accurate and more easily studied than microbial colonization of the gut lining [123]. While feces collection is a way of studying gut colonization, microbial contact with gut epithelium can only be studied using invasive, colonoscopic methods [124]. The experimental model developed by Löe and colleagues has led to a more complete understanding of biofilm formation, coaggregation, and host responsiveness to microbial challenges [125]. Most recently, this model has been amplified to examine chemokine and cytokine levels over the time course of the 3-week non-brushing model [68]. Unfortunately, many assumptions made about the host response to the immediate bacterial challenge in this model have only recently been documented. It is quite conceivable that microbial factors move through the subgingival epithelial barrier formed by the junctional and sulcular epithelium and that local host inflammation plays an important role in microbial dysbiosis [62,126].

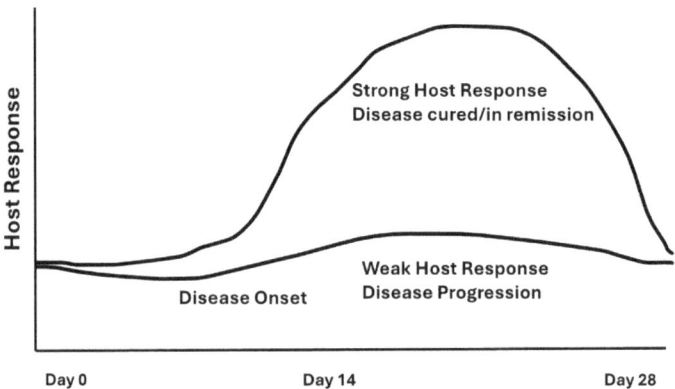

Figure 3. Diagram of Damage/Response. The solid upper line represents a normal healthy host response. At day zero an infection occurs driven by either a bacterial or viral challenge to the host. Following the microbial challenge after some delay the disease develops and the host response occurs. Disease resolves and the host response tapers to avoid furter tissue damage. The bolded straight line on the bottom represents an inadequate host response. Here tissue damage continues until an adequate host response occurs. Thus the bolded bottom line represents a muted host response and continued tissue damage.

(B)   Damage.

i.   Up until the mid-1980s, diagnostic microbiology, immunization, and antibiotic therapy have proven to provide a crucially important strategy used to control many prevalent infections caused by identifiable microorganisms [127]. However, since infections such as acquired immunodeficiency syndrome (AIDS), new insights into complex diseases that result from host modification leading to lethal progression due to secondary well-defined infections have taken center stage. These complex secondary infections required a holistic approach to diagnosis, prevention, and treatment of disease, hence the evolution of the damage/response framework [51].

Data acquired over the last 60 years of research in microbiology and immunology suggest that LAgP, in several ways, shows similarity to a local form of AIDS [29]. This realization contrasts with typical blood-borne mono-infections such as Syphilis (*Treponema pallidum*), Diphtheria (*Corynebacterium diphtheriae*), or Anthrax (*Bacillus anthracis*) or any blood-borne mono-infection that spreads disease-producing toxins [128]. In the localized immunomodulated AIDS-type scenario (LAgP/type scenario), once the barrier effect at the local site has been affected, bacteria from subgingival plaque weaken the local epithelial barrier and can enter the connective tissue, alter it, and then invade the bloodstream and translocate to distant sites [129,130].

In the context of this newly emerging concept of complex/host compromised/multi-species/multi-layered infection, the oral cavity provides an ideal environment to study diagnosis, initiation, and progression of diseases that involve multi-species microbial interactions and that produce altered host responses that fail to control shifting microbial challenges [119]. These sentiments are not meant to minimize post-infection host healing efforts to repair damage caused by infectious insults. On the contrary, because of access and exposure, the oral cavity can provide an ideal environment for studying disease initiation, metabolic processes, and disease progression in these complex multi-layered infections [131].

ii. *A. actinomycetemcomitans* is a pathobiont that is opportunistic in its own regard, but *Aa* also creates a perturbation of homeostasis by modulating PMNs, macrophages, lymphocytes, and other local immune functions [9,132–134]. Periodontitis, particularly LAgP, can be described as a disease that forms an acquired immunomodulated host response at the local level [135]. *Aa* and other microbes can be associated with disease susceptibility created by an imbalance between a dysbiotic microbiome, resulting in a perturbed host homeostasis [79]. The damage process can be further altered by subsets of other pathobionts, such as *P. gingivalis* [37] and *F. alocis* [136], such that exacerbated local damage can occur as a result of the overwhelming challenge due to the overgrowth of otherwise commensal/opportunistic microbes (*F. nucleatum, S. parasanguinis*) [29,94]. Overgrowth of these specific pathobionts and commensals in an otherwise compromised local immune response can now diminish the reparative capacity at the local site and enhance the resulting tissue damage [137]. The damage can remain localized, but in certain cases, an altered barrier can result in the movement of pathobionts and/or commensals to sites distant from the oral cavity [138]. Several experiments have replicated the early work of Okell and Elliott [129] showing transient bacteremias emanating from oral procedures can move many oral microbes to distant sites through the bloodstream [130,139]. Mechanical dental procedures such as scaling and root planning, as well as flossing, brushing, and eating an apple, can also induce transient bacteremias [140,141].

(C) Response.

i. Host: What we lack in this area of study is sufficient time course experiments that document host cellular changes that evolve from health to early, middle, and later stages of periodontal disease development [64]. Studies of these events have occurred more directly in experiments on endodontic lesions [142]. While different in some respects, oral biologists should be encouraged to examine the similarities and differences in periodontal and endodontic lesions. Just as the experimental gingivitis model enlightened our understanding of time-related events associated with microbial development in both the supragingival and subgingival environment, we still need to decipher the passage of substances from the "pocket" to and through the epithelial basement membrane to challenge the immediate area below the barrier membrane. It has taken 60 years from the inception of this classical gingivitis model to document interbacterial signaling distances and bacterial by-product host–cell interactions. However, we have now come to a time when technological advances have caught up to our theoretical understandings. We are now on the threshold of the merging of ideas and technological advances. DNA techniques [143], bar-coding [144], and CLASI_FISH [145] technologies now provide us with the tools required to study subgingival bacterial biogeography and cellular phenotypic responsiveness in a time-related manner [146]. In this quest for a more complete understanding of microbial–host interactions, we, as oral biologists, can now study these events in a sequential manner with easy access to microbial- and host-induced inflammatory response elements [39].

To re-iterate, early plaque development and initiation of gingivitis provided a straightforward path. Plaque could be collected easily, for example, from a tooth surrogate, which, when placed in the mouth, could serve as an aseptic surface for microbial associations over time [147–149]. Microbiological, immunological, and DNA technologies are now being used to catalog biogeography. A tooth analog can be placed at or just below the gum line to document the transition from supra to subgingival biofilm formation [150]. Documentation of subgingival plaque and the host response to supragingival plaque is more difficult. Early efforts to use mylar strips, cemental strips, and polyvinyl strips have yielded useful but incomplete information [147,148]. There have been several reports that have tried to document the complexity of subgingival plaque, but since this is the focal point for the spread of commensal oral microbes throughout the body, more must be done.

ii. Clinical Measurements as Determinants of Treatment Failure or Success. In the overall scheme of things, we have determined through both clinical observations and scientific testing that microbial plaque leads to gingival inflammation, which leads to tissue destruction, barrier alterations, pocketing, attachment loss, and then bone loss [151]. While this sequence of events has been observed in humans and replicated in animals, the timing of these events and their route of progression can be influenced and altered by a shifting microbiota as well as host responsiveness [63]. In the presence of sophisticated biological methodologies, our clinical measurement methods have remained stagnant and reliant on a periodontal probe and an X-ray.

It is hard to imagine that periodontitis is not due to a dysbiotic microbiome, which results in a disease defined by tissue destruction and weakened tooth support [151]. In most, if not all, diseases, successful treatment is typically measured by repair of altered tissue and/or alternatively in reduced recurrence or relapse of disease [30]. In most cases, treatment of periodontitis has relied on tissue repair as demonstrated by pocket depth reduction or attachment level gain [31]. However, in recent years, many studies have shown that oral microbes can travel through the bloodstream, and these oral bacteria can exacerbate systemic diseases at distant sites, such as colorectal cancer, heart disease, etc. [152]. In these cases, it might be prudent to look at treatment success in an alternative manner, such as the prevention of disease progression, recurrence, or relapse, as a way of reducing initiation of diseases at distant sites.

6. Distinct Characteristics of LAgP and an Alternative Approach for Assessing Treatment Success

(A)   Distinct Characteristics of LAgP: An Illustrative Case.

This case is presented to illustrate the distinctive nature of aggressive periodontal bone loss in a 20-year-old patient who reported to our clinic (RSDM) with extensive periodontal disease. After obtaining consent (IRB:PRO#012008035; year = 2009), we collected subgingival plaque, saliva, and buccal cells for analysis. The subgingival sample taken from various healthy and diseased sites had the "b" serotype of *Aa* with the JP2 promoter region. The patient had only one strain of *Aa* in his subgingival microbiome isolated from both healthy and diseased sites, with substantially more *Aa* isolated from diseased sites. We tested the *Aa* isolates for antibiotic sensitivity and for the presence of the hbpA-1, hpbA-2, and tbp-A pseudogenes using primers reported by Haubek et al. [153]. Saliva was assessed for salivary anti-*S. mutans* activity and buccal cells were used for the detection of the lactoferrin (LF) single nucleotide polymorphism associated with anti-*S. mutans* activity [154]. Our primary goal was to use our laboratory data to provide information about *Aa* antibiotic sensitivity, which could act as a supplement to treatment aimed at resolving this progressive disease in this young patient. The focus on *Aa* was pragmatic because our previous data had suggested that *Aa* was necessary but subsequently proved to be insufficient on its own to cause disease [29]; conversely, assessment of the complete consortia was impractical at that time. However, several of our other laboratory assessments proved useful.

While we recovered *Aa* from the diseased site, we cannot attribute disease to the presence of *Aa*. Microbial causation can only be implied if the bacterium preceded disease at the site of disease initiation [41]. Therefore, in this case, linking *Aa* to disease initiation and development can only be seen as speculative. Second, based on the complex patient history, it is reasonable to conclude that confounding social, psychological, and ecological modifiers could have contributed to a diminished host response, factors that could clearly be implicated in disease progression [42]. Based on antibiotic sensitivity testing, we ruled out the use of penicillin derivatives due to *Aa* insensitivity, which was a clinically useful finding. Furthermore, the age of the patient, the tooth loss attributed to periodontal disease, and the extent of bone loss indicated an aggressive nature of localized disease in this patient (Figure 4). We posit, based on tooth location and the patient's history, that the loss of two mandibular incisors was due to extensive periodontal disease (Figure 4). This conclusion appears to be a realistic appraisal of tooth loss as a consequence of (1) the dramatic level of bone loss in the existing molars and (2) the complete lack of caries in this subject's mouth (and the fact that the mandibular incisors lost are not typically vulnerable to caries) [155].

Testing for salivary anti-S. *mutans* activity gave an incomplete picture since several other oral microorganisms can also be related to caries [156]. The fact that anti-LF antibodies had no effect on *S. mutans* suggests that factors other than LF were responsible for the anti-*S. mutans* activity. This finding agrees with our previous data, where 20–30% of subjects tested showed factors independent of LF that also killed *S. mutans* [154]. The level of bone loss and lack of proximal decay reflects a pattern seen in many cases of LAgP [157,158]. Finally, point mutations in the hpbA-1 and tnp-B pseudogenes suggested that the patient was of West African descent [153].

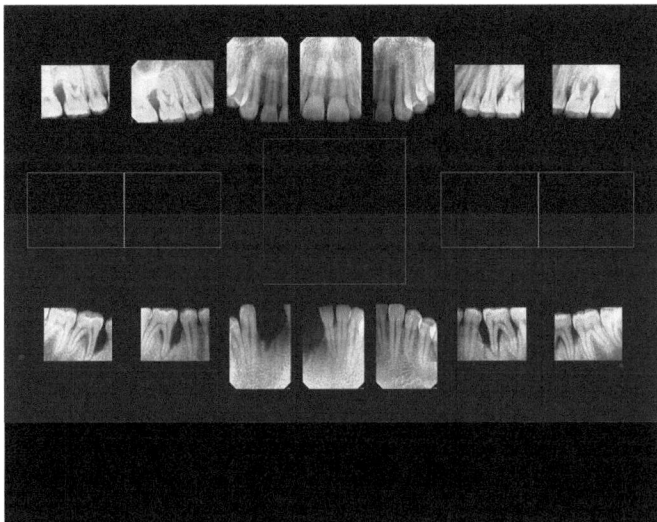

Figure 4. Radiographs of a patient with significant pocket depth and bone loss. Shows loss of two mandibular incisors and extensive bone loss in the first molar region,. Note the lack of carious lesions on radiographs throughout the dentition.

In summary, the clinical presentation, coupled with the presence of minimal plaque, the absence of proximal decay, severe periodontal disease, and the presence of *Aa*, all present a strong argument that LAgP is a disease uniquely distinguishable from periodontitis that occurs in adults (Figure 5).

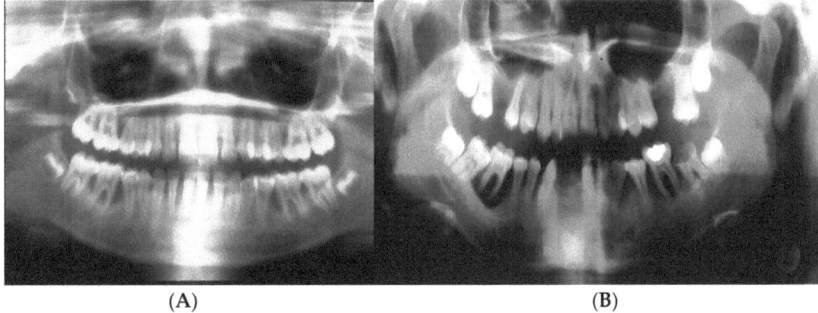

(A)   (B)

Figure 5. Panoramic radiographs of cases of aggressive periodontitis in adolescents. Panel (**A**) shows a panoramic view of excessive bone loss in the first molars and no carious lesions. Panel (**B**) shows more extensive disease in an adolescent with bone loss around the molars and missing molars and incisors with occlusal, but proximal decay is related to a blow-out occlusal lesion in the mandibular right second molar.

(B)   Another way of Assessing Periodontitis Treatment Success.

Many of our field's most revered longitudinal studies have relied on averaging pocket depth reduction or attachment level gain resulting from a specific treatment. Oftentimes, data are presented as a reduction of probing pocket depth or attachment gain over a 3-month to 1-year period after completion of treatment [31]. These measurements are usually averaged over 28 teeth, each tooth having six measured surfaces, thus yielding up to a total of 168 probable or measurable sites per mouth. To illustrate the issues related to averaging an overall dental response, we compared Cases A and B. Case A represents a patient that has two probable pockets, with each site having a 10 mm probing pocket depth on initial examination. Thus, we start with two 10 mm pockets on the distomesial and lingual–mesial surfaces of the left and right mandibular first molar or a total of 40 mm of pocketing at four diseased sites ($4 \times 10 = 40$). The remaining 164 probable sites have pockets of 3 mm. Cumulatively, these sites have a total of 492 mm (164 sites $\times$ 3 mm pockets per site = 492 mm of total probing depth). Overall, the patient presents with a total of 532 mm of pocketing in 168 probable sites ($492 + 40 = 532$ mm) over the whole mouth or an average of 3.17 mm of pocketing per site. After treatment, consisting of deep scaling and root planning, the four 10 mm pockets were reduced to 8 mm (now a total of 32 mm), while the remaining 164 sites remain at 3 mm ($164 \times 3 = 492$). After treatment, the total pocketing in the mouth is 492 mm + 32 mm = 524 mm. In this scenario, the average pocket depth is $524/168 = 3.12$ mm per site, a reduction of only 0.05 mm (3.17 mm to 3.12 mm). In case B pockets are reduced from 10 mm to 2 mm and thus pocket depth scores go from 3.17 to 2.97 ($492 + 2$ mm $\times 4 = 8$ mm or a total of 500 mm; $500/168 = 2.97$ mm). Thus in Case B a reduction of 20 mm is seen as compared to one of 0.05 mm. There has been some effort recently to focus on the categorization of changes in pocket depth reduction or attachment level gain in sites of low to moderate to high risk, but this has not been fully conceptualized or actuated [159].

When disease returns at specific sites, it is almost always associated with a dysbiotic microbiome [82,86]. Therefore, in contrast to measuring pocket depth reduction or attachment gain that we are accustomed to doing, a disease re-occurrence reduction or relapse to infection model is proposed. This can be applied independently or combined with standard measurements of improvement at the disease-affected sites. In this relapse model, we question how treatment has reduced the risk of re-occurrence of the disease. This disease re-occurrence reduction model implies that a goal of treatment is to enhance the local tissue barrier effect, such that the spreading of the infective oral bacteria from the site below the gum line to areas distant from the oral cavity is another goal of treatment. For example, in Case A, re-infection and return of deeply infected sites might likely occur 4 weeks post-treatment intervention, whereas in Case B, it might take 2 years or more for re-infection and reemergence of large pocket depths to re-occur. This pocket depth comparison presents an example of how oversight of re-infection in the oral dentition could provide a superior environment for patient overall health. The re-infection model takes into account the fact that while in our dental plaque model, we establish "good guys" and "bad guys" in a supra or subgingival plaque environment, we are fully aware of the fact that some of the so-called "good guys" become "bad guys" when they move past the local epithelial barrier and through the bloodstream such that they can then colonize heart valves, colon cells, lung or brain tissue [160]. Our proposed model moves away from the concept that infection and disease are a war between bacteria and the host and moves toward the concept that disease is the result of a damage/response ratio. The overall result appears to be dependent on coping mechanisms by the immune system that are designed to successfully reduce the consequences and spread of microbial/viral/fungal interactions from the local site to sites distant from their origin [161].

7. Conclusions: Future Challenges/Recommendations for the Clinical and Research Community

Consensus meetings in medicine and dentistry usually gather experts in the field with the goal of reviewing the current literature to define disease diagnoses and the most effective treatments [162]. The meetings are intended to generate a report that will be presented to the world of clinical scientists and practitioners with guidelines based on careful evaluation of information currently available. The resulting conclusions can have a profound influence on preventive, diagnostic, and treatment strategies for years into the future. The rules and regulations concerned with the conduct and presentation of material derived from consensus conferences vary widely and sometimes appear to be determined in a haphazard manner [162–164]. As such, the WWC organizers' re-classification of periodontitis case definitions is confounded by the use of overlapping and inaccurate clinical definitions that, in the case of LAgP, disregarded key clinical features that set it apart from other forms of periodontitis [21]. The decision to eliminate LAgP as a distinct form of periodontitis may have been partly because the population most often affected is not seen in some regions of the world.

While there is a great deal of inconsistency in the rules and regulations of consensus conferences, there are several examples that set standards for good practice. One example of a well-performed consensus conference required a vote of 70–80% or higher agreement by the experts involved to reach what could be labeled as a consensus [162–164]. Even with the 80% rule, consensus conference participants in the minority were required to publish the basis for their dissenting point of view so that readers could have a clear understanding as to how decisions were made, what the opposing views were, and the future directions projected [165]. This process should be used in the next WWCC.

To avoid problems that occurred in the most recent WWCC, it is recommended that future Consensus Conferences include the following characteristics: (1) A criteria statement made at the outset of the conference requiring that each foundational paper meet specific standards (e.g., use of the Delphi process, use of longitudinal data, clear case definitions, etc.); (2) a statement clearly articulating the percentage of participants that are required to agree with recommendations made by Conference attendees in order for the recommendation to be considered a consensus opinion (i.e., 70–80% agreement); (3) the presentation of dissenting points of view with explanations for such views so that readers of the report can gain an insight into the views of all participants; and (4) a concluding statement which should present realistic suggestions designed to improve case definitions in the future [165].

Finally, based on the data and examples presented in this review, we suggest that re-instating LAgP as a distinct disease entity should be carefully reconsidered. This would not in any manner replace Staging and Grading. However, for the reasons reviewed in this paper, the WWCC system should carefully consider making a distinction between this unique disease and the generally accepted adult form of periodontitis for the betterment of both research and clinical practice. In addition, as a result of the localized nature of this disease, we propose an expansion of treatment goals to include the reduction of re-emergence of new cycles of infection to serve as a supplementary way of assessing treatment success. This point speaks to the concern that re-infection of the local site may lead to the passage of either oral commensals or pathobionts from the local periodontal site to sites distant from the oral cavity. Therefore, the goals of treatment for periodontitis or any other dental infection are both to support local healing and repair coupled with the goal of reducing translocation of oral microbes throughout the body to limit the scope and extent of damage contributing to diseases occurring at sites distant from the oral cavity.

In an effort to engage our academic and clinical community in the process aimed at expanding the classification and therapeutic approaches as they relate to LAgP, we propose the following questions: Will the material we have presented in this review lead to a renewed enthusiasm for the reinstatement of LAgP as a distinct disease entity? (2) Will our community adopt the proposed addition of reduction in relapse of infection as an additional measure of treatment success in unique disease categories? For example, will the use of specifically targeted antibiotics typically used to reverse pocket depth and improve the gain of attachment also delay the time to relapse of infection and, as such, be considered as an additional measure of treatment success? (3) If this expanded assessment of treatment success is adopted, will this limit the potential for local dental infections to exacerbate systemic disease at sites distant from the oral cavity? The goal of this review has been to raise questions that can expand the horizons of dental research, diagnosis, and treatment so that clinicians and researchers can more effectively study how dental infections can be assessed and controlled for the benefit of the overall health and well-being of our patients.

Author Contributions: Each of the authors has contributed to the work described, has approved the submitted version of the paper, and agrees to be personally accountable for their own contributions to the paper. The paper was conceptualized by D.H.F. The original draft was written by D.H.F. and reviewed and revised by D.H.F., H.S. and S.R.D. All authors have read and agreed to the published version of the manuscript.

Funding: Funding for this work was partially obtained and supported by grants from the NIDCR; DE-13102, DE-016474, and DE-017968.

Institutional Review Board Statement: Information obtained for the case report presented was approved by the IRB of Rutgers University (PRO# 012008035) in 2009 and was conducted according to the guidelines of the Declaration of Helsinki 1975.

Informed Consent Statement: Informed consent was obtained from the subject material as described in the IRB statement above and presented in this paper. Other material regarding any subject material was waived and was not identifiable and, therefore, not applicable.

Acknowledgments: The authors would like to acknowledge contributions from Dipti Godboley, Kabilan Veliyagounder, and Senthil Velusamy. We would also like to thank Tom Bissell for his help with the case illustrated in the paper. In addition, we would like to thank the teachers, administrators, students, and parents from the Newark School System who participated in work that formed the basis of previously published studies of Localized Aggressive Periodontitis in adolescents.

Conflicts of Interest: None of the authors have any conflicts of interest that may be perceived as influencing the writing, representation, and/or interpretation of the research reported or summarized in this narrative review.

References

1. Papapanou, P.N.; Sanz, M.; Buduneli, N.; Dietrich, T.; Feres, M.; Fine, D.H.; Flemmig, T.F.; Garcia, R.; Giannobile, W.V.; Graziani, F.; et al. Periodontitis: Consensus report of workgroup 2 of the 2017 World Workshop on the Classification of Periodontal and Peri-Implant Diseases and Conditions. *J. Periodontol.* **2018**, *89* (Suppl. S1), S173–S182. [CrossRef] [PubMed]
2. Caton, J.G.; Armitage, G.; Berglundh, T.; Chapple, I.L.C.; Jepsen, S.; Kornman, K.S.; Mealey, B.L.; Papapanou, P.N.; Sanz, M.; Tonetti, M.S. A new classification scheme for periodontal and peri-implant diseases and conditions—Introduction and key changes from the 1999 classification. *J. Clin. Periodontol.* **2018**, *45* (Suppl. S20), S1–S8. [CrossRef] [PubMed]
3. Armitage, G.C. Periodontal diseases: Diagnosis. *Ann. Periodontol.* **1996**, *1*, 37–215. [CrossRef] [PubMed]
4. Greene, F.L. Cancer staging in outcomes assessment. *J. Surg. Oncol.* **2014**, *110*, 616–620. [CrossRef]
5. Park, B.K.; Schneider, J.; Suh, Y.J. Survival analysis for patients with metachronous contralateral breast cancer: Insights from a retrospective study. *Oncol. Lett.* **2024**, *28*, 390. [CrossRef]
6. Baer, P.N. The case for periodontosis as a clinical entity. *J. Periodontol.* **1971**, *42*, 516–520. [CrossRef]
7. Marazita, M.L.; Burmeister, J.A.; Gunsolley, J.C.; Koertge, T.E.; Lake, K.; Schenkein, H.A. Evidence for autosomal dominant inheritance and race-specific heterogeneity in early-onset periodontitis. *J. Periodontol.* **1994**, *65*, 623–630. [CrossRef]
8. Loe, H.; Brown, L.J. Early onset periodontitis in the United States of America. *J. Periodontol.* **1991**, *62*, 608–616. [CrossRef] [PubMed]
9. Fine, D.H.; Kaplan, J.B.; Kachlany, S.C.; Schreiner, H.C. How we got attached to Actinobacillus actinomycetemcomitans: A model for infectious diseases. *Periodontol. 2000* **2006**, *42*, 114–157. [CrossRef]
10. Fine, D.H.; Cohen, D.W.; Bimstein, E.; Bruckmann, C. A ninety-year history of periodontosis: The legacy of Professor Bernhard Gottlieb. *J. Periodontol.* **2015**, *86*, 1–6. [CrossRef]
11. Zambon, J.J. Authors' response. *J. Am. Dent. Assoc.* **2020**, *151*, 160–161. [CrossRef]
12. de Carvalho, F.M.; Tinoco, E.M.; Govil, M.; Marazita, M.L.; Vieira, A.R. Aggressive periodontitis is likely influenced by a few small effect genes. *J. Clin. Periodontol.* **2009**, *36*, 468–473. [CrossRef]

13. Fine, D.H.; Armitage, G.C.; Genco, R.J.; Griffen, A.L.; Diehl, S.R. Unique etiologic, demographic, and pathologic characteristics of localized aggressive periodontitis support classification as a distinct subcategory of periodontitis. *J. Am. Dent. Assoc.* **2019**, *150*, 922–931. [CrossRef] [PubMed]
14. Pallos, D.; Acevedo, A.C.; Mestrinho, H.D.; Cordeiro, I.; Hart, T.C. Novel cathepsin C mutation in a Brazilian family with Papillon-Lefevre syndrome: Case report and mutation update. *J. Dent. Child.* **2010**, *77*, 36–41.
15. Diehl, S.R.; Wu, T.; Michalowicz, B.S.; Brooks, C.N.; Califano, J.V.; Burmeister, J.A.; Schenkein, H.A. Quantitative measures of aggressive periodontitis show substantial heritability and consistency with traditional diagnoses. *J. Periodontol.* **2005**, *76*, 279–288. [CrossRef] [PubMed]
16. Yoo, H.W. Development of orphan drugs for rare diseases. *Clin. Exp. Pediatr.* **2024**, *67*, 315–327. [CrossRef]
17. Wade, D.N.; Kerns, D.G. Acute necrotizing ulcerative gingivitis-periodontitis: A literature review. *Mil. Med.* **1998**, *163*, 337–342. [CrossRef]
18. Albandar, J.M. Disparities and social determinants of periodontal diseases. *Periodontol. 2000* **2024**. [CrossRef]
19. Botelho, J.; Machado, V.; Proenca, L.; Mendes, J.J. The 2018 periodontitis case definition improves accuracy performance of full-mouth partial diagnostic protocols. *Sci. Rep.* **2020**, *10*, 7093. [CrossRef]
20. Fredman, G.; Oh, S.F.; Ayilavarapu, S.; Hasturk, H.; Serhan, C.N.; Van Dyke, T.E. Impaired phagocytosis in localized aggressive periodontitis: Rescue by Resolvin E1. *PLoS ONE* **2011**, *6*, e24422. [CrossRef]
21. Fine, D.H.; Patil, A.G.; Loos, B.G. Classification and diagnosis of aggressive periodontitis. *J. Periodontol.* **2018**, *89* (Suppl. S1), S103–S119. [CrossRef] [PubMed]
22. Endersby, J. Lumpers and splitters: Darwin, Hooker, and the search for order. *Science* **2009**, *326*, 1496–1499. [CrossRef] [PubMed]
23. Mukherjee, S. *The Emperor of All Maladies: A Biography of Cancer*; Scribner: New York, NY, USA, 2010.
24. Denoix, P.F. Présentation d'une nomenclature classification des cancers basee sur un atlas [Nomenclature and classification of cancers based on an atlas]. *Acta Unio Int. Contra Cancrum* **1953**, *9*, 769–771. [PubMed]
25. Snyderman, R. Personalized health care: From theory to practice. *Biotechnol. J.* **2012**, *7*, 973–979. [CrossRef] [PubMed]
26. Albandar, J.M. Aggressive periodontitis: Case definition and diagnostic criteria. *Periodontol. 2000* **2014**, *65*, 13–26. [CrossRef]
27. Cekici, A.; Kantarci, A.; Hasturk, H.; Van Dyke, T.E. Inflammatory and immune pathways in the pathogenesis of periodontal disease. *Periodontol. 2000* **2014**, *64*, 57–80. [CrossRef]
28. Billings, M.; Holtfreter, B.; Papapanou, P.N.; Mitnik, G.L.; Kocher, T.; Dye, B.A. Age-dependent distribution of periodontitis in two countries: Findings from NHANES 2009 to 2014 and SHIP-TREND 2008 to 2012. *J. Periodontol.* **2018**, *89* (Suppl. S1), S140–S158. [CrossRef]
29. Fine, D.H.; Markowitz, K.; Fairlie, K.; Tischio-Bereski, D.; Ferrendiz, J.; Furgang, D.; Paster, B.J.; Dewhirst, F.E. A consortium of *Aggregatibacter actinomycetemcomitans*, *Streptococcus parasanguinis*, and *Filifactor alocis* is present in sites prior to bone loss in a longitudinal study of localized aggressive periodontitis. *J. Clin. Microbiol.* **2013**, *51*, 2850–2861. [CrossRef]
30. Needleman, I.; Garcia, R.; Gkranias, N.; Kirkwood, K.L.; Kocher, T.; Iorio, A.D.; Moreno, F.; Petrie, A. Mean annual attachment, bone level, and tooth loss: A systematic review. *J. Periodontol.* **2018**, *89* (Suppl. S1), S120–S139. [CrossRef]
31. Leow, N.M.; Moreno, F.; Marletta, D.; Hussain, S.B.; Buti, J.; Almond, N.; Needleman, I. Recurrence and progression of periodontitis and methods of management in long-term care: A systematic review and meta-analysis. *J. Clin. Periodontol.* **2022**, *49* (Suppl. S24), 291–313. [CrossRef]
32. Fine, D.H.; Armitage, G.C.; Griffen, A.L.; Diehl, S.R. Authors' response. *J. Am. Dent. Assoc.* **2020**, *151*, 160. [CrossRef]
33. Bik, E.M.; Long, C.D.; Armitage, G.C.; Loomer, P.; Emerson, J.; Mongodin, E.F.; Nelson, K.E.; Gill, S.R.; Fraser-Liggett, C.M.; Relman, D.A. Bacterial diversity in the oral cavity of 10 healthy individuals. *ISME J.* **2010**, *4*, 962–974. [CrossRef] [PubMed]
34. Proctor, D.M.; Relman, D.A. The Landscape Ecology and Microbiota of the Human Nose, Mouth, and Throat. *Cell Host Microbe* **2017**, *21*, 421–432. [CrossRef] [PubMed]
35. Rubinstein, M.R.; Baik, J.E.; Lagana, S.M.; Han, R.P.; Raab, W.J.; Sahoo, D.; Dalerba, P.; Wang, T.C.; Han, Y.W. Fusobacterium nucleatum promotes colorectal cancer by inducing Wnt/beta-catenin modulator Annexin A1. *EMBO Rep.* **2019**, *20*. [CrossRef]
36. Han, Y.W.; Redline, R.W.; Li, M.; Yin, L.; Hill, G.B.; McCormick, T.S. Fusobacterium nucleatum Induces Premature and Term Stillbirths in Pregnant Mice: Implication of Oral Bacteria in Preterm Birth. *Infect. Immun.* **2004**, *72*, 2272–2279. [CrossRef] [PubMed]
37. Zambon, J.J. Periodontal diseases: Microbial factors. *Ann Periodontol* **1996**, *1*, 879–925. [CrossRef]
38. Darveau, R.P. Periodontitis: A polymicrobial disruption of host homeostasis. *Nat. Rev. Microbiol.* **2010**, *8*, 481–490. [CrossRef]
39. Lamont, R.J.; Koo, H.; Hajishengallis, G. The oral microbiota: Dynamic communities and host interactions. *Nat. Rev. Microbiol.* **2018**, *16*, 745–759. [CrossRef]
40. American Academy of Pediatric Dentistry Council on Clinical Affairs. Policy on use of a caries-risk assessment tool (CAT) for infants, children, and adolescents. *Pediatr. Dent.* **2005**, *27*, 25–27.
41. Loesche, W.J. Role of *Streptococcus mutans* in human dental decay. *Microbiol. Rev.* **1986**, *50*, 353–380. [CrossRef]
42. Marsh, P.D. Are dental diseases examples of ecological catastrophes? *Microbiology* **2003**, *149*, 279–294. [CrossRef] [PubMed]
43. Folayan, M.N.O.; Amalia, R.; Kemoli, A.; Sun, I.G.; Duangthip, D.; Abodunrin, O.; Virtanen, J.I.; Masumo, R.M.; Vukovic, A.; Al-Batayneh, O.B.; et al. Can the sustainable development goal 9 support an untreated early childhood caries elimination agenda? *BMC Oral Health* **2024**, *24*, 776. [CrossRef] [PubMed]
44. Sheykholeslam, Z.; Buonocore, M.G. Bonding of resins to phosphoric acid-etched enamel surfaces of permanent and deciduous teeth. *J. Dent. Res.* **1972**, *51*, 1572–1576. [CrossRef] [PubMed]

45. Li, K.; Chen, A.Y.; Geissler, K.H.; Dick, A.W.; Kranz, A.M. Clinician characteristics associated with fluoride varnish applications during well-child visits. *Am. J. Manag. Care* **2024**, *30*, e203–e209. [CrossRef]
46. Lumsden, C.L.; Edelstein, B.L.; Basch, C.E.; Wolf, R.L.; Koch, P.A.; McKeague, I.; Leu, C.S.; Andrews, H. Protocol for a family-centered behavioral intervention to reduce early childhood caries: The MySmileBuddy program efficacy trial. *BMC Oral Health* **2021**, *21*, 246. [CrossRef]
47. Lienhart, G.; Elsa, M.; Farge, P.; Schott, A.M.; Thivichon-Prince, B.; Chaneliere, M. Factors perceived by health professionals to be barriers or facilitators to caries prevention in children: A systematic review. *BMC Oral Health* **2023**, *23*, 767. [CrossRef]
48. Woodward, C.; Fisher, M.A. Drug treatment of common STDs: Part II. Vaginal infections, pelvic inflammatory disease and genital warts. *Am. Fam. Physician.* **1999**, *60*, 1716–1722. [PubMed]
49. Malhotra, M.; Sood, S.; Mukherjee, A.; Muralidhar, S.; Bala, M. Genital *Chlamydia trachomatis*: An update. *Indian J. Med. Res.* **2013**, *138*, 303–316.
50. Radu, O.; Pantanowitz, L. Kaposi sarcoma. *Arch. Pathol. Lab. Med.* **2013**, *137*, 289–294. [CrossRef]
51. Casadevall, A.; Pirofski, L.A. Host-pathogen interactions: Redefining the basic concepts of virulence and pathogenicity. *Infect. Immun.* **1999**, *67*, 3703–3713. [CrossRef]
52. Casadevall, A.; Pirofski, L.A. Microbiology: Ditch the term pathogen. *Nature* **2014**, *516*, 165–166. [CrossRef]
53. Casadevall, A.; Pirofski, L.A. What is a pathogen? *Ann. Med.* **2002**, *34*, 2–4. [CrossRef] [PubMed]
54. Pirofski, L.; Casadevall, A. The Damage-Response Framework as a Tool for the Physician-Scientist to Understand the Pathogenesis of Infectious Diseases. *J. Infect. Dis.* **2018**, *218*, S7–S11. [CrossRef] [PubMed]
55. Pirofski, L.A.; Casadevall, A. The meaning of microbial exposure, infection, colonisation, and disease in clinical practice. *Lancet Infect. Dis.* **2002**, *2*, 628–635. [CrossRef] [PubMed]
56. Miller, W.D. *The Micro-Organisms of the Human Mouth: The Local and General Diseases Which are Caused by Them*; Classics of Dentistry Library: Sydney, Australia, 1890.
57. Kritchevsky, B.; Seguin, P. The Pathogenesis and Treatment of Pyorrhea Alveolaris. *Dent. Cosm. A Mon. Rec. Dent. Sci.* **1918**, *60*, 781–784.
58. Beckwith, T.D.; Williams, A.; Rose, E.T. The role of bacteria in pyorrhea. *Med. J. Rec.* **1929**, *129*, 333–336.
59. Keyes, P.H.; Fitzgerald, R.J. Dental caries in the Syrian hamster. IX. *Arch. Oral. Biol.* **1962**, *7*, 267–277. [CrossRef]
60. Loe, H.; Theilade, E.; Jensen, S.B. Experimental Gingivitis in Man. *J. Periodontol.* **1965**, *36*, 177–187. [CrossRef]
61. Fine, D.H. Incorporating new technologies in periodontal diagnosis into training programs and patient care: A critical assessment and a plan for the future. *J. Periodontol.* **1992**, *63*, 383–393. [CrossRef]
62. Listgarten, M.A. Periodontal probing: What does it mean? *J. Clin. Periodontol.* **1980**, *7*, 165–176. [CrossRef]
63. Cugini, C.; Ramasubbu, N.; Tsiagbe, V.K.; Fine, D.H. Dysbiosis From a Microbial and Host Perspective Relative to Oral Health and Disease. *Front. Microbiol.* **2021**, *12*, 617485. [CrossRef] [PubMed]
64. Page, R.C.; Schroeder, H.E. Pathogenesis of inflammatory periodontal disease. A summary of current work. *Lab. Investig.* **1976**, *34*, 235–249. [PubMed]
65. Curtis, M.A.; Diaz, P.I.; Van Dyke, T.E. The role of the microbiota in periodontal disease. *Periodontol. 2000* **2020**, *83*, 14–25. [CrossRef] [PubMed]
66. Lang, N.P.; Kiel, R.A.; Anderhalden, K. Clinical and microbiological effects of subgingival restorations with overhanging or clinically perfect margins. *J. Clin. Periodontol.* **1983**, *10*, 563–578. [CrossRef]
67. Theilade, E.; Wright, W.H.; Jensen, S.B.; Loe, H. Experimental gingivitis in man. II. A longitudinal clinical and bacteriological investigation. *J. Periodontal. Res.* **1966**, *1*, 1–13. [CrossRef] [PubMed]
68. Bamashmous, S.; Kotsakis, G.A.; Kerns, K.A.; Leroux, B.G.; Zenobia, C.; Chen, D.; Trivedi, H.M.; McLean, J.S.; Darveau, R.P. Human variation in gingival inflammation. *Proc. Natl. Acad. Sci. USA* **2021**, *118*, e2012578118. [CrossRef]
69. Kolenbrander, P.E.; London, J. Adhere today, here tomorrow: Oral bacterial adherence. *J. Bacteriol.* **1993**, *175*, 3247–3252. [CrossRef]
70. Kolenbrander, P.E.; Palmer, R.J., Jr.; Periasamy, S.; Jakubovics, N.S. Oral multispecies biofilm development and the key role of cell-cell distance. *Nat. Rev. Microbiol.* **2010**, *8*, 471–480. [CrossRef]
71. Casadevall, A.; Pirofski, L.A. What is a host? Incorporating the microbiota into the damage-response framework. *Infect. Immun.* **2015**, *83*, 2–7. [CrossRef]
72. Loe, H.; Silness, J. Periodontal disease in pregancy. Prevalence and severity. *Acta Odontol Scand* **1963**, *21*, 533–551. [CrossRef]
73. Armitage, G.C. Learned and unlearned concepts in periodontal diagnostics: A 50-year perspective. *Periodontol. 2000* **2013**, *62*, 20–36. [CrossRef] [PubMed]
74. Newman, M.G.; Socransky, S.S.; Savitt, E.D.; Propas, D.A.; Crawford, A. Studies of the microbiology of periodontosis. *J. Periodontol.* **1976**, *47*, 373–379. [CrossRef] [PubMed]
75. Slots, J. The predominant cultivable organisms in juvenile periodontitis. *Scand. J. Dent. Res.* **1976**, *84*, 1–10. [CrossRef] [PubMed]
76. Loesche, W.J. Chemotherapy of dental plaque infections. *Oral. Sci. Rev.* **1976**, *9*, 65–107. [PubMed]
77. Loesche, W.J. Clinical and microbiological aspects of chemotherapeutic agents used according to the specific plaque hypothesis. *J. Dent. Res.* **1979**, *58*, 2404–2412. [CrossRef]
78. Klinger, R. Untersuchungen uber menschliche aktinomycose. *Zentralbl. Bakteriol.* **1912**, *62*, 191–200.

79. Marsh, P.D.; Zaura, E. Dental biofilm: Ecological interactions in health and disease. *J. Clin. Periodontol.* **2017**, *44* (Suppl. S18), S12–S22. [CrossRef]
80. Moore, W.E.; Moore, L.H.; Ranney, R.R.; Smibert, R.M.; Burmeister, J.A.; Schenkein, H.A. The microflora of periodontal sites showing active destructive progression. *J. Clin. Periodontol.* **1991**, *18*, 729–739. [CrossRef]
81. Socransky, S.S.; Haffajee, A.D.; Cugini, M.A.; Smith, C.; Kent, R.L., Jr. Microbial complexes in subgingival plaque. *J. Clin. Periodontol.* **1998**, *25*, 134–144. [CrossRef]
82. Socransky, S.S.; Haffajee, A.D. Periodontal microbial ecology. *Periodontol. 2000* **2005**, *38*, 135–187. [CrossRef]
83. Marsh, P.D. In Sickness and in Health-What Does the Oral Microbiome Mean to Us? An Ecological Perspective. *Adv. Dent. Res.* **2018**, *29*, 60–65. [CrossRef]
84. Gibbons, R.J.; Macdonald, J.B. Hemin and vitamin K compounds as required factors for the cultivation of certain strains of *Bacteroides melaninogenicus*. *J. Bacteriol.* **1960**, *80*, 164–170. [CrossRef] [PubMed]
85. Komiyama, K.; Khandelwal, R.L.; Heinrich, S.E. Glycogen synthetic and degradative activities by Actinomyces viscosus and Actinomyces naeslundii of root surface caries and noncaries sites. *Caries Res.* **1988**, *22*, 217–225. [CrossRef] [PubMed]
86. Moore, W.E.C.; Moore, L.V.H. The bacteria of periodontal disease. *Periodontol. 2000* **1994**, *5*, 66–77. [CrossRef]
87. Schachtele, C.F.; Loken, A.E.; Schmitt, M.K. Use of specifically labeled sucrose for comparison of extracellular glucan and fructan metabolism by oral streptococci. *Infect. Immun.* **1972**, *5*, 263–266. [CrossRef] [PubMed]
88. Kachlany, S.C.; Fine, D.H.; Figurski, D.H. Secretion of RTX leukotoxin by Actinobacillus actinomycetemcomitans. *Infect. Immun.* **2000**, *68*, 6094–6100. [CrossRef]
89. Pavloff, N.; Potempa, J.; Pike, R.N.; Prochazka, V.; Kiefer, M.C.; Travis, J.; Barr, P.J. Molecular cloning and structural characterization of the Arg-gingipain proteinase of Porphyromonas gingivalis. Biosynthesis as a proteinase-adhesin polyprotein. *J. Biol. Chem.* **1995**, *270*, 1007–1010. [CrossRef]
90. Chu, L.; Bramanti, T.E.; Ebersole, J.L.; Holt, S.C. Hemolytic activity in the periodontopathogen Porphyromonas gingivalis: Kinetics of enzyme release and localization. *Infect. Immun.* **1991**, *59*, 1932–1940. [CrossRef] [PubMed]
91. Gibbons, R.J.; Macdonald, J.B. Degradation of collagenous substrates by *Bacteroides melaninogenicus*. *J. Bacteriol.* **1961**, *81*, 614–621. [CrossRef]
92. Marsh, P.D. Microbial ecology of dental plaque and its significance in health and disease. *Adv. Dent. Res.* **1994**, *8*, 263–271. [CrossRef]
93. Usman, M.; Hameed, Y.; Ahmad, M. Does human papillomavirus cause human colorectal cancer? Applying Bradford Hill criteria postulates. *Ecancermedicalscience* **2020**, *14*, 1107. [CrossRef] [PubMed]
94. Wang, Q.; Wright, C.J.; Dingming, H.; Uriarte, S.M.; Lamont, R.J. Oral community interactions of *Filifactor alocis* in vitro. *PLoS ONE* **2013**, *8*, e76271. [CrossRef] [PubMed]
95. Johansson, A.; Claesson, R.; Aberg, C.H.; Haubek, D.; Lindholm, M.; Jasim, S.; Oscarsson, J. Genetic Profiling of *Aggregatibacter actinomycetemcomitans* Serotype B Isolated from Periodontitis Patients Living in Sweden. *Pathogens* **2019**, *8*, 153. [CrossRef]
96. Haffajee, A.D.; Patel, M.; Socransky, S.S. Microbiological changes associated with four different periodontal therapies for the treatment of chronic periodontitis. *Oral Microbiol. Immunol.* **2008**, *23*, 148–157. [CrossRef]
97. Socransky, S.S.; Haffajee, A.D. Microbial mechanisms in the pathogenesis of destructive periodontal diseases: A critical assessment. *J. Periodontal. Res.* **1991**, *26*, 195–212. [CrossRef]
98. Haubek, D.; Ennibi, O.K.; Poulsen, K.; Vaeth, M.; Poulsen, S.; Kilian, M. Risk of aggressive periodontitis in adolescent carriers of the JP2 clone of Aggregatibacter (*Actinobacillus*) actinomycetemcomitans in Morocco: A prospective longitudinal cohort study. *Lancet* **2008**, *371*, 237–242. [CrossRef]
99. Hoglund Aberg, C.; Kwamin, F.; Claesson, R.; Dahlen, G.; Johansson, A.; Haubek, D. Progression of attachment loss is strongly associated with presence of the JP2 genotype of *Aggregatibacter actinomycetemcomitans*: A prospective cohort study of a young adolescent population. *J. Clin. Periodontol.* **2014**, *41*, 232–241. [CrossRef]
100. Razooqi, Z.; Tjellstrom, I.; Hoglund Aberg, C.; Kwamin, F.; Claesson, R.; Haubek, D.; Johansson, A.; Oscarsson, J. Association of *Filifactor alocis* and its RTX toxin gene ftxA with periodontal attachment loss, and in synergy with *Aggregatibacter actinomycetemcomitans*. *Front. Cell. Infect. Microbiol.* **2024**, *14*, 1376358. [CrossRef] [PubMed]
101. Shaddox, L.M.; Huang, H.; Lin, T.; Hou, W.; Harrison, P.L.; Aukhil, I.; Walker, C.B.; Klepac-Ceraj, V.; Paster, B.J. Microbiological characterization in children with aggressive periodontitis. *J. Dent. Res.* **2012**, *91*, 927–933. [CrossRef]
102. Koo, S.S.; Fernandes, J.G.; Li, L.; Huang, H.; Aukhil, I.; Harrison, P.; Diaz, P.I.; Shaddox, L.M. Evaluation of microbiome in primary and permanent dentition in grade C periodontitis in young individuals. *J. Periodontol.* **2024**. [CrossRef]
103. Shenker, B.J.; Walker, L.P.; Zekavat, A.; Korostoff, J.; Boesze-Battaglia, K. *Aggregatibacter actinomycetemcomitans* Cytolethal Distending Toxin-Induces Cell Cycle Arrest in a Glycogen Synthase Kinase (GSK)-3-Dependent Manner in Oral Keratinocytes. *Int. J. Mol. Sci.* **2022**, *23*, 1831. [CrossRef] [PubMed]
104. Monteiro, M.F.; Altabtbaei, K.; Kumar, P.S.; Casati, M.Z.; Ruiz, K.G.S.; Sallum, E.A.; Nociti-Junior, F.H.; Casarin, R.C.V. Parents with periodontitis impact the subgingival colonization of their offspring. *Sci. Rep.* **2021**, *11*, 1357. [CrossRef] [PubMed]
105. Novak, M.J.; Stamatelakys, C.; Adair, S.M. Resolution of early lesions of juvenile periodontitis with tetracycline therapy alone: Long-term observations of 4 cases. *J. Periodontol.* **1991**, *62*, 628–633. [CrossRef] [PubMed]
106. Mandell, R.L.; Tripodi, L.S.; Savitt, E.; Goodson, J.M.; Socransky, S.S. The effect of treatment on Actinobacillus actinomycetemcomitans in localized juvenile periodontitis. *J. Periodontol.* **1986**, *57*, 94–99. [CrossRef]

107. Miller, K.A.; Branco-de-Almeida, L.S.; Wolf, S.; Hovencamp, N.; Treloar, T.; Harrison, P.; Aukhil, I.; Gong, Y.; Shaddox, L.M. Long-term clinical response to treatment and maintenance of localized aggressive periodontitis: A cohort study. *J. Clin. Periodontol.* **2017**, *44*, 158–168. [CrossRef]

108. Schreiner, H.C.; Sinatra, K.; Kaplan, J.B.; Furgang, D.; Kachlany, S.C.; Planet, P.J.; Perez, B.A.; Figurski, D.H.; Fine, D.H. Tight-adherence genes of *Actinobacillus actinomycetemcomitans* are required for virulence in a rat model. *Proc. Natl. Acad. Sci. USA* **2003**, *100*, 7295–7300. [CrossRef]

109. Schreiner, H.; Li, Y.; Cline, J.; Tsiagbe, V.K.; Fine, D.H. A comparison of *Aggregatibacter actinomycetemcomitans* (*Aa*) virulence traits in a rat model for periodontal disease. *PLoS ONE* **2013**, *8*, e69382. [CrossRef]

110. Parthiban, C.; Varudharasu, D.; Shanmugam, M.; Gopal, P.; Ragunath, C.; Thomas, L.; Nitz, M.; Ramasubbu, N. Structural and functional analysis of de-N-acetylase PgaB from periodontopathogen *Aggregatibacter actinomycetemcomitans*. *Mol. Oral Microbiol.* **2017**, *32*, 324–340. [CrossRef]

111. Ristow, L.C.; Welch, R.A. RTX Toxins Ambush Immunity's First Cellular Responders. *Toxins* **2019**, *11*, 720. [CrossRef]

112. Azzi-Martin, L.; Touffait-Calvez, V.; Everaert, M.; Jia, R.; Sifre, E.; Seeneevassen, L.; Varon, C.; Dubus, P.; Menard, A. Cytolethal Distending Toxin Modulates Cell Differentiation and Elicits Epithelial to Mesenchymal Transition. *J. Infect. Dis.* **2024**, *229*, 1688–1701. [CrossRef]

113. Ivanyi, L.; Challacombe, S.J.; Lehner, T. The specificity of serum factors in lymphocyte transformation in periodontal disease. *Clin. Exp. Immunol.* **1973**, *14*, 491–500. [PubMed]

114. Ebersole, J.L.; Dawson, D., 3rd; Emecen-Huja, P.; Nagarajan, R.; Howard, K.; Grady, M.E.; Thompson, K.; Peyyala, R.; Al-Attar, A.; Lethbridge, K.; et al. The periodontal war: Microbes and immunity. *Periodontol. 2000* **2017**, *75*, 52–115. [CrossRef]

115. Taubman, M.A.; Valverde, P.; Han, X.; Kawai, T. Immune response: The key to bone resorption in periodontal disease. *J. Periodontol.* **2005**, *76*, 2033–2041. [CrossRef]

116. Genco, R.J.; Sanz, M. Clinical and public health implications of periodontal and systemic diseases: An overview. *Periodontol. 2000* **2020**, *83*, 7–13. [CrossRef] [PubMed]

117. Taichman, N.S.; Dean, R.T.; Sanderson, C.J. Biochemical and morphological characterization of the killing of human monocytes by a leukotoxin derived from *Actinobacillus actinomycetemcomitans*. *Infect. Immun.* **1980**, *28*, 258–268. [CrossRef] [PubMed]

118. Taichman, N.S.; Wilton, J.M. Leukotoxicity of an extract from *Actinobacillus actinomycetemcomitans* for human gingival polymor-phonuclear leukocytes. *Inflammation* **1981**, *5*, 1–12. [CrossRef]

119. Proctor, D.M.; Shelef, K.M.; Gonzalez, A.; Davis, C.L.; Dethlefsen, L.; Burns, A.R.; Loomer, P.M.; Armitage, G.C.; Ryder, M.I.; Millman, M.E.; et al. Microbial biogeography and ecology of the mouth and implications for periodontal diseases. *Periodontol. 2000* **2020**, *82*, 26–41. [CrossRef]

120. Costello, E.K.; Stagaman, K.; Dethlefsen, L.; Bohannan, B.J.; Relman, D.A. The application of ecological theory toward an understanding of the human microbiome. *Science* **2012**, *336*, 1255–1262. [CrossRef]

121. Tabak, L.A.; Levine, M.J.; Mandel, I.D.; Ellison, S.A. Role of salivary mucins in the protection of the oral cavity. *J. Oral Pathol.* **1982**, *11*, 1–17. [CrossRef]

122. Mandel, I.D. The role of saliva in maintaining oral homeostasis. *J. Am. Dent. Assoc.* **1989**, *119*, 298–304. [CrossRef]

123. Socransky, S.S.; Manganiello, S.D. The oral microbiota of man from birth to senility. *J. Periodontol.* **1971**, *42*, 485–496. [CrossRef] [PubMed]

124. Lowe, A.M.; Yansouni, C.P.; Behr, M.A. Causality and gastrointestinal infections: Koch, Hill, and Crohn's. *Lancet Infect. Dis.* **2008**, *8*, 720–726. [CrossRef] [PubMed]

125. Ritz, H.L. Microbial population shifts in developing human dental plaque. *Arch. Oral Biol.* **1967**, *12*, 1561–1568. [CrossRef]

126. Hujoel, P.P.; White, B.A.; Garcia, R.I.; Listgarten, M.A. The dentogingival epithelial surface area revisited. *J. Periodontal Res.* **2001**, *36*, 48–55. [CrossRef]

127. Blaser, M.J. *Missing Microbes: How the Overuse of Antibiotics is Fueling our Modern Plagues*, 1st ed.; Henry Holt and Company: New York, NY, USA, 2014.

128. Del Romero, J.; Moreno Guillen, S.; Rodriguez-Artalejo, F.J.; Ruiz-Galiana, J.; Canton, R.; De Lucas Ramos, P.; Garcia-Botella, A.; Garcia-Lledo, A.; Hernandez-Sampelayo, T.; Gomez-Pavon, J.; et al. Sexually transmitted infections in Spain: Current status. *Rev. Esp. Quimioter.* **2023**, *36*, 444–465. [CrossRef] [PubMed]

129. Okell, C.C.; Elliott, S.D. Bacteriaaemia and oral sepsis with special reference to the aetiology of subacute endocarditis. *Lancet* **1935**, 869–872. [CrossRef]

130. Silver, J.G.; Martin, A.W.; McBride, B.C. Experimental transient bacteraemias in human subjects with varying degrees of plaque accumulation and gingival inflammation. *J. Clin. Periodontol.* **1977**, *4*, 92–99. [CrossRef]

131. Wells, P.M.; Sprockett, D.D.; Bowyer, R.C.E.; Kurushima, Y.; Relman, D.A.; Williams, F.M.K.; Steves, C.J. Influential factors of saliva microbiota composition. *Sci. Rep.* **2022**, *12*, 18894. [CrossRef] [PubMed]

132. Taichman, N.S.; Tsai, C.C.; Baehni, P.C.; Stoller, N.; McArthur, W.P. Interaction of inflammatory cells and oral microorganisms. IV. In vitro release of lysosomal constituents from polymorphonuclear leukocytes exposed to supragingival and subgingival bacterial plaque. *Infect. Immun.* **1977**, *16*, 1013–1023. [CrossRef]

133. Van Dyke, T.E.; Horoszewicz, H.U.; Genco, R.J. The polymorphonuclear leukocyte (PMNL) locomotor defect in juvenile periodontitis. Study of random migration, chemokinesis and chemotaxis. *J. Periodontol.* **1982**, *53*, 682–687. [CrossRef]

134. Fives-Taylor, P.M.; Meyer, D.H.; Mintz, K.P.; Brissette, C. Virulence factors of *Actinobacillus actinomycetemcomitans*. *Periodontol. 2000* **1999**, *20*, 136–167. [CrossRef] [PubMed]

135. Fine, D.H.; Schreiner, H. Oral microbial interactions from an ecological perspective: A narrative review. *Front. Oral Health* **2023**, *4*, 1229118. [CrossRef] [PubMed]

136. Aruni, W.; Chioma, O.; Fletcher, H.M. *Filifactor alocis*: The Newly Discovered Kid on the Block with Special Talents. *J. Dent. Res.* **2014**, *93*, 725–732. [CrossRef] [PubMed]

137. Fine, D.H.; Patil, A.G.; Velusamy, S.K. *Aggregatibacter actinomycetemcomitans* (*Aa*) under the Radar: Myths and Misunderstandings of *Aa* and Its Role in Aggressive Periodontitis. *Front. Immunol.* **2019**, *10*, 728. [CrossRef]

138. Offenbacher, S.; Katz, V.; Fertik, G.; Collins, J.; Boyd, D.; Maynor, G.; McKaig, R.; Beck, J. Periodontal infection as a possible risk factor for preterm low birth weight. *J. Periodontol.* **1996**, *67*, 1103–1113. [CrossRef]

139. Fine, D.H.; Furgang, D.; McKiernan, M.; Tereski-Bischio, D.; Ricci-Nittel, D.; Zhang, P.; Araujo, M.W. An investigation of the effect of an essential oil mouthrinse on induced bacteraemia: A pilot study. *J. Clin. Periodontol.* **2010**, *37*, 840–847. [CrossRef] [PubMed]

140. Kinane, D.F.; Riggio, M.P.; Walker, K.F.; MacKenzie, D.; Shearer, B. Bacteraemia following periodontal procedures. *J. Clin. Periodontol.* **2005**, *32*, 708–713. [CrossRef]

141. Shanson, D. New British and American guidelines for the antibiotic prophylaxis of infective endocarditis: Do the changes make sense? A critical review. *Curr. Opin. Infect. Dis.* **2008**, *21*, 191–199. [CrossRef]

142. Bergenholtz, G. Effect of bacterial products on inflammatory reactions in the dental pulp. *Scand. J. Dent. Res.* **1977**, *85*, 122–129.

143. Bik, E.M.; Eckburg, P.B.; Gill, S.R.; Nelson, K.E.; Purdom, E.A.; Francois, F.; Perez-Perez, G.; Blaser, M.J.; Relman, D.A. Molecular analysis of the bacterial microbiota in the human stomach. *Proc. Natl. Acad. Sci. USA* **2006**, *103*, 732–737. [CrossRef]

144. Black, S.; Phillips, D.; Hickey, J.W.; Kennedy-Darling, J.; Venkataraaman, V.G.; Samusik, N.; Goltsev, Y.; Schurch, C.M.; Nolan, G.P. CODEX multiplexed tissue imaging with DNA-conjugated antibodies. *Nat. Protoc.* **2021**, *16*, 3802–3835. [CrossRef] [PubMed]

145. Mark Welch, J.L.; Dewhirst, F.E.; Borisy, G.G. Biogeography of the Oral Microbiome: The Site-Specific Hyothesis. *Ann. Rev. Microbiol.* **2019**, *73*, 335–358. [CrossRef] [PubMed]

146. Lakschevitz, F.S.; Hassanpour, S.; Rubin, A.; Fine, N.; Sun, C.; Glogauer, M. Identification of neutrophil surface marker changes in health and inflammation using high-throughput screening flow cytometry. *Exp. Cell Res.* **2016**, *342*, 200–209. [CrossRef] [PubMed]

147. Oshrain, H.I.; Salind, A.; Mandel, I.D. A method for collection of subgingival plaque and calculus. *J. Periodontol.* **1968**, *39*, 322–325. [CrossRef] [PubMed]

148. Fine, D.H.; Greene, L.S. Microscopic evaluation of root surface associations in vivo. *J. Periodontal Res.* **1984**, *19*, 152–167. [CrossRef]

149. Wecke, J.; Wolf, V.; Fath, S.; Bernimoulin, J.P. The occurrence of treponemes and their spherical bodies on polytetrafluoroethylene membranes. *Oral Microbiol. Immunol.* **1995**, *10*, 278–283. [CrossRef] [PubMed]

150. Fine, D.H.; Markowitz, K.; Furgang, D.; Velliyagounder, K. *Aggregatibacter actinomycetemcomitans* as an early colonizer of oral tissues: Epithelium as a reservoir? *J. Clin. Microbiol.* **2010**, *48*, 4464–4473. [CrossRef]

151. Hajishengallis, G.; Lamont, R.J.; Koo, H. Oral polymicrobial communities: Assembly, function, and impact on diseases. *Cell Host Microbe* **2023**, *31*, 528–538. [CrossRef]

152. Hajishengallis, G. Interconnection of periodontal disease and comorbidities: Evidence, mechanisms, and implications. *Periodontol. 2000* **2022**, *89*, 9–18. [CrossRef]

153. Haubek, D.; Poulsen, K.; Kilian, M. Microevolution and patterns of dissemination of the JP2 clone of *Aggregatibacter* (*Actinobacillus*) *actinomycetemcomitans*. *Infect. Immun.* **2007**, *75*, 3080–3088. [CrossRef]

154. Fine, D.H.; Toruner, G.A.; Velliyagounder, K.; Sampathkumar, V.; Godboley, D.; Furgang, D. A lactotransferrin single nucleotide polymorphism demonstrates biological activity that can reduce susceptibility to caries. *Infect. Immun.* **2013**, *81*, 1596–1605. [CrossRef] [PubMed]

155. Esmaeilyfard, R.; Bonyadifard, H.; Paknahad, M. Dental Caries Detection and Classification in CBCT Images Using Deep Learning. *Int. Dent. J.* **2024**, *74*, 328–334. [CrossRef] [PubMed]

156. Pitts, N.B.; Twetman, S.; Fisher, J.; Marsh, P.D. Understanding dental caries as a non-communicable disease. *Br. Dent. J.* **2021**, *231*, 749–753. [CrossRef]

157. Sioson, P.B.; Furgang, D.; Steinberg, L.M.; Fine, D.H. Proximal caries in juvenile periodontitis patients. *J. Periodontol.* **2000**, *71*, 710–716. [CrossRef] [PubMed]

158. Zambon, J.J. *Actinobacillus actinomycetemcomitans* in human periodontal disease. *J. Clin. Periodontol.* **1985**, *12*, 1–20. [CrossRef]

159. Holtfreter, B.; Kuhr, K.; Borof, K.; Tonetti, M.S.; Sanz, M.; Kornman, K.; Jepsen, S.; Aarabi, G.; Volzke, H.; Kocher, T.; et al. ACES: A new framework for the application of the 2018 periodontal status classification scheme to epidemiological survey data. *J. Clin. Periodontol.* **2024**, *51*, 512–521. [CrossRef]

160. Herzberg, M.C. Platelet-streptococcal interactions in endocarditis. *Crit. Rev. Oral Biol. Med.* **1996**, *7*, 222–236. [CrossRef]

161. Peters, J.; Robinson, F.; Dasco, C.; Gentry, L.O. Subacute bacterial endocarditis due to *Actinobacillus actinomycetemcomitans*. *Am. J. Med. Sci.* **1983**, *286*, 35–41. [CrossRef]

162. Diamond, I.R.; Grant, R.C.; Feldman, B.M.; Pencharz, P.B.; Ling, S.C.; Moore, A.M.; Wales, P.W. Defining consensus: A systematic review recommends methodologic criteria for reporting of Delphi studies. *J. Clin. Epidemiol.* **2014**, *67*, 401–409. [CrossRef]

163. Hutchinson, P.J.; Kolias, A.G.; Tajsic, T.; Adeleye, A.; Aklilu, A.T.; Apriawan, T.; Bajamal, A.H.; Barthelemy, E.J.; Devi, B.I.; Bhat, D.; et al. Consensus statement from the International Consensus Meeting on the Role of Decompressive Craniectomy in the Management of Traumatic Brain Injury: Consensus statement. *Acta Neurochir.* **2019**, *161*, 1261–1274. [CrossRef]

164. Pelosi, L.; Aranyi, Z.; Beekman, R.; Bland, J.; Coraci, D.; Hobson-Webb, L.D.; Padua, L.; Podnar, S.; Simon, N.; van Alfen, N.; et al. Expert consensus on the combined investigation of ulnar neuropathy at the elbow using electrodiagnostic tests and nerve ultrasound. *Clin. Neurophysiol.* **2021**, *132*, 2274–2281. [CrossRef] [PubMed]

165. Clyne, B.; Sharp, M.K.; O'Neill, M.; Pollock, D.; Lynch, R.; Amog, K.; Ryan, M.; Smith, S.M.; Mahtani, K.; Booth, A.; et al. An international modified Delphi process supported updating the web-based "right review" tool. *J. Clin. Epidemiol.* **2024**, *170*, 111333. [CrossRef] [PubMed]

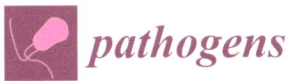

MDPI

Review

Grade C Molar-Incisor Pattern Periodontitis in Young Adults: What Have We Learned So Far?

Manuela Maria Viana Miguel [1] and Luciana Macchion Shaddox [1,2,*]

1   Center for Oral Health Research, College of Dentistry, University of Kentucky, Lexington, KY 40508, USA; vianamiguel.manuela@gmail.com
2   Department of Oral Health Practice, Periodontology Division, College of Dentistry, University of Kentucky, Lexington, KY 40508, USA
*   Correspondence: lshaddox@uky.edu; Tel.: +1-859-323-8269; Fax: +1-859-257-6566

Abstract: Grade C molar-incisor pattern periodontitis (C-MIP) is a disease that affects specific teeth with an early onset and aggressive progression. It occurs in systemically healthy patients, mostly African descendants, at an early age, with familial involvement, minimal biofilm accumulation, and minor inflammation. Severe and rapidly progressive bone loss is observed around the first molars and incisors. This clinical condition has been usually diagnosed in children and young adults with permanent dentition under 30 years of age. However, this disease can also affect the primary dentition, which is not as frequently discussed in the literature. Radiographic records have shown that most patients diagnosed in the permanent dentition already presented disease signs in the primary dentition. A hyperresponsive immunological profile is observed in local (gingival crevicular fluid-GCF) and systemic environments. Siblings have also displayed a heightened inflammatory profile even without clinical signs of disease. *A. actinomycetemcomitans* has been classified as a key pathogen in C-MIP in both dentitions. Scaling and root planning associated with systemic antibiotics is the current gold standard to treat C-MIP, leading to GCF biomarker reduction, some systemic inflammatory response modulation and microbiome profile changes to a healthy-site profile. Further studies should focus on other possible disease-contributing risk factors.

Keywords: periodontitis; aggressive; immunological factors; microbiota; genetics

Citation: Miguel, M.M.V.; Shaddox, L.M. Grade C Molar-Incisor Pattern Periodontitis in Young Adults: What Have We Learned So Far? *Pathogens* **2024**, *13*, 580. https://doi.org/10.3390/pathogens13070580

Academic Editor: Daniel H. Fine

Received: 8 June 2024
Revised: 26 June 2024
Accepted: 9 July 2024
Published: 12 July 2024

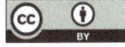
1. Clinical Overview

Periodontitis is a biofilm-dependent condition characterized by a shift in the resident microbiota, leading to increased host response to its challenge [1]. As a result of this dysbiosis and host immunological profile, destruction of the tooth-supporting apparatus [2] can clinically be detected in different progression and severity patterns. According to the 1999 classification of periodontal diseases and conditions [3], Localized Aggressive Periodontitis (LAP) was characterized to occur in systemically healthy patients at an early age with familial involvement, minimal biofilm accumulation, and low gingival margin inflammation, severe bone loss along with rapid clinical attachment loss (CAL) progression, specifically in first molars and incisors. According to the new periodontitis classification based on stages and grades, LAP was then named Grade C molar-incisor pattern periodontitis (C-MIP) [4]. Epidemiological data have provided evidence that early onset aggressive periodontal condition oscillates in different populations, where higher prevalences can be observed in African descendants (up to 6% of prevalence) and the lowest in Caucasians (less than 1%) [5,6]. Along with the African continent, South America comprises a prevalence of 0.3–5% of the disease [5,7] which may be correlated to locations with a mixed-race population. This pattern suggests a specific geographic distribution of the disease. This clinical condition has been frequently diagnosed in older children and young adults in permanent dentition under 30–35 years of age [6,8]. However, it is important to highlight that primary dentition can also be affected by Grade C Periodontitis [9–12]. The lack of periodontal assessment in pediatric dental examination may overlook this disease's initial development, jeopardizing the actual timing of onset, and may contribute to the development of the disease in the permanent dentition, as suggested before [13–16]. In general, Grade C periodontitis in primary dentition can mostly be detected in primary molars and may be diagnosed late at severe stages or by early exfoliation due to disproportional bone loss occurring around these teeth in relation to the rate of physiological apical root resorption [10,16]. In addition, external and internal root resorptions in primary dentition are conditions that have also been reported in this disease [10,16] (Figure 1A). Early diagnosis in primary dentition displays a pivotal role in treatment success, along with strict periodontal maintenance follow-up to prevent the development of the disease in the permanent dentition (Figure 1B) [9,15–17]. Gender influence in LAP/C-MIP prevalence has been studied; however, inconsistent evidence has been reported [18]. Literature has shown similar [19] or higher [20] disease prevalence in females. However, due to some differences found in the inflammatory response in this disease between sexes [18], sex hormones may be the key to a better understanding of how gender may impact this disease (see further discussion below regarding host response).

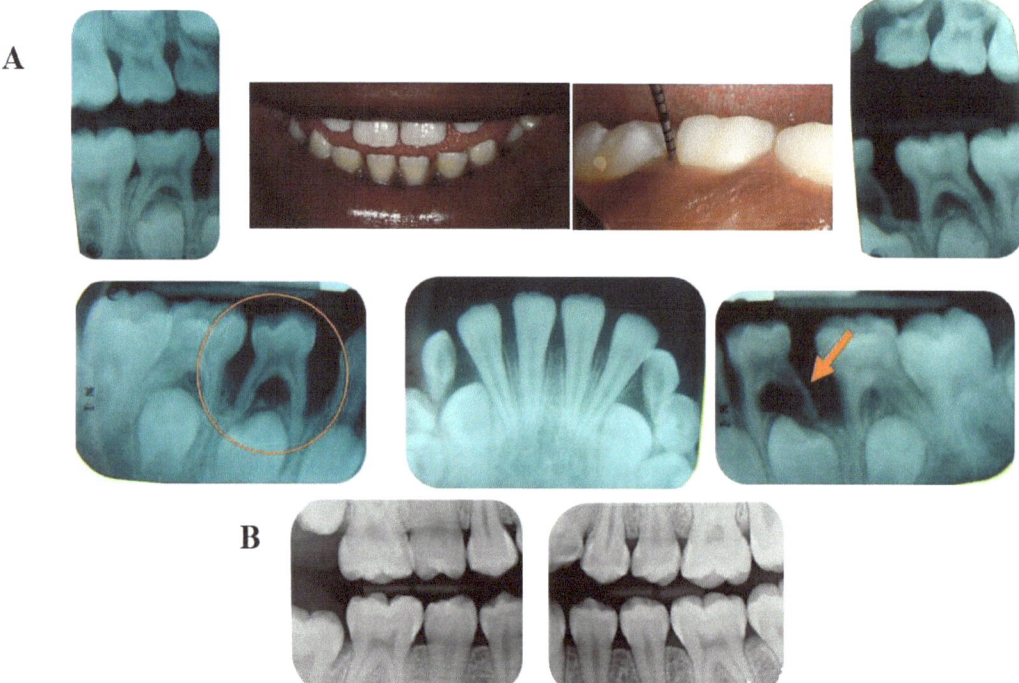

Figure 1. Clinical Case: 8-year-old African American female diagnosed with C-MIP in primary dentition. Patient smiles with low gingival margin inflammation; however, probing depth > 5 mm in the first molar. In the X-ray, severe bone loss in the lower first primary molars (orange arrow and circle) along with internal and external resorption of the lower left primary first molar in the primary dentition (orange arrow) (**A**). Permanent dentition in healthy conditions following therapy (SRP+ABX) in the primary dentition (**B**). (Source of the image [10]).

2. Immunological Aspects

Local inflammation. Focusing on host immunological response complexity to a low biofilm aggregation, Branco-de-Almeida et al. [21] and Shaddox et al. [22] reported high levels of IL-12p40, GMCSF, TNF-α, IL-6, IL-12p70, IL-2, INFγ, IL1β, and MIP-1α gingival crevicular fluid (GCF) of LAP patients diseased sites when compared to health sites from the same patients [22] and/or health siblings and healthy unrelated controls [21,22] Interestingly, a significant differential profile of these markers was observed among these sites, where most differences fall between diseased and healthy sites, however, the healthy sites from healthy individuals tended to cluster more closely together (Figure 2). For instance, higher GCF concentrations of Eotaxin, GM-CSF, IL-10, IL-12p70, and IL-2 were observed in health sites from LAP patients when compared to their health siblings [21]. Additionally, healthy siblings of LAP subjects displayed an increase in IFN-γ and OPG without any clinical evidence of disease [21]. Interestingly, Martins et al. [23] showed similarity of some biomarker's expression (IL1β, ICAM-1, and GMCSF) either in C-MIP or generalized aggressive forms of periodontitis (GAgP; CAL > 4 mm affecting at least three permanent teeth other than the first molars and incisors), at baseline to health controls. A current systematic review and meta-analysis [24] confirm that most of the cited biomarkers above were highly expressed in the GCF of C-MIP patients; however, the literature still needs more evidence to use this approach as a diagnosis tool. Some of these biomarkers have a pivotal role in stimulating cells' environment towards osteoclastic activity and sustaining proinflammatory profile by chemotaxis. Thus, these differentiated local levels of inflammatory markers may contribute to local microbial dysbiosis and possible site breakdown in these individuals (see microbial discussion below).

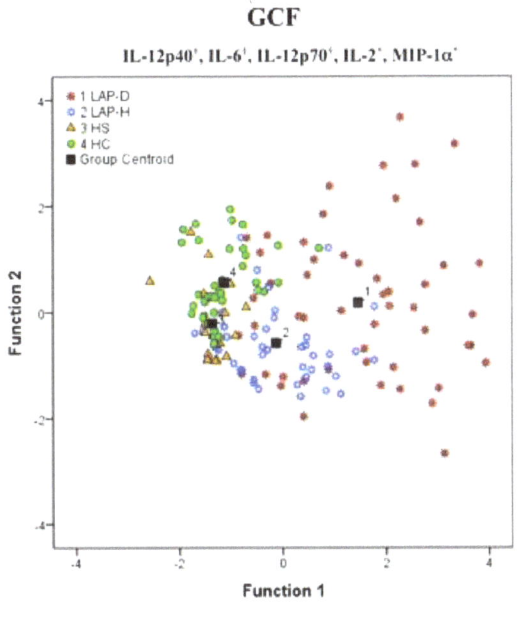

Figure 2. Discriminatory gingival crevicular fluid (GCF) in localized aggressive periodontitis (LAP) subjects, their healthy siblings (HS), and unrelated healthy controls (HC) displaying four different group centroids (1–4). The separation between LAP diseased sites (LAP−D) and LAP healthy sites (LAP−H) is clearly observed in the graphic along with a closely related profile (although statistically different) for HS sites and HC sites by a biomarker group of IL−12p−40, IL−6, IL−12p70, IL−2, and MIP−1α (Wilks's lambda < 0.001 in canonical functions 1 and 2). * Significant biomarker in function 1. † Significant biomarker in function 2. (Source of the image [21]).

Systemic inflammation. Peripheral blood from C-MIP stimulated either with LPS or biofilm from healthy and diseased sites has shown a hyperinflammatory responsiveness profile with increased levels of G-CSF, IFNγ, IL-10, IL12(p40), IL1β, IL-6, IL-8, MCP-1, MIP-1α, and TNFα when compared healthy control patients [25,26]. Interestingly, the similar response, regardless of the specific biofilm used for stimulation, highlights the role of host response in this unique disease. Tabaa et al. [27] have shown a similar pattern of proinflammatory response (IL-6, IL-8, IL-10, MIP1α, MCP1, and IL-1β) among affected siblings after peripheral blood LPS stimulation (Figure 3). Similarly, both *E. coli* and *P. gingivalis* LPS-stimulated peripheral blood from healthy siblings of LAP subjects has shown a tendency of hyperresponsiveness with IL2, IL12p40, TNFα, IFNγ, and IL6 elevated levels compared to unrelated health controls [25]. In fact, healthy siblings of LAP individuals tend to show a high peripheral response to diseased biofilms, showing increased levels of IL-6 and INFγ. In fact, even in response to healthy biofilm stimulation, this group had a higher concentration of INFγ compared to unrelated healthy patients [26]. This evidence collectively can point to two reasonable hypotheses. First, there seems to be a familial aggregation associated with this hyper-inflammatory response to bacterial stimuli in families with this disease [27]. Second, it can be hypothesized that inflammatory response could potentially precede or exacerbate bacterial dysbiosis in susceptible individuals in this clinical condition since both healthy and pathogenic biofilms have been shown to elicit a hyper-inflammatory host response in these individuals [26]. In addition, healthy sites in diseased patients display biomarkers featuring a differentiated and proinflammatory local profile [26].

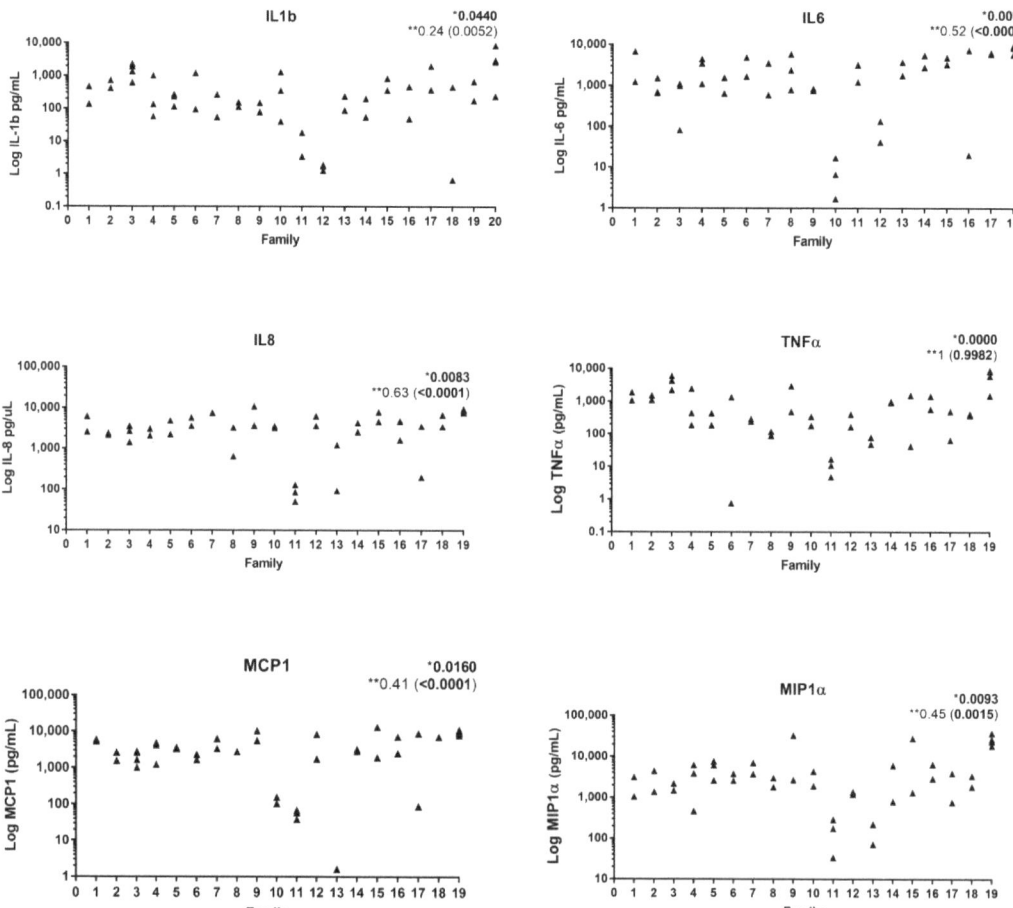

Figure 3. Significant correlations of host response to bacterial lipopolysaccharides within and among families with C-MIP. * Overall covariance *p*-value among families; ** Within families intraclass correlation coefficient followed by within family *p*-value in parenthesis. (Source of the image [27]).

The first line of defense in individuals who suffer from an aggressive form of periodontitis can be compromised due to either neutrophil hyperactivity [28] or dysfunction [29,30]. Van Dyke et al. [29] showed a deficiency in neutrophil chemotaxis in 26 out of 32 patients diagnosed with C-MIP/LAP compared to age and sex-matched healthy controls. This pattern remains even in those whose disease has already been treated. According to the same study, 7 out of 10 patients displayed neutrophil chemotaxis deficiency after 6 months to 2 years post-therapy [29]. Thus, it seems that a genetic determination may be associated with this neutrophil role. Van Dyke et al. [30] have shown neutrophil dysfunction in 90% of healthy siblings under 12 years old featuring a familial aggregation. This deficiency can be considered a predictor of aggressive forms of periodontitis since some of the healthy siblings detected with neutrophils at the beginning of the mentioned studies developed the disease during the study [30]. Focusing on humoral response, high levels of immunoglobulin G2 (IgG2 antibody) have also been observed in LAP patients [31]. Studies are controversial if this immunological response is specific to *A. actinomycetemcomitans* [32,33]; however, a racial influence was observed in this immunoglobulin levels [34], where higher concentrations of IgG2 serum was observed in African American descendants diagnosed with LAP when compared to Caucasians [34].

Gender and host response. Although the literature is still controversial about gender influence in C-MIP, local and systemic inflammatory biomarkers are differently expressed in males and females. Tavakoli et al. [18] reported increased GCF levels of TNFα, IFNγ, MCP1, and MIP-1α in diseased sites of males. Interestingly, healthy sites in male patients diagnosed with LAP/C-MIP also presented high levels of IFNγ and a tendency to higher G-CSF levels as well. On the other hand, peripheral blood from C-MIP females stimulated with *P. gingivalis* e *E. coli* LPS showed an increase in systemic biomarkers, such as Eotaxin, IFNγ, and GM-CSF, compared to C-MIP males [18]. Considering the age range of disease initiation in the permanent dentition, sex hormones may indeed have an impact on both the local and systemic inflammatory response. In fact, high testosterone levels in males have been correlated to periodontitis prevalence and severity [35], while estrogen reduction in a woman's lifetime may increase the risk of periodontal issues due to its protective role [36]. However, based on the results above regarding systemic responses, it can be inferred that females diagnosed with C-MIP have a hyperresponsive tendency to biofilm challenge (LPS), which may impact faster periodontal apparatus loss [18]. Thus, hormonal imbalances during puberty in both males and females and their impact on C-MIP predisposition or initiation certainly warrant further investigation.

Genetic influence on host response. Genetic aspects could also have an impact on the host inflammatory response [37–39]. Toll-like receptors (TLR), e.g., TLR-2 and TLR-4, have been associated with LAP/C-MIP hyper-inflammatory response [25]. This transmembrane glycoprotein pathway has shown more than a two-fold-increase in specific gene expression correlated to inflammation, such as TICAM-1 (TRIF), FOS, IRAK1, TLR2, and CCL2 in LAP/C-MIP patients compared to healthy unrelated controls [40]. IRAK1 displayed a significantly increased expression in these subjects, which may be explained by IL-1β increase in these patients [41]. Epigenetic regulation plays an important role in host immunological response via the TLR pathway. According to Shaddox et al. [42], up- (e.g., MYD88, MAP3K7, RIPK2, IL6R) and downregulation (e.g., FADD, PPARA, IRAK1BP1) of several genes can be explained by DNA methylation in specific sites. For example, methylation in FADD position 5 was positively correlated with LPS-stimulated levels of IL-6 and TNF-α systemically. Conversely, MYD88 methylation in position 4 presented a negative correlation with IL-10, IP-10, and MCP-1 [42].

Several gene single nucleotide polymorphisms (SNP) can influence immunological patterns and susceptibility in aggressive forms of periodontitis. IL-1α (rs1800587) and IL-1-β (rs1143634) polymorphisms have been correlated to generalized aggressive periodontitis [43]. SNP in the Lactoferrin gene, the iron-binding protein with antimicrobial activity related to host first-line defense (G-allele), was detected in young African Americans [44] and Taiwanese [45] diagnosed with aggressive forms of periodontitis. Similarly, cathepsin C SNP (rs3888798), a cysteine protease involved in neutrophil maturation and its activity in immune response, was also associated with this disease, along with lower PMN function, enhancing the risk of aggressive periodontitis development [46]. Several reviews of the literature evaluating the role of genetics in aggressive periodontitis have been published [37,47–51]. Given the several genes potentially associated with the disease and its inflammatory pathways, it is likely that several genetic polymorphisms are associated with susceptibility to this disease. There is also some evidence that indicates a possible genetic predisposition to specific microbial colonization [52,53]. Thus, comprehensive genomic studies with a high number of diseased individuals from different populations need to be conducted to clarify specific genes and their role in this disease.

Finally, some studies have investigated the roles of small RNAs, known as microRNAs, or miRNAs, in periodontitis [40,54,55] and other inflammatory diseases [56]. In our cohort of LAP individuals, several miRNAs, including miR-9-5p, 155-5p, and 147a, all presented elevated expression (2-fold up-regulated) in our LAP/C-MIP cohort [40]. Interestingly, increased miR-9-5p levels were previously found in inflamed gingival tissue from patients diagnosed with periodontitis [54] and also in neutrophils and monocytes post-TLR2-4 activation [57], and both miR155-5 and 147a have also been found elevated post-LPS stimulation, promoting further inflammatory cascade [58–60]. There seems to be an important role for miRNA regulation in TLR responsiveness in this disease, which deserves to be further explored by comprehensive next-generation sequencing approaches at different disease stages.

3. Microbiological Aspects

Literature has shown a microbial profile associated with localized early-onset periodontitis [61–65]. Microorganisms such as *A. actinomycetemcomitans*, *T. lecithinolyticum*, and *T. forsythia* have been strongly associated with this condition [62,64]. Moreover, studies have shown that *P. gingivalis*, *P. intermedia*, *T. denticola*, *C. gracilis*, *E. nodatum*, and *F. nucleatum* are highly correlated with active disease and its prevalence [63,66]. *A. actinomycetemcomitans* has been classified as a key pathogen in young adults diagnosed with LAP/C-MIP [63–69] and even with sites with progressive bone loss [70,71]. This microorganism has different mechanisms of action including direct and indirect ways of influence in host response [72–74]. Seven serotypes can be linked with this species (a–g) based on membrane polysaccharides surface. A particular JP2 Genotype from serotype "b" has been highly associated with a severe form of periodontal disease [12,75,76] and in sites with progressive bone loss as well [76,77]. In the beginning, this species was identified in subjects from North and West Africa. Due to the transatlantic slave trade, new colonization was spread out in North and South America [75], which could explain the higher prevalence of this disease in African descendants in both these regions. In fact, JP2 clone has been reported in aggressive periodontitis in both North [78] and South American populations [67]. One of the main virulence factors from this genotype/serotype "b" is the expressive release of leukotoxin (LtxA), intensifying leukotoxic and cell death in high doses [79]. Not only does LtxA depreciate leukocyte activity, but it also increases lysosomal release in macrophages reducing its phagocytic profile [80].

Tissue invasion is a well-known propriety from *A. actinomycetemcomitans*, and it has already been identified in periodontal tissues from young adults [81], even at a very young age [82]. Several virulence factors in relation to this action have been described in in vitro and in vivo analysis [83]. Outer membrane protein 100 (Omp100) present in *A. actinomycetemcomitans* membrane surface composition has the capacity to bind in human epithelial cells [84]. After its adhesion, other Omp protein class groups act specifically in tissue invasion. Omp29 allows microorganism diffusion into epithelial cells, enhancing permeability due to F-actin rearrangement via FAK signaling cascade [85]. In the same way, cytolethal distending toxin (CDT) produced by this bacterium has the capacity to impact the cell cycle, leading to epithelial layer organization disruption due to the dissolution of cell junctions (e.g., cadherin) [86]. This scenario results in soft tissue collapse, allowing microorganisms and their toxins to make intimate contact with the connective tissue below [86].

Early *A. actinomycetemcomitans* acquisition can be correlated with C-MIP in primary and mixed dentition [64,71,75,87]. A longitudinal study reported that individuals containing *A. actinomycetemcomitans*, *S. parasanguinis*, and *F. alocis* are more prone to develop LAP/C-MIP disease [71]. In fact, a higher risk for bone loss was observed when the three microorganisms coexisted [71]. Jensen et al. have shown that healthy Moroccan toddlers between 7–10 years presented a higher CAL in mixed dentition when the JP2 genotype of *A. actinomycetemcomitans* was detected in their biofilm at incisor and molars [12]. Indeed, studies have reported a higher risk of bone loss when either non- or JP2 genotype is part of their microbiota in advance [76,77]. Aberg et al. [77] evaluated a 2-year progression of CAL based on the presence of JP2 and non-JP2 genotypes of *A. actinomycetemcomitans* in 500 adolescents (from 10 to 19 years of age). After the longitudinal follow-up, it was possible to predict a higher progression of CAL $\geq$ 3 mm when JP2 (OR = 14.3) and non-JP2 genotypes (OR = 3.4) were detected in subgingival biofilm. Moreover, an increasing risk of disease development followed by CAL $\geq$ 3 mm (RR = 7.3) was detected in healthy individuals at baseline with JP2 identification in subgingival biofilm. This evidence emphasizes the role of specific microorganisms in aggressive forms of periodontitis [77].

One of the possible explanations for this precocious colonization is family aggregation. Monteiro et al. [88] have reported a vertical pathogenic microbiome transmission between parents diagnosed with grade C periodontitis and their progeny. In fact, offspring' subgingival biofilm from parents diagnosed with periodontal disease has shown exclusive microorganisms such as *Filifactor alocis*, *Porphyromonas gingivalis*, *Streptococcus parasanguinis*, *Fusobacterium nucleatum subsp. nucleatum* when compared to progeny from parents who do not suffer from grade C periodontitis. Moreover, even after biofilm maintenance, several periodontopathogenic species remain stable and in higher abundance in offspring from periodontal diagnosed families, including *A. actinomycetemcomitans*, *P. gingivalis*, *T. denticola*, and *T. forsythia* [88].

Microbiome profiles in diagnosed C-MIP subjects can distinguish between primary and permanent dentition. According to a recent study (Koo et al. [89]), a partial overlap was observed between the two types of dentitions in disease conditions with the detection of distinguished microorganisms in primary and permanent affected sites (Figure 4). *Capnocytophaga ochracea*, *Leptotrichia buccalis*, *goodfellowii*, and *Sneathia sanguinegens* were found more frequently in primary teeth-affected sites when compared to the permanent ones. On the other hand, *Filifactor alocis*, *Tannerella forsythia*, and *Synergistetes sp* were elevated at C-MIP permanent sites, whereas *A. actinomycetemcomitans*, *Campylobacter*, *Fusobacterium nucleatum*, and *Gemella morbillorum* were identified in both primary and permanent affected sites characterizing the overlapping between them. In fact, *A. actinomycetemcomitans* was highly abundant in both affected dentitions (85% and 71%, respectively), corroborating its important role in this disease, both in primary and permanent dentitions. It seems that a more mature microbiome is developed in permanent diseased sites. However, the identification of some periodontopathogens, such as *Campylobacter gracilis* and *F. nucletum ss nucleatum* were also observed early in the primary dentition [89], which has been reported by the literature in early-onset periodontitis [90,91]. Thus, despite their low abundance, primary dentition already exhibits an identification of microorganisms that potentially increase the risk of disease development in the latest detention. Moreover, the high abundance of *A. actinomycetemcomitans*, regardless of dentition, highlights this species' role in C-MIP disease.

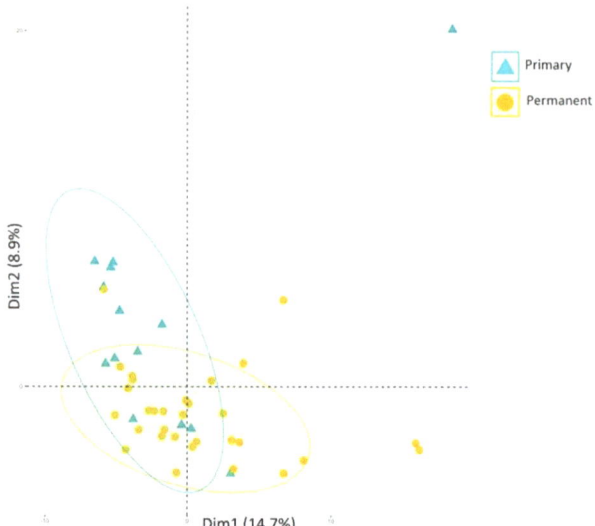

Figure 4. Beta-diversity analysis of C-MIP sites in children affected in the primary and permanent dentitions based on detection levels for all taxa in the HOMIM microarray. Principal component 1 (PC1, x-axis, 14.7%) vs. principal component 2 (PC2, y-axis, 8.9%) account for 23.6% of the total data variability. Ellipses represent 90% of the data variability within each group. Primary and Permanent groups differed when compared (PERMANOVA $p < 0.01$) and after adjusting for probing depth (PD) (PERMANOVA $p < 0.05$). (Source of the image [89]).

An important point to consider is intrafamilial transmission and its role in the acquisition of periodontopathogens. It has been shown that individuals from the same family harbored the same biotype and serotype of *A. actinomycetemcomitans* [92], and Christersson also found that members of the same family with LAP also harbored the same biotype and serotype of *A. actinomycetemcomitans* [93]. Haubek et al. also reported the same isolates of JP2 clones in African LAP families and suggested that the strong familial aggregation of this disease was due to intrafamilial transmission of this virulent strain [94]. The most likely route of transmission is via the saliva and could be vertical (parent to child) or horizontal (partner to partner or sibling to sibling) [95,96]. Transmission theories have been reinforced by sequencing studies of specific strains [97–99]. However, it is possible that transient transmission does not lead to persistent colonization of the organism, as this will also depend on the host, bacterium characteristics, and the abundance of the transferred species, among others. There may also be genetic influence of colonization patterns, as the periodontal flora of identical twins has been shown to be more similar than that of fraternal ones [100,101].

4. Diseases Initial Time-Point

In reviewing the topics discussed above, it is possible to question whether C-MIP actually starts in the primary dentition. If left untreated, the persistent presence of the pathogen *A. actinomycetemcomitans* within tissues [93,102,103] may allow this species to recolonize the pockets around permanent dentition and within sites of hyper-inflammatory host predisposition, may lead to rapid periodontal destruction in these individuals, as studies show that treatment of this disease early in the primary dentition seems to reduce disease recurrence in the permanent dentition [15–17]. This microorganism can act in tissue breakdown in indirect and direct ways jeopardizing the host first-line response (PMN recruitment) all together with microorganism selectivity in the subgingival environment, respectively [72]. Other more recent retrospective analyses [10,16] were carried out evaluating radiograph bone loss patterns, external/internal root resorption, enlarged chamber pulp, and exfoliation patterns in primary dentition records from patients diagnosed with LAP/C-MIP in permanent teeth. The first study [16] had access to 39 patient's radiographic records (20 C-MIP diagnosed and 19 healthy siblings). Ninety percent of those who had C-MIP in the permanent dentition also presented signs of radiographic bone loss around their first and second primary molars in the retrospective evaluation (Figure 5). Moreover, six of the 19 siblings who were healthy in their permanent dentition presented bone loss in primary radiographic records retrospectively, and two of them went on to develop the disease in the study follow-up [16] (Figure 6). Likewise, the second study [10] evaluated 49 periapical radiographs in 33 patients who presented the disease in the primary dentition. The first primary molar was the most affected teeth, followed by the second primary molar [10] (Figure 7). The authors suggest there seems to be a pattern of progression from the first to the second primary molar, and this could potentially lead to colonization of the first permanent molar if left untreated. Thus, it seems reasonable to infer that it is possible that C-MIP may indeed start in the primary dentition and, if left undiagnosed and untreated, may lead to disease in the permanent dentition. Thus, the role of pediatric dentists in the diagnosis and management of this disease early becomes essential for the proper treatment of this disease and prevention of possible breakdown of the permanent dentition [104]. The Academy of Pediatric Dentistry's latest recommendation for the diagnosis of periodontal disease in children is to perform a full mouth periodontal examination as soon as the first permanent molar erupts, around 6 years of age [105], or earlier if clinical signs of disease or radiographic bone loss are detected or suspected.

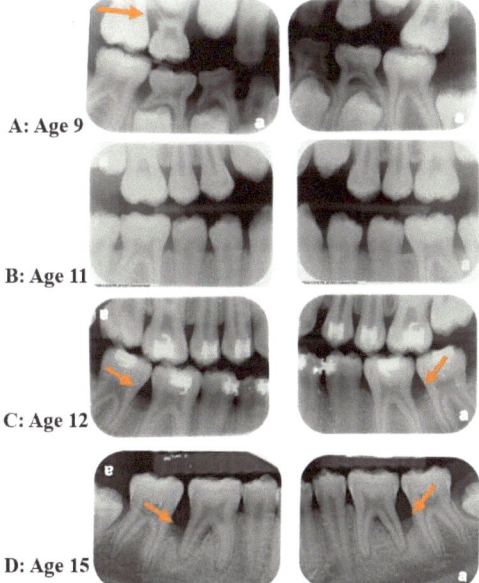

Figure 5. Clinical Case: The patient was referred to periodontal treatment at age 15 with significant vertical bone loss on #19 and 30. Retrospective radiographic analyses of the permanent and primary dentitions show evidence of bone loss in the upper (orange arrow) and lower primary molars at age 9 (**A**), healthy permanent dentition at age 11 (**B**), and beginning of bone defects in permanent dentition at age 12 and 15 (**C,D**); #19 and 30 distal surfaces) (Source of the image [10]).

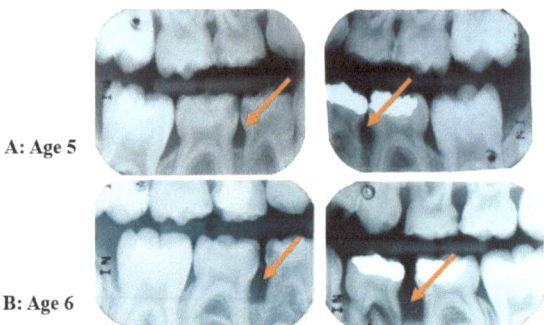

A: Age 5

B: Age 6

Figure 6. Retrospective evaluation of radiographs of a sibling of a C-MIP patient. Childhood radiographic records show initial bone loss at the first primary molars at five years old (**A**). The disease progressed fast and spread to the second primary molars at age 6 (orange arrows) (**B**). (Source of the image [16]).

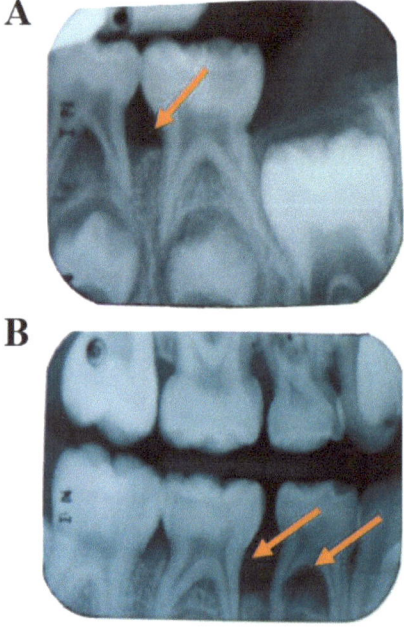

A

B

Figure 7. Seven-year-old African American male diagnosed with C-MIP in primary dentition. Severe bone loss on lower left primary first molar (orange arrow) (**A**). Severe bone loss of lower right first and second primary molars along with external root resorption (orange arrows) (**B**). (Source of the image [10]).

5. Treatment Aspects

Scaling and root planning (SRP) associated with systemic antibiotic therapy (Amoxicillin and Metronidazole) is the current gold standard for treating C-MIP [62,106–109]. According to most clinical studies, this therapy can provide significant probing depth (PD) reduction, clinical attachment level (CAL) gain, along with positive modulation in host proinflammatory profile (GCF), maintaining microbial compatibility with health sites in the short and long term (Figure 8) [62,106–109]. However, it is important to highlight that although patients respond well to this therapy, patients who present a high LPS responsiveness may not achieve equal outcomes to the ones presenting a lower responsiveness, even under the same clinical approach [110].

Baseline

2 years

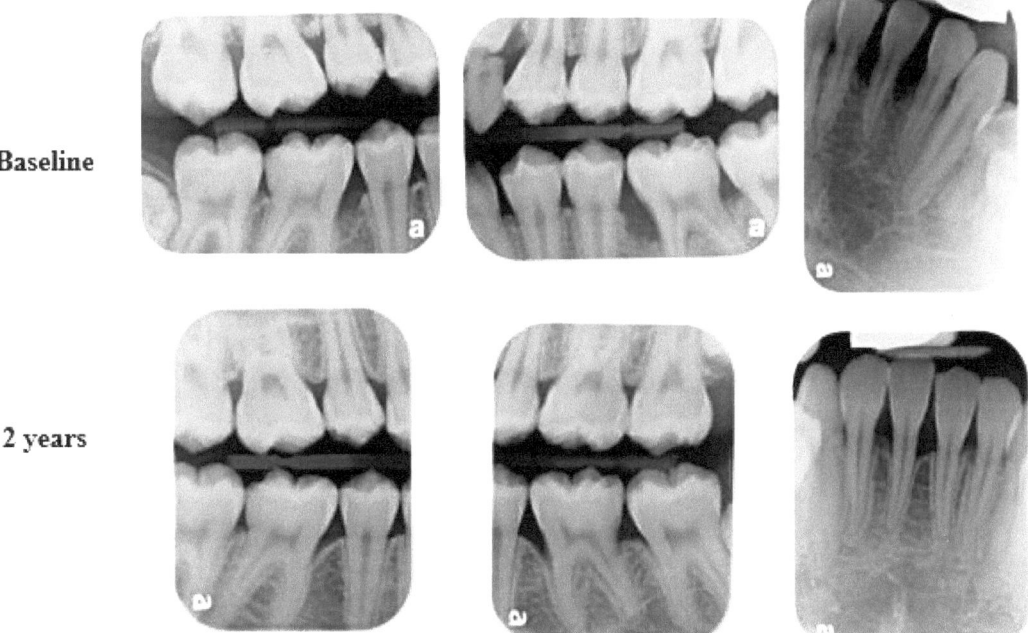

Figure 8. Female patient diagnosed with C-MIP presenting bone loss in the incisors (25) and 1st permanent molars (baseline-upper). After SRP + ABX treatment, bone fill and stability were achieved at 2 years of follow-up (bottom).

Branco de Almeida et al. [109] and Miller et al. [16] showed great PD reduction and clinical attachment gain in diagnosed LAP/C-MIP patients when a regimen of full mouth debridement associated with systemic antibiotic therapy (ABX at baseline: Metronidazole-250 mg and Amoxicillin-500 mg, 3× per day for 7 days) immediately after the clinical debridement was the treatment of choice. Positive clinical parameter reductions were observed in the short-term (6 months) and maintained in the long-term (2 years), while Miller et al. [16] showed this reduction in clinical parameters was maintained for up to 4 years post-treatment. Moreover, several biomarkers in diseased and health sites from LAP/C-MIP patients were reduced in at least one time point when compared to baseline levels [109]. Most of these decreased biomarkers have been characterized as disease features in discriminative analysis [21]. Thus, it seems that this type of approach can lead to clinical stability and local host modulation in the long term. Despite the positive and sustained modulation in GCF biomarkers after the non-surgical periodontal therapy combined with ABX, serum biomarkers modulation does not provide the same outcome [111]. Limited cytokines/chemokines are reduced in some post-treatment time points, while others seem to rebound, especially after 6 months [112]. In fact, some studies have shown that serum inflammatory biomarkers persist at higher rates compared to diagnosed patients even after treatment [113] or return to their baseline levels after long-term follow-up [114]. Comparing C-MIP and GAgP response after 1-year long-term follow under the ABX approach, it is possible to observe similarities between both disease types of outcomes regarding serum and GCF levels [23].

From a microbiological perspective, the same clinical approach (SRP+ABX) can modify host microbiota, reducing putative species correlated to C-MIP disease [114]. Velsko et al. [62] have shown that this protocol (debridement with a 7-day course of ABX) maintained a healthy microbial environment in a 2-year long-term, decreasing *A. actinomycetemcomitans*, *F. alocis*, *T. forsythia*, and *C. gracilis* while health-associated species, such *S. anginosus/gordonii* and *S. parasanguinis*, increased (Figure 9A). A statistical difference in community profile could be observed between healthy and diseased sites before therapy, and a closer cluster (more similar profile) between health and disease profiles could be observed in C-MIP patients post-treatment compared to baseline (Figure 9B) [62]. Burgess et al. [78] also reported a drastic reduction in the initially high prevalence of JP2 genotype post-treatment, and this significant reduction was maintained for 12 months post-treatment, with one course of ABX at baseline and proper periodontal maintenance. In diseased sites, JP2 genotype prevalence was reduced to 3.23% (1/31 site detection) after 1 year of treatment compared to baseline, while no detection was observed in the health sites of African American patients diagnosed with LAP/C-MIP [78]. A different regiment of ABX (Metronidazole-400 mg and Amoxicilin-500 mg, 3× per day for 14 days) along with SRP also decreased JP2 genotype in LAP/C-MIP patients after 1 year. Additionally, serum IgG against Omp29 was also decreased, which is one of the virulence factors correlated to tissue invasion [106].

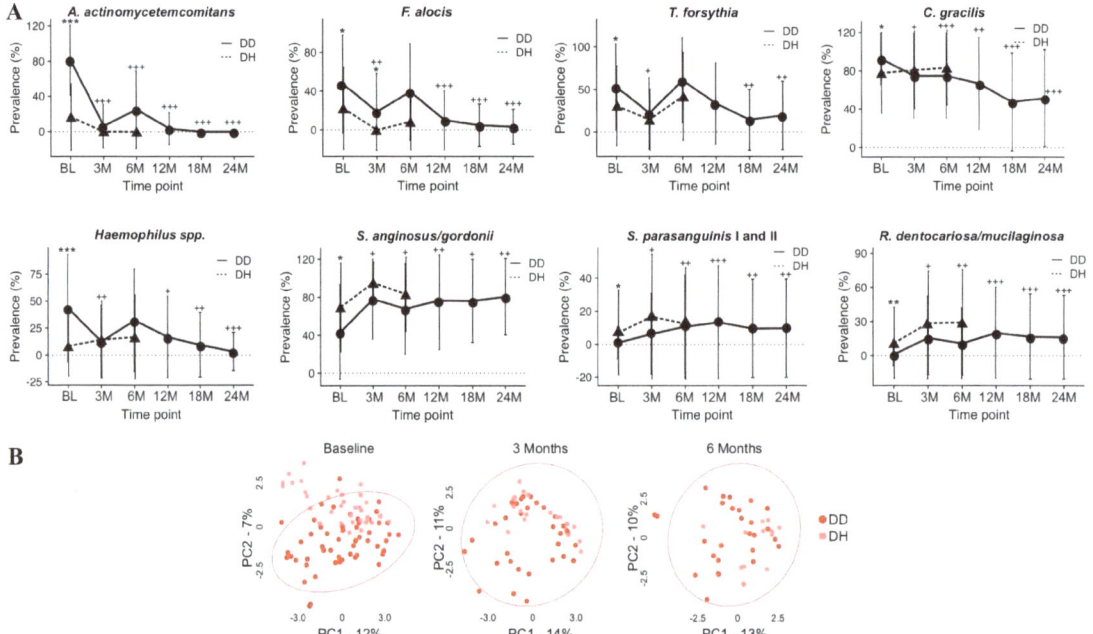

Figure 9. Prevalence of disease- and healthy-associated species after treatment (mechanical debridement with systemic antibiotics —metronidazole 250 mg + amoxicillin 500 mg per 7 days) of C/MIP patients over time (**A**). Principal coordinates analysis (PCoA) shows visibly separated clusters at baseline disease (DD) and healthy (DH) sites than after treatment with an overlap in bacterial profiles of DD and DH sites at 6 months ($p < 0.05$). Ellipses show 95% confidence intervals (**B**). Values are mean ± SD. * $p < 0.05$, ** $p < 0.01$, *** $p < 0.001$ between DD and DH. + $p < 0.05$, ++ $p < 0.01$, +++ $p < 0.001$ in DD compared to baseline. (Source of the image [62]).

Considering dentition type under SRP+ABX clinical approach, Merchant et al. [9] have shown a better clinical attachment gain in primary dentition at 3, 6, and 12 months compared to the permanent dentition, although both dentitions presented a significant reduction in all clinical parameters post-treatment. These results were encouraging regarding early treatment of disease and indicated that younger patients may be more likely to have disease resolution [9]. This can be associated with a few conditions, such as low inflammatory rates in younger children [115], as well as precocious disease diagnosis and intervention under a less complex dysbiotic environment [89]. Depending on the amount of bone level compromised due to disease progression, primary tooth extraction may be an alternative, especially in cases with extensive mobility, pain/abscess, or loss of function impact on quality of life [116].

There is no study confirming disease prevention in permanent teeth in patients diagnosed and treated in the primary dentition. However, the few longitudinal studies following patients diagnosed with LAP/C-MIP in primary dentition indicate a favorable response to treatment and a low incidence of disease in permanent dentition with proper maintenance. According to Mros and Berglundh [15], no bone loss was detected in 7 out of 13 subjects previously diagnosed with the disease in early dentition under proper periodontal maintenance. Miller et al. did not report a recurrence of the disease in permanent dentition in a long-term follow-up of the Florida cohort [16]. Despite the small sample size, low rates of disease recurrence were also observed by Bimstein [17] and Merchant et al. [9]. Thus, it seems reasonable to reinforce periodontal screening in pediatric dental appointments focusing on early diagnosis, especially when cases of aggressive periodontitis are reported in the family.

6. Conclusions

C-MIP is an oral disease more prevalent in African descendants and young systemically healthy adults (under 35 years old) that affects the tooth-supporting apparatus of very specific teeth and features rapid alveolar bone loss. Most cases are associated with low biofilm accumulation, bone loss affecting first molars and incisors, along with familial aggregation. Although less studied, this disease can also be diagnosed in the primary dentition, which may lead to more successful treatment and possibly prevent the occurrence of the disease in the permanent dentition. Studies evaluating primary dentition records have shown that most patients diagnosed in the permanent dentition had disease signs (i.e., bone loss) in the primary dentition.

A heightened inflammatory response to bacteria can be observed in these patients, and healthy siblings also present a tendency of high inflammatory response even without a clinical diagnosis, which may be a result of a genetic predisposition to the disease, given the similar patterns of host response seen in families. The immunological response to biofilm is high regardless of the stimuli used. Periodontal therapy has been shown to successfully manage the local inflammatory profile and clinical response to treatment; however, the modulation of serum biomarkers is not as consistent, and some markers seem to remain high or rebound in the long term despite clinical response remaining positive.

A. actinomycetemcomitans is a key pathogen either in primary or permanent dentition affected with this disease, characterized by special tools for tissue invasion and more virulent genotypes (e.g., JP2). *A. actinomycetemcomitans* early acquisition was also reported as a possible predictor to disease initiation. The colonization of *A. actinomycetemcomitans* in primary dentition can be explained by familial aggregation and possible pathogenic transmission within families. Similar subgingival biofilm composition between parents diagnosed with an aggressive type of periodontitis and their offspring has been reported in the literature. In fact, the bacterial community in these children seems to be resistant even after periodontal maintenance. After periodontal therapy, periodontopathogens are significantly reduced, and this profile can be maintained for a long period with proper supportive periodontal therapy.

SRP + ABX is the gold standard for treating C-MIP, supported by several studies and systematic reviews. Most studies report amoxicillin and metronidazole as the regimen of choice as adjuncts to SRP/full mouth debridement. The disease affecting both primary and permanent dentition presents a favorable clinical response to treatment. However, higher gains in clinical attachment levels seem to happen in younger children. This may be explained by a lower inflammatory profile in young children [115] and a less mature microbial community compared to permanent dentition [89]

7. Future Directions

There are still many gaps to be investigated in C-MIP, such as sex hormones (androgens, estrogens, and progestogens) and other cofactors during childhood development that may influence the disease incidence. Moreover, epigenetic studies and other comprehensive analyses using integrative -omics analysis (e.g., proteomic, metagenomic, genomics) should be carried out focusing on better understanding the biomolecular features of this disease in different time points and in different populations. In addition, there is not yet a group of feature inflammatory biomarkers to control diagnosis, progression, and disease severity over time. A better understanding and correlation between serum, GCF, and saliva biomarkers may guide research and clinical practitioners to a more assertive approach to this disease. Despite the great success under SRP+ABX therapy, host modulation, e.g., pro-resolving lipid mediators, may be an alternative option in future studies [117–119], given the increase in ABX resistance and the heightened inflammatory response seen in these individuals. Considering the current classification system, it is important to include clinical characteristics that have been discussed and published in the past for this disease in different stages so that studies with specific inclusion criteria are conducted, and knowledge continues to be developed for this particular disease in the future. Moreover, given the fact that some evidence indicates a possible disease initiation in the primary dentition, periodontal screening during pediatric appointments remains crucial for early disease diagnosis and treatment and possible prevention of disease at later stages.

Author Contributions: Conceptualization, L.M.S.; Methodology, L.M.S. and M.M.V.M.; Writing—Original Draft Preparation, L.M.S. and M.M.V.M.; Writing—Review and Editing, L.M.S. and M.M.V.M.; Supervision, L.M.S.; Funding Acquisition, L.M.S. All authors have read and agreed to the published version of the manuscript.

Funding: National Institutes of Health: R01DE019456 and 1U01DE031223.

Institutional Review Board Statement: Not applicable.

Informed Consent Statement: Not applicable.

Data Availability Statement: Not applicable.

Conflicts of Interest: The authors declare no conflicts of interest.

References

1. Scannapieco, F.A.; Dongari-Bagtzoglou, A. Dysbiosis Revisited: Understanding the Role of the Oral Microbiome in the Pathogenesis of Gingivitis and Periodontitis: A Critical Assessment. *J. Periodontol.* **2021**, *92*, 1071–1078. [CrossRef] [PubMed]
2. Ebersole, J.L.; Dawson, D.R.; Morford, L.A.; Peyyala, R.; Miller, C.S.; Gonzaléz, O.A. Periodontal Disease Immunology: "double Indemnity" in Protecting the Host. *Periodontology 2000* **2013**, *62*, 163–202. [CrossRef] [PubMed]
3. Armitage, G.C. Development of a Classification System for Periodontal Diseases and Conditions. *Ann. Periodontol.* **1999**, *4*, 1–6. [CrossRef] [PubMed]
4. Papapanou, P.N.; Sanz, M.; Buduneli, N.; Dietrich, T.; Feres, M.; Fine, D.H.; Flemmig, T.F.; Garcia, R.; Giannobile, W.V.; Graziani, F.; et al. Periodontitis: Consensus Report of Workgroup 2 of the 2017 World Workshop on the Classification of Periodontal and Peri-Implant Diseases and Conditions. *J. Periodontol.* **2018**, *89* (Suppl. S1), S173–S182. [CrossRef] [PubMed]
5. Susin, C.; Haas, A.N.; Albandar, J.M. Epidemiology and Demographics of Aggressive Periodontitis. *Periodontology 2000* **2014**, *65*, 27–45. [CrossRef] [PubMed]
6. Albandar, J.M.; Tinoco, E.M.B. Global Epidemiology of Periodontal Diseases in Children and Young Persons. *Periodontology 2000* **2002**, *29*, 153–176. [CrossRef] [PubMed]
7. Bouziane, A.; Hamdoun, R.; Abouqal, R.; Ennibi, O. Global Prevalence of Aggressive Periodontitis: A Systematic Review and Meta-analysis. *J. Clin. Periodontol.* **2020**, *47*, 406–428. [CrossRef] [PubMed]
8. Lang, N.; Bartold, P.M.; Cullinan, M.; Jeffcoat, M.; Mombelli, A.; Murakami, S.; Page, R.; Papapanou, P.; Tonetti, M.; Van Dyke, T. Consensus Report: Aggressive Periodontitis. *Ann. Periodontol.* **1999**, *4*, 53. [CrossRef]

9. Merchant, S.N.; Vovk, A.; Kalash, D.; Hovencamp, N.; Aukhil, I.; Harrison, P.; Zapert, E.; Bidwell, J.; Varnado, P.; Shaddox, L.M. Localized Aggressive Periodontitis Treatment Response in Primary and Permanent Dentitions. *J. Periodontol.* **2014**, *85*, 1722–1729. [CrossRef]

10. Miller, K.; Treloar, T.; Guelmann, M.; Rody, W.J.; Shaddox, L.M. Clinical Characteristics of Localized Aggressive Periodontitis in Primary Dentition. *J. Clin. Pediatr. Dent.* **2018**, *42*, 95–102. [CrossRef]

11. Bimstein, E. Radiographic Description of the Distribution of Aggressive Periodontitis in Primary Teeth. *J. Clin. Pediatr. Dent.* **2018**, *42*, 91–94. [CrossRef] [PubMed]

12. Jensen, A.B.; Ennibi, O.K.; Ismaili, Z.; Poulsen, K.; Haubek, D. The JP2 Genotype of Aggregatibacter Actinomycetemcomitans and Marginal Periodontitis in the Mixed Dentition. *J. Clin. Periodontol.* **2016**, *43*, 19–25. [CrossRef] [PubMed]

13. Cogen, R.B.; Wright, J.T.; Tate, A.L. Destructive Periodontal Disease in Healthy Children. *J. Periodontol.* **1992**, *63*, 761–765. [CrossRef] [PubMed]

14. Mandell, R.L.; Siegal, M.D.; Umland, E. Localized Juvenile Periodontitis of the Primary Dentition. *ASDC J. Dent. Child.* **1986**, *53*, 193–196. [PubMed]

15. Mros, S.T.; Berglundh, T. Aggressive Periodontitis in Children: A 14–19-Year Follow-Up. *J. Clin. Periodontol.* **2010**, *37*, 283–287. [CrossRef] [PubMed]

16. Miller, K.A.F.S.; Branco-de-Almeida, L.S.; Wolf, S.; Hovencamp, N.; Treloar, T.; Harrison, P.; Aukhil, I.; Gong, Y.; Shaddox, L.M. Long-Term Clinical Response to Treatment and Maintenance of Localized Aggressive Periodontitis: A Cohort Study. *J. Clin. Periodontol.* **2017**, *44*, 158–168. [CrossRef] [PubMed]

17. Bimstein, E. Seven-Year Follow-up of 10 Children with Periodontitis. *Pediatr. Dent.* **2003**, *25*, 389–396.

18. Tavakoli, T.T.; Gholami, F.; Huang, H.; Gonçalves, P.F.; Villasante-Tezanos, A.; Aukhil, I.; de Oliveira, R.C.G.; Hovencamp, N.; Wallet, S.; Ioannidou, E.; et al. Gender Differences in Immunological Response of African-American Juveniles with Grade C Molar Incisor Pattern Periodontitis. *J. Periodontol.* **2022**, *93*, 392–402. [CrossRef] [PubMed]

19. Melvin, W.L.; Sandifer, J.B.; Gray, J.L. The Prevalence and Sex Ratio of Juvenile Periodontitis in a Young Racially Mixed Population. *J. Periodontol.* **1991**, *62*, 330–334. [CrossRef]

20. Nassar, M.M.; Afifi, O.; Deprez, R.D. The Prevalence of Localized Juvenile Periodontitis in Saudi Subjects. *J. Periodontol.* **1994**, *65*, 698–701. [CrossRef]

21. Branco-De-Almeida, L.S.; Cruz-Almeida, Y.; Gonzalez-Marrero, Y.; Huang, H.; Aukhil, I.; Harrison, P.; Wallet, S.M.; Shaddox, L.M. Local and Plasma Biomarker Profiles in Localized Aggressive Periodontitis. *JDR Clin. Trans. Res.* **2017**, *2*, 258–268. [CrossRef] [PubMed]

22. Shaddox, L.M.; Wiedey, J.; Calderon, N.L.; Magnusson, I.; Bimstein, E.; Bidwell, J.A.; Zapert, E.F.; Aukhil, I.; Wallet, S.M. Local Inflammatory Markers and Systemic Endotoxin in Aggressive Periodontitis. *J. Dent. Res.* **2011**, *90*, 1140–1144. [CrossRef] [PubMed]

23. Martins, E.S.; César-Neto, J.B.; Albuquerque-Souza, E.; Rebeis, E.S.; Holzhausen, M.; Pannuti, C.M.; Mayer, M.P.A.; Saraiva, L. One-Year Follow-up of the Immune Profile in Serum and Selected Sites of Generalized and Localized Aggressive Periodontitis. *Cytokine* **2019**, *116*, 27–37. [CrossRef] [PubMed]

24. Alamri, M.M.; Antonoglou, G.N.; Proctor, G.; Balsa-Castro, C.; Tomás, I.; Nibali, L. Biomarkers for Diagnosis of Stage III, Grade C with Molar Incisor Pattern Periodontitis in Children and Young Adults: A Systematic Review and Meta-Analysis. *Clin. Oral Investig.* **2023**, *27*, 4929–4955. [CrossRef] [PubMed]

25. Shaddox, L.; Wiedey, J.; Bimstein, E.; Magnuson, I.; Clare-Salzler, M.; Aukhil, I.; Wallet, S.M. Hyper-Responsive Phenotype in Localized Aggressive Periodontitis. *J. Dent. Res.* **2010**, *89*, 143–148. [CrossRef] [PubMed]

26. Shaddox, L.M.; Spencer, W.P.; Velsko, I.M.; Al-Kassab, H.; Huang, H.; Calderon, N.; Aukhil, I.; Wallet, S.M. Localized Aggressive Periodontitis Immune Response to Healthy and Diseased Subgingival Plaque. *J. Clin. Periodontol.* **2016**, *43*, 746–753. [CrossRef] [PubMed]

27. Tabaa, M.; Adatowovor, R.; Shabila, A.; Morford, L.; Dawson, D.; Harrison, P.; Aukhil, I.; Huang, H.; Stromberg, A.; Goncalves, J.; et al. Pattern of Grade C Molar-Incisor Pattern Periodontitis in Families. *J. Periodontol.* **2023**, *94*, 811–822. [CrossRef]

28. Kantarci, A.; Oyaizu, K.; Van Dyke, T.E. Neutrophil-Mediated Tissue Injury in Periodontal Disease Pathogenesis: Findings from Localized Aggressive Periodontitis. *J. Periodontol.* **2003**, *74*, 66–75. [CrossRef] [PubMed]

29. Van Dyke, T.E.; Horoszewicz, H.U.; Cianciola, L.J.; Genco, R.J. Neutrophil Chemotaxis Dysfunction in Human Periodontitis. *Infect. Immun.* **1980**, *27*, 124–132. [CrossRef]

30. Van Dyke, T.E.; Schweinebraten, M.; Cianciola, L.J.; Offenbacher, S.; Genco, R.J. Neutrophil Chemotaxis in Families with Localized Juvenile Periodontitis. *J. Periodontal Res.* **1985**, *20*, 503–514. [CrossRef]

31. Schenkein, H.A.; Barbour, S.E.; Tew, J.G. Cytokines and Inflammatory Factors Regulating Immunoglobulin Production in Aggressive Periodontitis. *Periodontology 2000* **2007**, *45*, 113–127. [CrossRef] [PubMed]

32. Wilson, M.E.; Hamilton, R.G. Immunoglobulin G Subclass Response of Localized Juvenile Periodontitis Patients to Actinobacillus Actinomycetemcomitans Y4 Lipopolysaccharide. *Infect. Immun.* **1992**, *60*, 1806–1812. [CrossRef] [PubMed]

33. Ling, T.Y.; Sims, T.J.; Chen, H.A.; Whitney, C.W.; Moncla, B.J.; Engel, L.D.; Page, R.C. Titer and Subclass Distribution of Serum IgG Antibody Reactive with Actinobacillus Actinomycetemcomitans in Localized Juvenile Periodontitis. *J. Clin. Immunol.* **1993**, *13*, 101–112. [CrossRef] [PubMed]

34. Lu, H.; Wang, M.; Gunsolley, J.C.; Schenkein, H.A.; Tew, J.G. Serum Immunoglobulin G Subclass Concentrations in Periodontally Healthy and Diseased Individuals. *Infect. Immun.* **1994**, *62*, 1677–1682. [CrossRef] [PubMed]
35. Steffens, J.P.; Wang, X.; Starr, J.R.; Spolidorio, L.C.; Van Dyke, T.E.; Kantarci, A. Associations Between Sex Hormone Levels and Periodontitis in Men: Results From NHANES III. *J. Periodontol.* **2015**, *86*, 1116–1125. [CrossRef] [PubMed]
36. Boyapati, R.; Cherukuri, S.A.; Bodduru, R.; Kiranmaye, A. Influence of Female Sex Hormones in Different Stages of Women on Periodontium. *J. Midlife Health* **2021**, *12*, 263–266. [CrossRef] [PubMed]
37. Shaddox, L.M.; Morford, L.A.; Nibali, L. Periodontal Health and Disease: The Contribution of Genetics. *Periodontology 2000* **2021**, *85*, 161–181. [CrossRef] [PubMed]
38. Gonçalves, P.F.; Harris, T.H.; Elmariah, T.; Aukhil, I.; Wallace, M.R.; Shaddox, L.M. Genetic Polymorphisms and Periodontal Disease in Populations of African Descent: A Review. *J. Periodontal Res.* **2018**, *53*, 164–173. [CrossRef]
39. Harris, T.H.; Wallace, M.R.; Huang, H.; Li, H.; Mohiuddeen, A.; Gong, Y.; Kompotiati, T.; Harrison, P.; Aukhil, I.; Shaddox, L.M. Association of P2RX7 Functional Variants with Localized Aggressive Periodontitis. *J. Periodontal Res.* **2020**, *55*, 32–40. [CrossRef]
40. Gonçalves Fernandes, J.; Morford, L.A.; Harrison, P.L.; Kompotiati, T.; Huang, H.; Aukhil, I.; Wallet, S.M.; Macchion Shaddox, L. Dysregulation of Genes and MicroRNAs in Localized Aggressive Periodontitis. *J. Clin. Periodontol.* **2020**, *47*, 1317–1325. [CrossRef]
41. Vollmer, S.; Strickson, S.; Zhang, T.; Gray, N.; Lee, K.L.; Rao, V.R.; Cohen, P. The Mechanism of Activation of IRAK1 and IRAK4 by Interleukin-1 and Toll-like Receptor Agonists. *Biochem. J.* **2017**, *474*, 2027–2038. [CrossRef] [PubMed]
42. Shaddox, L.M.; Mullersman, A.F.; Huang, H.; Wallet, S.M.; Aukhil, I. Epigenetic Regulation of Inflammation in Localized Aggressive Periodontitis. *Clin. Epigenetics* **2017**, *9*, 94. [CrossRef] [PubMed]
43. Diehl, S.R.; Wang, Y.; Brooks, C.N.; Burmeister, J.A.; Califano, J.V.; Wang, S.; Schenkein, H.A. Linkage Disequilibrium of Interleukin-1 Genetic Polymorphisms with Early-Onset Periodontitis. *J. Periodontol.* **1999**, *70*, 418–430. [CrossRef] [PubMed]
44. Jordan, W.J.; Eskdale, J.; Lennon, G.P.; Pestoff, R.; Wu, L.; Fine, D.H.; Gallagher, G. A Non-Conservative, Coding Single-Nucleotide Polymorphism in the N-Terminal Region of Lactoferrin Is Associated with Aggressive Periodontitis in an African-American, but Not a Caucasian Population. *Genes Immun.* **2005**, *6*, 632–635. [CrossRef]
45. Wu, Y.M.; Juo, S.H.; Ho, Y.P.; Ho, K.Y.; Yang, Y.H.; Tsai, C.C. Association between Lactoferrin Gene Polymorphisms and Aggressive Periodontitis among Taiwanese Patients. *J. Periodontal Res.* **2009**, *44*, 418–424. [CrossRef] [PubMed]
46. Noack, B.; Görgens, H.; Hempel, U.; Fanghänel, J.; Hoffmann, T.; Ziegler, A.; Schackert, H.K. Cathepsin C Gene Variants in Aggressive Periodontitis. *J. Dent. Res.* **2008**, *87*, 958–963. [CrossRef] [PubMed]
47. Vieira, A.R.; Albandar, J.M. Role of Genetic Factors in the Pathogenesis of Aggressive Periodontitis. *Periodontology 2000* **2014**, *65*, 92–106. [CrossRef] [PubMed]
48. Kinane, D.F.; Hart, T.C. Genes and Gene Polymorphisms Associated with Periodontal Disease. *Crit. Rev. Oral Biol. Med.* **2003**, *14*, 430–449. [CrossRef] [PubMed]
49. Meng, H.; Xu, L.; Li, Q.; Han, J.; Zhao, Y. Determinants of Host Susceptibility in Aggressive Periodontitis. *Periodontology 2000* **2007**, *43*, 133–159. [CrossRef]
50. de Carvalho, F.M.; Tinoco, E.M.B.; Govil, M.; Marazita, M.L.; Vieira, A.R. Aggressive Periodontitis Is Likely Influenced by a Few Small Effect Genes. *J. Clin. Periodontol.* **2009**, *36*, 468–473. [CrossRef]
51. Nibali, L. Aggressive Periodontitis: Microbes and Host Response, Who to Blame? *Virulence* **2015**, *6*, 223–228. [CrossRef]
52. Nibali, L.; Henderson, B.; Tariq Sadiq, S.; Donos, N. Genetic Dysbiosis: The Role of Microbial Insults in Chronic Inflammatory Diseases. *J. Oral Microbiol.* **2014**, *6*, 22962. [CrossRef]
53. Zoheir, N.; Kurushima, Y.; Lin, G.-H.; Nibali, L. Periodontal Infectogenomics: A Systematic Review Update of Associations between Host Genetic Variants and Subgingival Microbial Detection. *Clin. Oral Investig.* **2022**, *26*, 2209–2221. [CrossRef] [PubMed]
54. Lee, Y.H.; Na, H.S.; Jeong, S.Y.; Jeong, S.H.; Park, H.R.; Chung, J. Comparison of Inflammatory MicroRNA Expression in Healthy and Periodontitis Tissues. *Biocell* **2011**, *35*, 43–49. [CrossRef] [PubMed]
55. Li, Y.; Liu, X.; Du, A.; Zhu, X.; Yu, B. MiR-203 Accelerates Apoptosis and Inflammation Induced by LPS via Targeting NFIL3 in Cardiomyocytes. *J. Cell. Biochem.* **2019**, *120*, 6605–6613. [CrossRef]
56. Luan, X.; Zhou, X.; Naqvi, A.; Francis, M.; Foyle, D.; Nares, S.; Diekwisch, T.G.H. MicroRNAs and Immunity in Periodontal Health and Disease. *Int. J. Oral Sci.* **2018**, *10*, 24. [CrossRef] [PubMed]
57. Bazzoni, F.; Rossato, M.; Fabbri, M.; Gaudiosi, D.; Mirolo, M.; Mori, L.; Tamassia, N.; Mantovani, A.; Cassatella, M.A.; Locati, M. Induction and Regulatory Function of MiR-9 in Human Monocytes and Neutrophils Exposed to Proinflammatory Signals. *Proc. Natl. Acad. Sci. USA* **2009**, *106*, 5282–5287. [CrossRef]
58. Tang, B.; Xiao, B.; Liu, Z.; Li, N.; Zhu, E.-D.; Li, B.-S.; Xie, Q.-H.; Zhuang, Y.; Zou, Q.-M.; Mao, X.-H. Identification of MyD88 as a Novel Target of MiR-155, Involved in Negative Regulation of Helicobacter Pylori-Induced Inflammation. *FEBS Lett.* **2010**, *584*, 1481–1486. [CrossRef]
59. Tili, E.; Michaille, J.-J.; Cimino, A.; Costinean, S.; Dumitru, C.D.; Adair, B.; Fabbri, M.; Alder, H.; Liu, C.G.; Calin, G.A.; et al. Modulation of MiR-155 and MiR-125b Levels Following Lipopolysaccharide/TNF-Alpha Stimulation and Their Possible Roles in Regulating the Response to Endotoxin Shock. *J. Immunol.* **2007**, *179*, 5082–5089. [CrossRef]
60. Liu, G.; Friggeri, A.; Yang, Y.; Park, Y.-J.; Tsuruta, Y.; Abraham, E. MiR-147, a MicroRNA That Is Induced upon Toll-like Receptor Stimulation, Regulates Murine Macrophage Inflammatory Responses. *Proc. Natl. Acad. Sci. USA* **2009**, *106*, 15819–15824. [CrossRef]

61. Amado, P.P.P.; Kawamoto, D.; Albuquerque-Souza, E.; Franco, D.C.; Saraiva, L.; Casarin, R.C.V.; Horliana, A.C.R.T.; Mayer, M.P.A. Oral and Fecal Microbiome in Molar-Incisor Pattern Periodontitis. *Front. Cell. Infect. Microbiol.* **2020**, 10, 583761. [CrossRef] [PubMed]
62. Velsko, I.M.; Harrison, P.; Chalmers, N.; Barb, J.; Huang, H.; Aukhil, I.; Shaddox, L. Grade C Molar-Incisor Pattern Periodontitis Subgingival Microbial Profile before and after Treatment. *J. Oral Microbiol.* **2020**, 12, 1814674. [CrossRef] [PubMed]
63. Darby, I.; Curtis, M. Microbiology of Periodontal Disease in Children and Young Adults. *Periodontology 2000* **2001**, 26, 33–53. [CrossRef] [PubMed]
64. Shaddox, L.M.; Huang, H.; Lin, T.; Hou, W.; Harrison, P.L.; Aukhil, I.; Walker, C.B.; Klepac-Ceraj, V.; Paster, B.J. Microbiological Characterization in Children with Aggressive Periodontitis. *J. Dent. Res.* **2012**, 91, 927–933. [CrossRef]
65. Könönen, E.; Müller, H. Microbiology of Aggressive Periodontitis. *Periodontology 2000* **2014**, 65, 46–78. [CrossRef] [PubMed]
66. Faveri, M.; Figueiredo, L.C.; Duarte, P.M.; Mestnik, M.J.; Mayer, M.P.A.; Feres, M. Microbiological Profile of Untreated Subjects with Localized Aggressive Periodontitis. *J. Clin. Periodontol.* **2009**, 36, 739–749. [CrossRef]
67. Cortelli, J.R.; Cortelli, S.C.; Jordan, S.; Haraszthy, V.I.; Zambon, J.J. Prevalence of Periodontal Pathogens in Brazilians with Aggressive or Chronic Periodontitis. *J. Clin. Periodontol.* **2005**, 32, 860–866. [CrossRef]
68. Slots, J.; Ting, M. Actinobacillus Actinomycetemcomitans and Porphyromonas Gingivalis in Human Periodontal Disease: Occurrence and Treatment. *Periodontology 2000* **1999**, 20, 82–121. [CrossRef]
69. Åberg, C.H.; Kelk, P.; Johansson, A. Aggregatibacter Actinomycetemcomitans: Virulence of Its Leukotoxin and Association with Aggressive Periodontitis. *Virulence* **2015**, 6, 188–195. [CrossRef]
70. Fine, D.H.; Markowitz, K.; Furgang, D.; Fairlie, K.; Ferrandiz, J.; Nasri, C.; McKiernan, M.; Gunsolley, J. Aggregatibacter Actinomycetemcomitans and Its Relationship to Initiation of Localized Aggressive Periodontitis: Longitudinal Cohort Study of Initially Healthy Adolescents. *J. Clin. Microbiol.* **2007**, 45, 3859–3869. [CrossRef]
71. Fine, D.H.; Markowitz, K.; Fairlie, K.; Tischio-Bereski, D.; Ferrendiz, J.; Furgang, D.; Paster, B.J.; Dewhirst, F.E. A Consortium of Aggregatibacter Actinomycetemcomitans, Streptococcus Parasanguinis, and Filifactor Alocis Is Present in Sites Prior to Bone Loss in a Longitudinal Study of Localized Aggressive Periodontitis. *J. Clin. Microbiol.* **2013**, 51, 2850–2861. [CrossRef] [PubMed]
72. Fine, D.H.; Patil, A.G.; Velusamy, S.K. Aggregatibacter Actinomycetemcomitans (Aa) Under the Radar: Myths and Misunderstandings of Aa and Its Role in Aggressive Periodontitis. *Front. Immunol.* **2019**, 10, 728. [CrossRef] [PubMed]
73. Herbert, B.A.; Novince, C.M.; Kirkwood, K.L. Aggregatibacter Actinomycetemcomitans, a Potent Immunoregulator of the Periodontal Host Defense System and Alveolar Bone Homeostasis. *Mol. Oral Microbiol.* **2016**, 31, 207–227. [CrossRef] [PubMed]
74. Raja, M. Aggregatibacter Actinomycetemcomitans—A Tooth Killer? *J. Clin. Diagn. Res.* **2014**, 8, ZE13–6. [CrossRef] [PubMed]
75. Haubek, D.; Poulsen, K.; Kilian, M. Microevolution and Patterns of Dissemination of the JP2 Clone of Aggregatibacter (Actinobacillus) Actinomycetemcomitans. *Infect. Immun.* **2007**, 75, 3080–3088. [CrossRef] [PubMed]
76. Haubek, D.; Ennibi, O.-K.; Poulsen, K.; Vaeth, M.; Poulsen, S.; Kilian, M. Risk of Aggressive Periodontitis in Adolescent Carriers of the JP2 Clone of Aggregatibacter (Actinobacillus) Actinomycetemcomitans in Morocco: A Prospective Longitudinal Cohort Study. *Lancet* **2008**, 371, 237–242. [CrossRef] [PubMed]
77. Höglund Åberg, C.; Kwamin, F.; Claesson, R.; Dahlén, G.; Johansson, A.; Haubek, D. Progression of Attachment Loss Is Strongly Associated with Presence of the JP2 Genotype of Aggregatibacter Actinomycetemcomitans: A Prospective Cohort Study of a Young Adolescent Population. *J. Clin. Periodontol.* **2014**, 41, 232–241. [CrossRef] [PubMed]
78. Burgess, D.K.; Huang, H.; Harrison, P.; Kompotiati, T.; Aukhil, I.; Shaddox, L.M. Non-Surgical Therapy Reduces Presence of JP2 Clone in Localized Aggressive Periodontitis. *J. Periodontol.* **2017**, 88, 1263–1270. [CrossRef] [PubMed]
79. Höglund Åberg, C.; Haubek, D.; Kwamin, F.; Johansson, A.; Claesson, R. Leukotoxic Activity of Aggregatibacter Actinomycetemcomitans and Periodontal Attachment Loss. *PLoS ONE* **2014**, 9, e104095. [CrossRef]
80. Johansson, A.; Claesson, R.; Hänström, L.; Sandström, G.; Kalfas, S. Polymorphonuclear Leukocyte Degranulation Induced by Leukotoxin from Actinobacillus Actinomycetemcomitans. *J. Periodontal Res.* **2000**, 35, 85–92. [CrossRef]
81. Saglie, F.R.; Marfany, A.; Camargo, P. Intragingival Occurrence of Actinobacillus Actinomycetemcomitans and Bacteroides Gingivalis in Active Destructive Periodontal Lesions. *J. Periodontol.* **1988**, 59, 259–265. [CrossRef] [PubMed]
82. Lamell, C.W.; Griffen, A.L.; McClellan, D.L.; Leys, E.J. Acquisition and Colonization Stability of Actinobacillus Actinomycetemcomitans and Porphyromonas Gingivalis in Children. *J. Clin. Microbiol.* **2000**, 38, 1196–1199. [CrossRef] [PubMed]
83. Oscarsson, J.; Claesson, R.; Lindholm, M.; Åberg, C.H.; Johansson, A. Tools of Aggregatibacter Actinomycetemcomitans to Evade the Host Response. *J. Clin. Med.* **2019**, 8, 1079. [CrossRef] [PubMed]
84. Asakawa, R.; Komatsuzawa, H.; Kawai, T.; Yamada, S.; Goncalves, R.B.; Izumi, S.; Fujiwara, T.; Nakano, Y.; Suzuki, N.; Uchida, Y.; et al. Outer Membrane Protein 100, a Versatile Virulence Factor of Actinobacillus Actinomycetemcomitans. *Mol. Microbiol.* **2003**, 50, 1125–1139. [CrossRef] [PubMed]
85. Kajiya, M.; Komatsuzawa, H.; Papantonakis, A.; Seki, M.; Makihira, S.; Ouhara, K.; Kusumoto, Y.; Murakami, S.; Taubman, M.A.; Kawai, T. Aggregatibacter Actinomycetemcomitans Omp29 Is Associated with Bacterial Entry to Gingival Epithelial Cells by F-Actin Rearrangement. *PLoS ONE* **2011**, 6, e18287. [CrossRef] [PubMed]
86. DiRienzo, J.M. Breaking the Gingival Epithelial Barrier: Role of the Aggregatibacter Actinomycetemcomitans Cytolethal Distending Toxin in Oral Infectious Disease. *Cells* **2014**, 3, 476–499. [CrossRef] [PubMed]
87. Alaluusua, S.; Saarela, M.; Jousimies-Somer, H.; Asikainen, S. Ribotyping Shows Intrafamilial Similarity in Actinobacillus Actinomycetemcomitans Isolates. *Oral Microbiol. Immunol.* **1993**, 8, 225–229. [CrossRef] [PubMed]

88. Monteiro, M.F.; Altabtbaei, K.; Kumar, P.S.; Casati, M.Z.; Ruiz, K.G.S.; Sallum, E.A.; Nociti-Junior, F.H.; Casarin, R.C.V. Parents with Periodontitis Impact the Subgingival Colonization of Their Offspring. *Sci. Rep.* **2021**, *11*, 1357. [CrossRef]

89. Koo, S.S.; Fernandes, J.G.; Li, L.; Huang, H.; Aukhil, I.; Harrison, P.; Diaz, P.I.; Shaddox, L.M. Evaluation of Microbiome in Primary and Permanent Dentition in Grade C Periodontitis in Young Individuals. *J. Periodontol.* 2024; *Epub ahead of print*. [CrossRef]

90. Dibart, S.; Chapple, I.L.; Skobe, Z.; Shusterman, S.; Nedleman, H.L. Microbiological Findings in Prepubertal Periodontitis. A Case Report. *J. Periodontol.* **1998**, *69*, 1172–1175. [CrossRef]

91. Yoshida-Minami, I.; Kishimoto, K.; Suzuki, A.; Fujiwara, T.; Shintani, S.; Morisaki, I.; Sobue, S.; Miyamoto, M.; Nagai, A.; Kurihara, H. Clinical, Microbiological and Host Defense Parameters Associated with a Case of Localized Prepubertal Periodontitis. *J. Clin. Periodontol.* **1995**, *22*, 56–62. [CrossRef]

92. Zambon, J.J.; Christersson, L.A.; Slots, J. Actinobacillus Actinomycetemcomitans in Human Periodontal Disease. Prevalence in Patient Groups and Distribution of Biotypes and Serotypes within Families. *J. Periodontol.* **1983**, *54*, 707–711. [CrossRef] [PubMed]

93. Christersson, L.A. Actinobacillus Actinomycetemcomitans and Localized Juvenile Periodontitis. Clinical, Microbiologic and Histologic Studies. *Swed. Dent. J. Suppl.* **1993**, *90*, 1–46. [PubMed]

94. Haubek, D.; Poulsen, K.; Westergaard, J.; Dahlèn, G.; Kilian, M. Highly Toxic Clone of Actinobacillus Actinomycetemcomitans in Geographically Widespread Cases of Juvenile Periodontitis in Adolescents of African Origin. *J. Clin. Microbiol.* **1996**, *34*, 1576–1578. [CrossRef] [PubMed]

95. van Steenbergen, T.J.; van der Velden, U.; Abbas, F.; de Graaff, J. Microbiological and Clinical Monitoring of Non-Localized Juvenile Periodontitis in Young Adults: A Report of 11 Cases. *J. Periodontol.* **1993**, *64*, 40–47. [CrossRef] [PubMed]

96. Sixou, M.; Duffaut-Lagarrigue, D.; Lodter, J.P. [The Distribution and Prevalence of Haemophilus Actinomycetemcomitans in the Oral Cavity]. *J. Biol. Buccale* **1991**, *19*, 221–228. [PubMed]

97. Saarela, M.; Mättö, J.; Asikainen, S.; Jousimies-Somer, H.; Torkko, H.; Pyhälä, L.; Stucki, A.M.; Hannula, J.; Hölttä, P.; Alaluusua, S. Clonal Diversity OfActinobacillus Actinomycetemcomitans, Porphyromonas GingivalisandPrevotella Intermedia/Nigrescensin Two Families: CLINICAL MICROBIOLOGY. *Anaerobe* **1996**, *2*, 19–27. [CrossRef]

98. Petit, M.D.; van Steenbergen, T.J.; Scholte, L.M.; van der Velden, U.; de Graaff, J. Epidemiology and Transmission of Porphyromonas Gingivalis and Actinobacillus Actinomycetemcomitans among Children and Their Family Members. A Report of 4 Surveys. *J. Clin. Periodontol.* **1993**, *20*, 641–650. [CrossRef] [PubMed]

99. DiRienzo, J.M.; Slots, J.; Sixou, M.; Sol, M.A.; Harmon, R.; McKay, T.L. Specific Genetic Variants of Actinobacillus Actinomycetemcomitans Correlate with Disease and Health in a Regional Population of Families with Localized Juvenile Periodontitis. *Infect. Immun.* **1994**, *62*, 3058–3065. [CrossRef] [PubMed]

100. Hodge, P.; Michalowicz, B. Genetic Predisposition to Periodontitis in Children and Young Adults. *Periodontology 2000* **2001**, *26*, 113–134. [CrossRef] [PubMed]

101. Moore, W.E.; Burmeister, J.A.; Brooks, C.N.; Ranney, R.R.; Hinkelmann, K.H.; Schieken, R.M.; Moore, L. V Investigation of the Influences of Puberty, Genetics, and Environment on the Composition of Subgingival Periodontal Floras. *Infect. Immun.* **1993**, *61*, 2891–2898. [CrossRef]

102. Wennström, J.L.; Dahlén, G.; Svensson, J.; Nyman, S. *Actinobacillus Actinomycetemcomitans*, Bacteroides *Gingivalis* and Bacteroides *Intermedius*: Predictors of Attachment Loss? *Oral Microbiol. Immunol.* **1987**, *2*, 158–163. [CrossRef] [PubMed]

103. Christersson, L.A.; Albini, B.; Zambon, J.J.; Wikesjö, U.M.E.; Genco, R.J. Tissue Localization of Actinobacillus Actinomycetemcomitans in Human Periodontitis. *J. Periodontol.* **1987**, *58*, 529–539. [CrossRef] [PubMed]

104. Clerehugh, V.; Tugnait, A. Diagnosis and Management of Periodontal Diseases in Children and Adolescents. *Periodontology 2000* **2001**, *26*, 146–168. [CrossRef] [PubMed]

105. American Academy of Pediatric Dentistry. Periodontal Diseases of Children and Adolescents. *J. Periodontol.* **2003**, *74*, 1696–1704. [CrossRef] [PubMed]

106. Rebeis, E.S.; Albuquerque-Souza, E.; Paulino da Silva, M.; Giudicissi, M.; Mayer, M.P.A.; Saraiva, L. Effect of Periodontal Treatment on Aggregatibacter Actinomycetemcomitans Colonization and Serum IgG Levels against A. Actinomycetemcomitans Serotypes and Omp29 of Aggressive Periodontitis Patients. *Oral Dis.* **2019**, *25*, 569–579. [CrossRef] [PubMed]

107. Rabelo, C.C.; Feres, M.; Gonçalves, C.; Figueiredo, L.C.; Faveri, M.; Tu, Y.-K.; Chambrone, L. Systemic Antibiotics in the Treatment of Aggressive Periodontitis. A Systematic Review and a Bayesian Network Meta-Analysis. *J. Clin. Periodontol.* **2015**, *42*, 647–657. [CrossRef] [PubMed]

108. Keestra, J.A.J.; Grosjean, I.; Coucke, W.; Quirynen, M.; Teughels, W. Non-Surgical Periodontal Therapy with Systemic Antibiotics in Patients with Untreated Chronic Periodontitis: A Systematic Review and Meta-Analysis. *J. Periodontal Res.* **2015**, *50*, 294–314. [CrossRef] [PubMed]

109. Branco-de-Almeida, L.S.; Cruz-Almeida, Y.; Gonzalez-Marrero, Y.; Kudsi, R.; de Oliveira, I.C.V.; Dolia, B.; Huang, H.; Aukhil, I.; Harrison, P.; Shaddox, L.M. Treatment of Localized Aggressive Periodontitis Alters Local Host Immunoinflammatory Profiles: A Long-Term Evaluation. *J. Clin. Periodontol.* **2021**, *48*, 237–248. [CrossRef] [PubMed]

110. Allin, N.; Cruz-Almeida, Y.; Velsko, I.; Vovk, A.; Hovemcamp, N.; Harrison, P.; Huang, H.; Aukhil, I.; Wallet, S.M.; Shaddox, L.M. Inflammatory Response Influences Treatment of Localized Aggressive Periodontitis. *J. Dent. Res.* **2016**, *95*, 635–641. [CrossRef]

111. Branco-de-Almeida, L.S.; Velsko, I.M.; de Oliveira, I.C.V.; de Oliveira, R.C.G.; Shaddox, L.M. Impact of Treatment on Host Responses in Young Individuals with Periodontitis. *J. Dent. Res.* **2023**, *102*, 473–488. [CrossRef]

112. Shaddox, L.M.; Gonçalves, P.F.; Vovk, A.; Allin, N.; Huang, H.; Hou, W.; Aukhil, I.; Wallet, S.M. LPS-Induced Inflammatory Response after Therapy of Aggressive Periodontitis. *J. Dent. Res.* **2013**, *92*, 702–708. [CrossRef] [PubMed]
113. Cifcibasi, E.; Koyuncuoglu, C.; Ciblak, M.; Badur, S.; Kasali, K.; Firatli, E.; Cintan, S. Evaluation of Local and Systemic Levels of Interleukin-17, Interleukin-23, and Myeloperoxidase in Response to Periodontal Therapy in Patients with Generalized Aggressive Periodontitis. *Inflammation* **2015**, *38*, 1959–1968. [CrossRef] [PubMed]
114. Tinoco, E.M.B.; Beldi, M.I.; Campedelli, F.; Lana, M.; Loureiro, C.A.; Bellini, H.T.; Rams, T.E.; Tinoco, N.M.B.; Gjermo, P.; Preus, H.R. Clinical and Microbiological Effects of Adjunctive Antibiotics in Treatment of Localized Juvenile Periodontitis. A Controlled Clinical Trial. *J. Periodontol.* **1998**, *69*, 1355–1363. [CrossRef] [PubMed]
115. Shaddox, L.; Hu, J.; Vovk, A.; Huang, H.; Wallet, S.; Harrison, P.; Aukhil, I.L. Hyper-Inflammatory Response between Primary and Permanent Dentition with Aggressive Periodontitis. *Int. Assoc. Dent. Res.-J. Den. Res.* **2012**, *91*, 941.
116. Suzuki, J.; Okada, M.; Wang, Y.; Nii, N.; Miura, K.; Kozai, K. Localized Aggressive Periodontitis in Primary Dentition: A Case Report. *J. Periodontol.* **2003**, *74*, 1060–1066. [CrossRef] [PubMed]
117. Castro dos Santos, N.C.; Furukawa, M.V.; Oliveira-Cardoso, I.; Cortelli, J.R.; Feres, M.; Van Dyke, T.; Rovai, E.S. Does the Use of Omega-3 Fatty Acids as an Adjunct to Non-surgical Periodontal Therapy Provide Additional Benefits in the Treatment of Periodontitis? A Systematic Review and Meta-analysis. *J. Periodontal Res.* **2022**, *57*, 435–447. [CrossRef] [PubMed]
118. Castro dos Santos, N.C.; Andere, N.M.R.B.; Araujo, C.F.; de Marco, A.C.; Kantarci, A.; Van Dyke, T.E.; Santamaria, M.P. Omega-3 PUFA and Aspirin as Adjuncts to Periodontal Debridement in Patients with Periodontitis and Type 2 Diabetes Mellitus: Randomized Clinical Trial. *J. Periodontol.* **2020**, *91*, 1318–1327. [CrossRef]
119. El-Sharkawy, H.; Aboelsaad, N.; Eliwa, M.; Darweesh, M.; Alshahat, M.; Kantarci, A.; Hasturk, H.; Van Dyke, T.E. Adjunctive Treatment of Chronic Periodontitis With Daily Dietary Supplementation With Omega-3 Fatty Acids and Low-Dose Aspirin. *J. Periodontol.* **2010**, *81*, 1635–1643. [CrossRef]

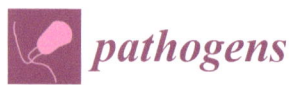

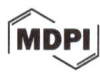

Review

From Global to Nano: A Geographical Perspective of *Aggregatibacter actinomycetemcomitans*

Mark I. Ryder [1,2,*], Daniel H. Fine [3] and Annelise E. Barron [1]

1   Department of Bioengineering, School of Medicine and School of Engineering, Stanford University, Stanford, CA 94143, USA; aebarron@stanford.edu
2   Division of Periodontology, Department of Orofacial Sciences, School of Dentistry, University of California San Francisco, San Francisco, CA 94143, USA
3   Department of Oral Biology, Rutgers School of Dental Medicine, 443 Via Ortega, Stanford, CA 94305, USA
*   Correspondence: mryder@stanford.edu

Abstract: The periodontal disease pathobiont *Aggregatibacter actinomycetemcomitans* (*A. actinomycetemcomitans*) may exert a range of detrimental effects on periodontal diseases in general and, more specifically, with the initiation and progression of Localized Stage III Grade C periodontitis (molar–incisor pattern). In this review of the biogeography of this pathobiont, the full range of geographical scales for *A. actinomycetemcomitans*, from global origins and transmission to local geographical regions, to more locally exposed probands and families, to the individual host, down to the oral cavity, and finally, to spatial interactions with other commensals and pathobionts within the plaque biofilms at the micron/nanoscale, are reviewed. Using the newest technologies in genetics, imaging, in vitro cultures, and other research disciplines, investigators may be able to gain new insights to the role of this pathobiont in the unique initial destructive patterns of Localized Stage III Grade C periodontitis. These findings may incorporate the unique features of the microbiome that are influenced by variations in the geographic environment within the entire mouth. Additional insights into the geographic distribution of molar–incisor periodontal breakdown for Localized Stage III Grade C periodontitis may derive from the spatial interactions between *A. actinomycetemcomitans* and other pathobionts such as *Porphyromonas gingivalis*, *Filifactor aclocis*, and commensals such as *Streptococcus gordonii*. In addition, while the association of *A. actinomycetemcomitans* in systemic diseases is limited at the present time, future studies into possible periodontal disease–systemic disease links may also find *A. actinomycetemcomitans* and its geographical interactions with other microbiome members to provide important clues as to implications of pathobiological communications.

Keywords: *Aggregatibacter actinomycetemcomitans*; aggressive periodontitis; *Porphyromonas gingivalis*; biogeography; biofilms; Localized Stage III Grade C periodontitis

Citation: Ryder, M.I.; Fine, D.H.; Barron, A.E. From Global to Nano: A Geographical Perspective of *Aggregatibacter actinomycetemcomitans*. *Pathogens* **2024**, *13*, 837. https://doi.org/10.3390/pathogens13100837

Academic Editor: Marat R. Sadykov

Received: 13 August 2024
Revised: 23 September 2024
Accepted: 24 September 2024
Published: 27 September 2024

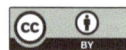

1. Introduction

The series of papers in this monograph present an extensive review of the range of pathological effects of *Aggregatibacter actinomycetemcomitans* (*A. actinomycetemcomitans*), a periodontal pathobiont, with the focus on Localized Stage III Grade C periodontitis (AKA Localized Molar–Incisor Grade III Stage C periodontitis, Localized Juvenile periodontitis, or Localized Aggressive periodontitis). The role of this pathobiont through its prevalence in dysbiotic microbial communities, suppression effects on the host response, toxicity to periodontal tissues, and stimulation of the destructive arms of the inflammatory response has been extensively investigated [1]. The arsenal of destructive weapons of *A. actinomycetemcomitans* include toxins within the fimbriae on the surface of the bacteria, secreted cytolethal distending toxins, and lipopolysaccharides [1]. These detrimental effects of *A. actinomycetemcomitans* can be modified in periodontal diseases on the smallest geographical scale by the spatial proximity to other periodontal pathobionts, as well as commensal bacteria [2]. In addition, when discussing the broader definition of geography for a pathobiont such as *A. actinomycetemcomitans*, one can expand the range of scales from the largest origins and transmission on a global scale to local geographical regions, to more locally exposed probands, and to within families. From a geographical perspective, we can then consider the oral cavity as a whole, the plaque biofilm structure, and finally, at the smallest scale of individual interactions between *A. actinomycetemcomitans* and adjacent or nearby commensal organisms and pathobionts at the sub-micron/nanoscale in supragingival, subgingival, and systemically affected environments.

In this geographical tour of *A. actinomycetemcomitans* and Localized Stage III Grade C periodontitis, we start at these largest global scales and work down to the smallest nanometer scales to address how this pathobiont may play a key role to this rapidly progressing form of periodontal disease, as well as in the exacerbation of systemic diseases. Studies of the geography of *A. actinomycetemcomitans* may help answer central questions regarding the ethnic, racial, and familial distributions of this rapidly progressing periodontal disease, as well as the specific intraoral geographical location of this disease to first molars and incisors. While some of these questions on the global to nanoscale remain unanswered, and theories arising from published observations are yet to be confirmed, a broad range of techniques used in these approaches described in this review may yield new insights into these global to nanoscale geographical questions.

2. Global Origins

In examining geography at the "widest field of vision", a variety of genetic tools have been used to trace the global migration of the potential geographic origins of this pathobiont, as well as the divergence of this pathobiont from the species level to serotypes and strains [3,4]. Initially, genetic signatures have been employed to determine both the common origin and routes of dissemination and divergence [5]. Aside from microbiology, there are interesting parallels of such approaches in fields of study such as epidemiology, anthropology, genetics, and even in disciplines as far afield as linguistics [6].

Geographical concepts can be addressed at the broad cultural level that can include language and anatomical appearances. The broader cultural and biological structures of language and gross anatomical appearance can then be assessed at a finer level of resolution using genomic data [7]. For example, in order to determine the geographic origin for the migration patterns of the Polynesian people, both linguists and human and animal anatomists and geneticists have used the "language tools" of their respective disciplines to propose that the origin of these migrations were from early civilizations from the southern tip of Taiwan [8,9]. Similarly, using the genetics of primate mitochondria, anthropologists working with geneticists have postulated a "Mitochondrial Eve" originating in defined areas of East Africa as the geographic origin of migrating *Homo sapiens* populations [10]. By analogy to this type of geographical genetic tracing, we can draw interesting parallels to the more rapid evolution, divergence, and migration patterns of SARS-CoV-2 strains [11]. In particular, the emergence of a particular SARS-CoV-2 strain variant and its initial predominance and probable origins from South Africa, then spreading to more northern locations in the African continent, has been demonstrated using these tools [12].

For the geographic origins of *A. actinomycetemcomitans*, similar back tracing approaches have determined in part why the spread of this pathobiont is more common in African American populations [13]. For example, studies restricted to limited regions such as Africa and Scandinavia and analysis of clones prevalent in these populations indicate that the origin of one or more of the more pathogenic strains of *A. actinomycetemcomitans* (the JP 2 clone) may have been in Mediterranean Africa [14] around present day Morocco; after which, it spread to Western Africa and then to the Americas, due in part to migration patterns of the slave trade [15] (Figure 1). In Scandinavia, the migration patterns may have resulted in the presence of the JP 2 clone in smaller, discrete geographical areas. For example, in two studies in Sweden, this pathogenic clone was detected in two studies [16,17], while, in Denmark, a study of younger subjects did not detect the prevalence of this clone [18].

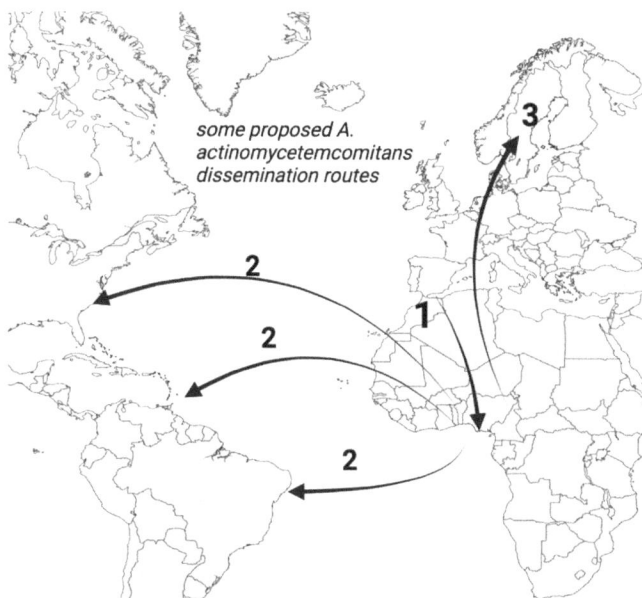

Figure 1. A proposed geographical origin and pathway of dissemination of *A. actinomycetemcomitans* in the African American population through genetic back tracing: 1. Origin from North Africa to West Central Africa and then to 2. North and South America through the slave trade [14–16]. 3. Regarding the spread to other parts of the world where *A. actinomycetemcomitans* may have disseminated and been detected, these geographical routes have yet to be determined but may include discrete geographic zones, such as regions of Sweden [16,17] (original image created by the author for this manuscript with Biorender.com).

3. Smaller Populations and the Individual

At a higher magnification of the geographical level, it is well established that cases of Localized Stage III Grade C periodontitis cluster within certain racial/ethnic groups and within families [13,19]. In addition to the local exposure from close geographical proximity, a genetic component may play an important role in this pattern [19]. From a microbiological perspective, the roles of both genetics and host response elements raise questions as to whether *A. actinomycetemcomitans* transmission occurs primarily within the smaller physical spaces of families or whether geographically adjacent probands may also play a role.

The use of various genetic fingerprinting techniques have demonstrated that there is strong evidence for the physical/geographical transmission of *A. actinomycetemcomitans* within the closer physical confines of families, even to members that do not show evidence of the disease [20]. While a developing fetus may not be expected to acquire *A. actinomycetemcomitans* in the womb, the initial passage of the child through the birth canal can potentially expose the child first to the mother's microbiome [21,22]. While prior studies have not demonstrated *A. actinomycetemcomitans* per se in the birth canal pathway, other periodontal pathobionts have been detected in these anatomical regions [23]. Nevertheless, acquisition of *A. actinomycetemcomitans* as a risk factor in the initiation of localized Stage III Grade C periodontitis [24–27] could occur from mother to child immediately postpartum with exposure to the close geographic environment [28]. Evidence for this earlier physical acquisition of *A. actinomycetemcomitans* before clinical signs of this rapid form of periodontitis is supported by studies that have shown similar patterns of rapid destruction in the primary teeth in the same geographical areas of the mouth as the future affected first molars [29]. Once established within a closely geographically associated proband such as family or community, there may be the retention of specific species and strains of pathogenic microbiota such as *A. actinomycetemcomitans* and *Porphyromonas gingivalis* (*P. gingivalis*) [20]. Evidence to support this persistence of specific microbial profiles of periodontal pathobionts in the form of dysbiotic communities has been confirmed from early studies that demonstrated the retention of the same species and strains of species of periodontal pathobionts [30], including *P. gingivalis*, as well as *A. actinomycetemcomitans*, even after attempts at debridement and maintenance [31,32], and since these pathobionts may reside in multiple inaccessible geographical areas in the mouth, their complete elimination from the oral cavity is not possible. Therefore, there is a risk of recolonization into their originally colonized intraoral geographical areas.

One of the most extensively studied areas in dental and medical research is the potential for periodontal pathobionts to translocate to other parts of the body and thereby induce both local inflammatory and destructive responses, as well as an elevated state of systemic inflammation. These pathways of microbial translocation include invasion of pathobionts into the bloodstream and lymphatic system through the breakdown of the epithelial barrier between the gingival tissue and sulcus microbiota spread along neural pathways, and direct invasion of pathobionts into tissue [33–35]. In addition, periodontal pathobionts can directly invade host cells such as epithelial cells and immune cells in the periodontal tissue and then be carried as "Trojan horses" to distal sites of the body [36]. This proposed translocation pathway mechanism has been extensively studied and observed for the periodontal pathobiont *P. gingivalis* [34,36]. For both *A. actinomycetemcomitans* and *P. gingivalis*, epithelial cell mechanisms for adhesion and rearranging the actin cytoskeleton of the host cell function have been shown to facilitate ingestion into the cell [37].

To date, there has been some published evidence that has focused on the clinical implications of the geographic translocation of *A. actinomycetemcomitans* to other parts of the body. Individual case reports or series of case reports have noted the presence of *A. actinomycetemcomitans* in various pulmonary infections [38], non-oral abscesses [39], and general septicemia. For *A. actinomycetemcomitans*, the most studied of these non-oral infections to distal sites in the body is for cardiovascular disease—in particular, endocarditis [40–42] and atherosclerosis [43]. The detection rates of this pathobiont in endocarditis have been reported to range from 0.6% for *A. actinomycetemcomitans* per se to 3% for pathobionts in a related group of eight species found in periodontal disease plaques (HACEK group) [5] that may include *A. actinomycetemcomitans*. These apparently low rates for *A. actinomycetemcomitans* detection from these earlier studies may actually be higher when using newer big data and high-throughput approaches with more detailed and sensitive 16S ribotyping techniques [44–46]. This is particularly relevant because *A. actinomycetemcomitans* is not as elevated in subgingival plaque and, in general, is more prevalent in specific segments of the population [47,48]. In addition, since the new World Workshop Classification meeting in 2017, there has been a highly significant decrease in the ratio of publications that feature *A. actinomycetemcomitans* as compared to *P. gingivalis*. Importantly, an extensive series of case reports provided evidence that *A. actinomycetemcomitans* can translocate to a variety of organs [39]. More specifically, an extensive review of 26 studies related to the recovery of oral pathobionts from atherosclerotic cardiovascular samples has shown 8 out of 26 where *P. gingivalis* recovery was the most prevalent, whereas 7 studies showed *A. actinomycetemcomitans* to be the most prevalent [43]. None of the other six reputed pathobionts reached a higher level than *A. actinomycetemcomitans* or *P. gingivalis* in any samples taken [43]. Furthermore, in addition to the potential translocation of whole *A. actinomycetemcomitans*, mouse models have shown that *A. actinomycetemcomitans*, like the more extensively studied *P. gingivalis* [49], can secrete outer membrane vesicles (OMV's) that can potentially cross the blood–brain barrier and induce neuroinflammation [36,50,51]. Whether this phenomenon of OMV's from *A. actinomycetemcomitans* also exists in humans has yet to be investigated. As demonstrated in previous studies with OMVs from *P. gingivalis* [34,52], if such a translocation for *A. actinomycetemcomitans* does occur, it may have broad implications for the initiation and progression of Alzheimer's disease and other forms of dementia. It should, however, be noted that, unlike the increased levels of the detection of *P. gingivalis* in the periodontal disease microbiome in older adults, it appears that levels of *A. actinomycetemcomitans* may decrease in the periodontal disease microbiome in older adults [53]. Nevertheless, it is possible that any translocation of a periodontal pathobiont at an earlier age may contribute to the upstream chain of events that may become clinically detectable diseases and conditions later in life.

4. The Oral Cavity

These aforementioned examples provide evidence for the geographic origins, transmission, and strain diversity of *A. actinomycetemcomitans* on the global, familial, and whole individual scales. When we refocus at the smaller geographical scale on the central role of *A. actinomycetemcomitans* in Localized Stage III grade C periodontitis, a central question arises as follows: Since this condition is initially localized to the region of the first molars and incisor teeth in the permanent dentition and corresponding areas of the primary dentition, can the local microbial geography and ecology of the mouth explain, in part, the initial localization and rapid bone loss in the first molar and incisor regions in both the primary and permanent dentition? These local geographic factors within the mouth can interact with the larger scale systemic variations and risk factors such as variations in the systemic host response to *A. actinomycetemcomitans*. These overarching factors are presented in other papers of this monograph.

Over the past several decades, there have been investigations into the influence of regional variations of the conditions in the mouth that may affect regional differences in the microbiome, which have been taken into consideration: (1) the location of the microbiome by tooth type and position in the mouth [54,55]; (2) temperature gradients within the oral cavity [56]; (3) soft tissue type and surface; (4) location of the salivary glands and overall levels of salivary flow, which may have both diurnal variation and variation before, during, and after mastication and in hyposalivation conditions such as Sjogren's syndrome [57]; (5) differences in the levels of salivary flow from the front and back of the mouth and around salivary duct openings [58]; (6) physical effects of mastication, including forces of the musculature of the cheek and tongue on the teeth during periods of mastication and periods where the mastication of food is not occurring; (7) differences in the plaque mass per se around teeth in different regions of the mouth [59]; and (8) the chemical nature and physical consistency of their diet [44,57,60–62] (Figure 2).

In a review by Proctor et al. [60], the principles that may govern the regional distribution and profile of the periodontopathic microflora within a small geographic niche were more extensively reviewed using the principles of selection, physical dispersal, and genetic drift within an individual species and increased or decreased species diversity [60]. There have been several studies that demonstrated a preferential colonization and high recovery rate of *A. actinomycetemcomitans* in the first molar regions both with and without rapid periodontal breakdown at the time of sample collection [63–65]. One early study by Mombelli et al. demonstrated a high predictive rate of the presence of *A. actinomycetemcomitans* on a first mandibular molar on one side of the mouth and the presence of *A. actinomycetemcomitans* on the contralateral first mandibular molar, thereby supporting the concept of bilateral symmetry of microbial profiles in periodontal disease [66]. Furthermore, Haffajee et al. demonstrated that, when compared to the broader distribution of *P. gingivalis* in a wider area of the dentition of periodontal diseases, *A. actinomycetemcomitans* was detected in more limited locations, such as the first molar region [67]. These detection rates for *A. actinomycetemcomitans* are seen in more discrete areas as constituents of complex supragingival and subgingival biofilms in contrast to other surfaces of the oral cavity, which may be explained in part by a relatively smaller proportion of *A. actinomycetemcomitans* in these complex biofilms. These findings could be due to older, less sensitive culturing techniques or DNA checkboard techniques [68].

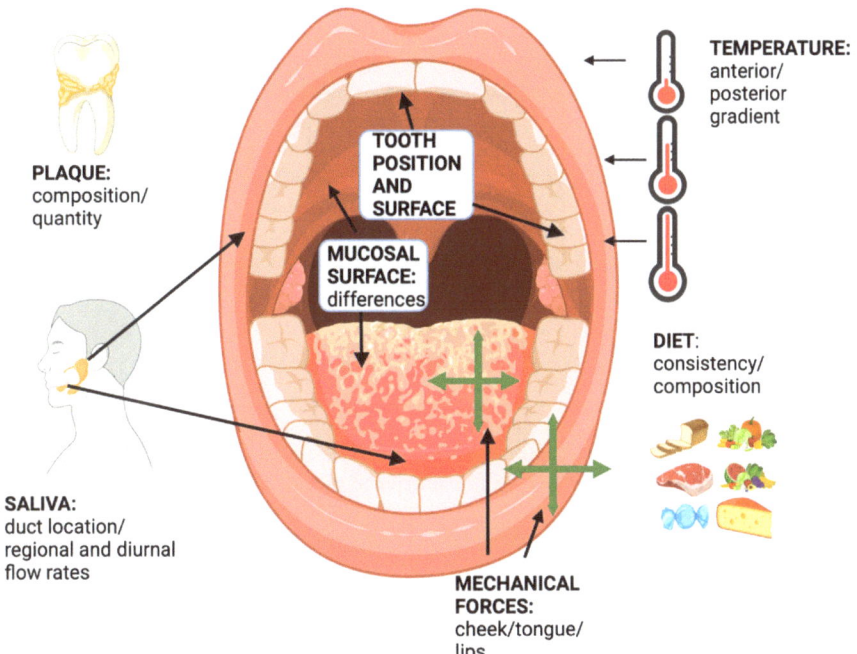

Figure 2. Differences in physical geography of the oral cavity that may affect regional variations of the location and distribution of *A. actinomycetemcomitans* may include tooth location, tooth type, and tooth surface; temperature gradients from the anterior to posterior oral cavity; attachment to different mucosal surfaces; location of the salivary ducts, salivary composition, and differences in salivary flow; effects of the cheek, tongue, and masticatory musculature; regional variations in the quantity of plaque accumulation; and chemical and physical characteristics of the diet (original image created by the author for this manuscript with Biorender.com).

However, using new bioinformatics and big data approaches, future studies that characterize the microbiome on a tooth-by-tooth and site-by-site basis for both supra and subgingival biofilms in deciduous, mixed, and permanent dentitions, which show the clinical hallmarks of Localized Stage III grade C patients, may shed light on the influence of the eight factors listed above on the geographic variations in the total microbial environment. In addition, eruption patterns of the permanent teeth could be another factor for *A. actinomycetemcomitans* localization [69]. The new technologies could lead to an increased understanding of the presence and/or pathogenic potential of *A. actinomycetemcomitans* to these molar/incisor sites. Furthermore, comparing these distributions with the tooth-by-tooth microbial profiles of periodontally healthy subjects and with subjects with less severe periodontitis in Stage I or II/Grade A or B classes may further our understanding of the unique localized periodontal breakdown patterns in subjects with Localized Stage III Grade C periodontitis.

The promise of these approaches that focus on the site-by-site location of bacterial species and distribution patterns for the entire mouth is supported by recent work [57,60,61] designed to examine the effects of hyposalivation on gradients in the patterns, diversity, and spatial connections of the microbiome. These approaches have included the collection of supragingival samples from each buccal and lingual tooth surface, selected subgingival samples, and intraoral soft tissue surface sites including exfoliated epithelial cells (which may serve as an early reservoir for *A. actinomycetemcomitans* [70]). These investigations have shown different gradients in phyla distribution with different corresponding levels of salivary flow and strong similarities in phyla distribution based on closer geographical distancing as opposed to inter-arch or bilateral geographical distances. From these observations on phyla and diversity distributions based on salivary flow, such distribution mapping may aid researchers and clinicians in identifying patients at risk for caries and periodontal diseases. By using these tools at finer resolution to the genus, species, and strain levels, investigators may also gain new insights into the next higher geographical magnification of different tooth environments that can identify interactions of *A. actinomycetemcomitans* with the total local microflora in individual sulcus sites. These tools could be used to study the biofilm adherent to the tooth surface, the overlying planktonic suspension of bacteria in the gingival sulcus, local invasion of bacteria into the periodontal tissues and within tissue, and host response cells within the tissue. The promise of studying such interactions using the approaches described in this section can examine this microbial geography at the highest resolution.

5. Microbial Communities and Biofilms

There is compelling evidence that the survival and pathogenic potential of *A. actino-mycetemcomitans* is dependent on the local interactions of this pathobiont with the complex communities of both the supra gingival and sub gingival biofilms. These interactions occur geographically on the micro and nanoscales and include interactions with microbial extracellular matrices, quorum sensing, exchange of genetic material, exchange of nutrients, and neutralization of host defense molecules [71–73]. While extensive studies have been published on such interactions to the whole biofilm for individual pathobiont species such as *P. gingivalis*, *T. denticola*, and *Fusobacterium nucleatum* (*F. nucleatum*), there is a dearth of studies that focused on *A. actinomycetemcomitans* from this high magnification geographical viewpoint. Such studies are important, as sampling studies from sites with Localized Stage III Grade C periodontitis have shown recovery rates of *A. actinomycetemcomitans* with other periodontal pathobionts such as *Filofactor alocis* (*F. alocis*) and *P. gingivalis* [74]. Two newer approaches that take into account the geographical proximity of *A. actinomycetemcomitans* to these other pathobionts have the potential to yield new insights into the pathogenic role of this species in these Localized Stage III grade C lesions [75,76].

The first of these approaches stem from the elegant studies employing novel immunofluorescent techniques to identify multiple pathobionts in the biofilm using a combination of two florescent probes out of a library of individual colors of a defined spectrum [75,76]. These imaging approaches have enabled investigators to develop multicolored maps of the development of bacterial communities in the biofilm [75,77,78] and the phylum to the species level. Of particular interest for the spatial organization of *A. actinomycetem-comitans* at the phylum level is the demonstration of complexes of *A. actinomycetemcomitans* in a defined area consisting of a "hedgehog-shaped" core of corynebacteria connected by *F. nucleatum* [76] (Figure 3). These hedgehogs are studded at the surface by commensals such as streptococcus species and pathobionts such as *P. gingivalis* in a corncob appearance and then surrounded by pathobionts of the same phyla as *A. actinomycetemcomitans*, which may be attached to these corncobs [76,78] (Figure 3).

In this complex structure, the role of *F. nucleatum* is of particular interest, as it appears to serve as a geographical "isthmus" between bacterial species at the core and surface through several types of adhesins [79]. In addition, other images of different sectional views using this staining technique demonstrated the presence of the pathobionts in discrete patches [76]. Since the specifics of *A. actinomycetemcomitans* binding to *F. nucleatum* have not been studied at this molecular level, further studies are required. It is difficult to study *A. actinomycetemcomitans* and its ability to become an early colonizer of teeth in humans [70]. One such study tested for the presence of *A. actinomycetemcomitans* on buccal epithelial cells in volunteers prior to entering them into a longitudinal in vivo study [70]. Six sterile hydroxyapatite squares were placed into an acrylic stent, and one square was removed at intervals ranging from 5 min to 7 h after placement, sonicated, and screened for early colonizing bacteria. *A. actinomycetemcomitans* was found in volunteers 4, 6, and 7 h after placement and only in volunteers with *A. actinomycetemcomitans* prior to square placement. Streptococci and Actinomyces were found at all time points and in both *A. actinomycetemcomitans*-positive and *A. actinomycetemcomitans*-negative volunteers. Fusobacteria were also found at later time points.

Turning to *P. gingivalis* and its effects on the biogeography of *A. actinomycetemcomitans* within the biofilm, a major pathogenic product of *P. gingivalis* is the family of gingipains, which are required for the breakdown of healthy surrounding tissue for essential nutrients [80]. The geographic proximity of *A. actinomycetemcomitans* and *P. gingivalis* as described in the immunofluorescent approaches described above [76] raises interesting questions as to the negative effects of these gingipains on the colonization of *A. actinomycetemcomitans* within the plaque biofilm (Figure 3). While recent studies have shown that these gingipains also have adhesin binding sites to various hard and soft tissue surfaces in the oral cavity [81], in vitro studies have demonstrated that these gingipains can promote the detachment of *A. actinomycetemcomitans* from hard tissue surfaces and an inhibition of the aggregation of *A. actinomycetemcomitans* [82,83]. However, it is important to point out that *P. gingivalis* is a more fastidious anaerobe and occurs at later stages of plaque development [48].

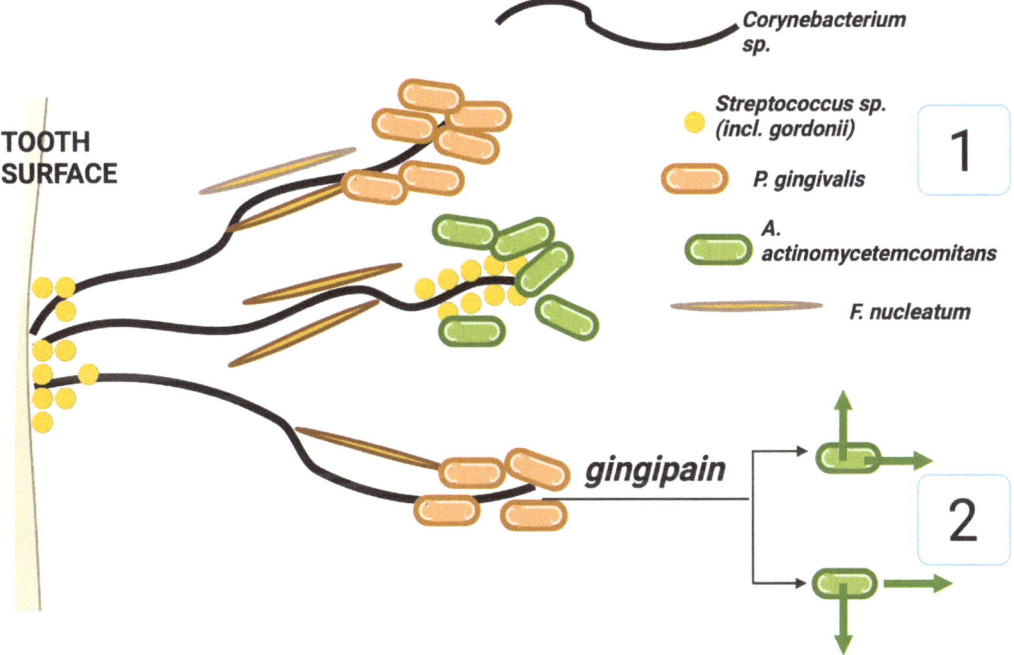

Figure 3. A proposed geographical model distribution of *A. actinomycetemcomitans* in the plaque biofilm based on diverse prior imaging studies and in vitro studies [76,81–83]. (**1**) *A. actinomycetemcomitans* may cluster around streptococcus "corncob" formations at the end of the filamentous corynebacterium species and may also form clusters near other pathobionts such as *P. gingivalis*. (**2**) However, gingipain enzymes from *P. gingivalis* may also exclude *A. actinomycetemcomitans* from areas of the plaque biofilm and prevent aggregation within the biofilm (original image created by the author for this manuscript with Biorender.com).

A second interesting geographical interaction at the micro/nanoscale between two species within biofilms is between *A. actinomycetemcomitans* and *Streptococcus gordonii* (*S. gordonii*) in what has been described as a "fight or flight interaction" (Figure 4). *S. gordonii* can also play a role in the chain of formation of biofilms in the adhesion and colonization of *P. gingivalis* within the biofilm of some periodontal lesions [5,84]. In addition, as noted above, in the absence of gingipains from *P. gingivalis* or other factors, *A. actinomycetemcomitans* may form strong adhesions to saliva-treated surfaces [1] and promote a local pathogenic colony formation of pathobionts within the biofilm [85]. For *A. actinomycetemcomitans*, per se, the close geographical proximity to *S. gordonii* benefits its growth due to the production of lactate by *S. gordonii*, which contributes to the survival and pathogenicity of *A. actinomycetemcomitans* [86–88]. However, since *S. gordonii* also produces hydrogen peroxide (H_2O_2), which is toxic to *A. actinomycetemcomitans* at higher concentrations, a direct adherence would be potentially toxic to *A. actinomycetemcomitans*. To ensure a safe working distance between these two species, *A. actinomycetemcomitans* produces an enzyme, dispersin B, that promotes movement of this bacteria a short distance away from a higher concentration of this H_2O_2 in a "flight" response. *A. actinomycetemcomitans* also produces catalase to neutralize the lower concentrations of H_2O_2 at this safer distance [87]. At the same time, during this process, the exposure of *A. actinomycetemcomitans* to H_2O_2 produced in part by *S. gordonii* may aid in the formation of surface membrane receptors on *A. actinomycetemcomitans* that increase the resistance to complement-mediated destruction in yet another "fight" response. One additional geographical interaction that is less understood is that of *A. actinomycetemcomitans* and *F. alocis* [74,89,90]. While supported by both in vivo and in vitro studies, these interactions appear to be strain-dependent, and most evidence suggests that *F. alocis*, another leukotoxin producer, appears to occur after *A. actinomycetemcomitans* is present in deep subgingival pockets [91].

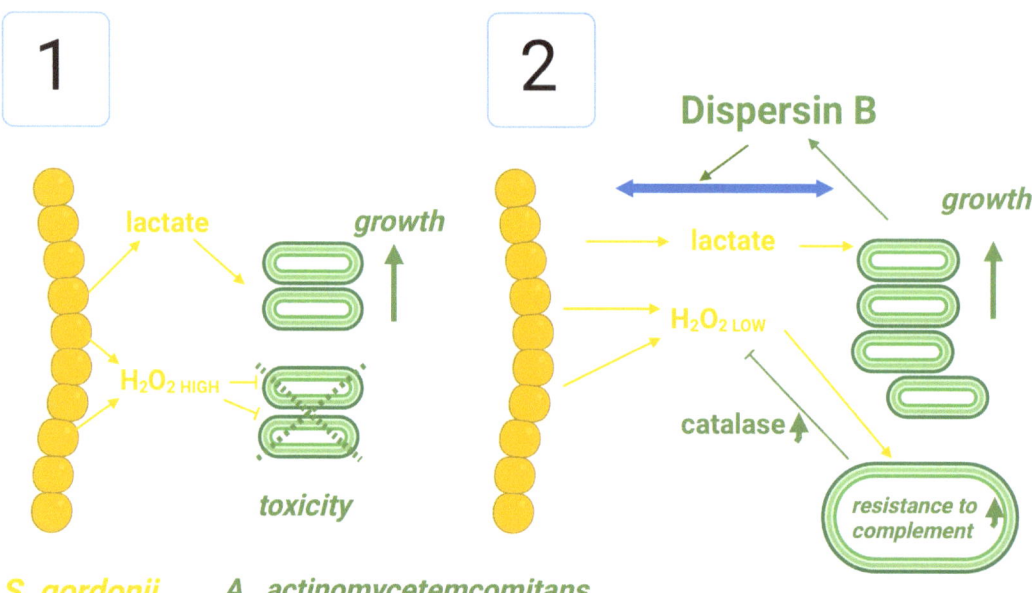

Figure 4. "Fight/Flight interactions between *A. actinomycetemcomitans* and *S. gordonii*. (**1**) At the closest geographical distances between these two microbial species, the beneficial effects of lactate production from *S. gordonii* on the growth of *A actinomycetemcomitans* are offset by the higher toxic concentrations of H_2O_2. (**2**) However, the production of dipersin B by *A. actinomycetemcomitans* facilitates a separation from *S. gordonii* and an exposure to a lower and less toxic concentration of H_2O_2, which can be neutralized by catalases from *A. actinomycetemcomitans*, stimulate resistance to complement from the host response, and maintain some of the nutritional benefits of *S. gordonii* produced lactate (original image created by the author for this manuscript with Biorender.com).

6. Conclusions

On this tour of microbial geography of *A. actinomycetemcomitans* from the global to nanoscale, we have presented the range of tools used to answer questions regarding (1) the origins and spread of this pathobiont; (2) the establishment, survival, and pathogenicity of this pathobiont; and (3) the complexity of biofilms and other oral microbial communities. Each of these tools can be considered a form of communication, with some common and unique features of grammar, syntax, and vocabulary down to the morphemes and phonemes in the genetic, environmental, and biochemical realm. Questions of the historical origin of *A. actinomycetemcomitans* and its spread to communities around the world and to families and close geographic probands have been answered in part by these approaches. Nevertheless, several central questions remain at a higher magnification level. These include the higher detection rates of *A. actinomycetemcomitans* within those localized areas of first molars and incisors typical of patients with the now defined Localized Stage III Grade C periodontitis and features of the microbiome as a whole in these areas of localized destruction of the periodontal support that can be explained by the variations in the geographical environment within the entire mouth and within the individual microbiomes and biofilms around tooth types and locations. The broad range of newer techniques described in this paper may provide novel hypotheses and answers to these questions. On the whole-mouth scale, a study of the variations in the "climate and ecology" of different geographical environments may provide some answers. In addition, studies that focus on the geographical proximity of *A. actinomycetemcomitans* to other biofilm species, including other pathobionts and commensals, followed by investigations of potential beneficial and biochemical reactions may yield new insights into the role of geography in the role of *A. actinomycetemcomitans* in this unique periodontal disease pattern. While the association of *A. actinomycetemcomitans* in systemic diseases is limited at the present time when compared to the more extensive work with other periodontal pathobionts such as *P. gingivalis*, future studies looking at other possible periodontal disease–systemic links may find that *A. actinomycetemcomitans* possesses important properties that permit translocation and exacerbate systemic diseases, particularly coronary heart diseases.

Author Contributions: Conceptualization—M.I.R., D.H.F. and A.E.B.; Methodology—M.I.R.; Writing—Original Draft Preparation—M.I.R.; Writing—Review and Editing—M.I.R., D.H.F. and A.E.B.; Funding Acquisition—A.E.B. All authors have read and agreed to the published version of the manuscript.

Funding: 1 DP1 AG072438, the Stanford's Discovery Innovation Fund, the Cisco University Research Program Fund, the Silicon Valley Community Foundation, and James J. Truchard & the Truchard Foundation.

Institutional Review Board Statement: Not applicable.

Informed Consent Statement: Not applicable.

Data Availability Statement: Not applicable.

Acknowledgments: Stephen Dominy for review and suggestions for this manuscript.

Conflicts of Interest: The authors declare no conflicts of interest.

References

1. Fine, D.H.; Schreiner, H.; Velusamy, S.K. Aggregatibacter, A Low Abundance Pathobiont That Influences Biogeography, Microbial Dysbiosis, and Host Defense Capabilities in Periodontitis: The History of A Bug, And Localization of Disease. *Pathogens* **2020**, *9*, 179. [CrossRef] [PubMed]
2. Murray, J.L.; Connell, J.L.; Stacy, A.; Turner, K.H.; Whiteley, M. Mechanisms of synergy in polymicrobial infections. *J. Microbiol.* **2014**, *52*, 188–199. [CrossRef] [PubMed]
3. Kittichotirat, W.; Bumgarner, R.E.; Chen, C. Evolutionary Divergence of *Aggregatibacter actinomycetemcomitans*. *J. Dent. Res.* **2016**, *95*, 94–101. [CrossRef] [PubMed]
4. Kittichotirat, W.; Bumgarner, R.E.; Chen, C. Genomic Islands Shape the Genetic Background of Both JP2 and Non-JP2 *Aggregatibacter actinomycetemcomitans*. *Pathogens* **2022**, *11*, 1037. [CrossRef] [PubMed]

5. Asikainen, S.; Chen, C.; Saarela, M.; Saxen, L.; Slots, J. Clonal specificity of *Actinobacillus actinomycetemcomitans* in destructive periodontal disease. *Clin. Infect. Dis.* **1997**, *25* (Suppl. S2), S227–S229. [CrossRef]
6. Adsera, A.; Pytlikova, M. The role of language in shaping international migration. *Econ. J.* **2015**, *125*, F49–F81. [CrossRef]
7. Nielsen, R.; Akey, J.M.; Jakobsson, M.; Pritchard, J.K.; Tishkoff, S.; Willerslev, E. Tracing the peopling of the world through genomics. *Nature* **2017**, *541*, 302–310. [CrossRef]
8. Diamond, J.M. Taiwan's gift to the world. *Nature* **2000**, *403*, 709–710. [CrossRef]
9. Larson, G.; Cucchi, T.; Fujita, M.; Matisoo-Smith, E.; Robins, J.; Anderson, A.; Rolett, B.; Spriggs, M.; Dolman, G.; Kim, T.H.; et al. Phylogeny and ancient DNA of Sus provides insights into neolithic expansion in Island Southeast Asia and Oceania. *Proc. Natl. Acad. Sci. USA* **2007**, *104*, 4834–4839. [CrossRef]
10. Maier, P.A.; Runfeldt, G.; Estes, R.J.; Vilar, M.G. African mitochondrial haplogroup L7: A 100,000-year-old maternal human lineage discovered through reassessment and new sequencing. *Sci. Rep.* **2022**, *12*, 10747. [CrossRef]
11. Markov, P.V.; Ghafari, M.; Beer, M.; Lythgoe, K.; Simmonds, P.; Stilianakis, N.I.; Katzourakis, A. The evolution of SARS-CoV-2. *Nat. Rev. Microbiol.* **2023**, *21*, 361–379. [CrossRef] [PubMed]
12. Tegally, H.; San, J.E.; Cotten, M.; Moir, M.; Tegomoh, B.; Mboowa, G.; Martin, D.P.; Baxter, C.; Lambisia, A.W.; Diallo, A.; et al. The evolving SARS-CoV-2 epidemic in Africa: Insights from rapidly expanding genomic surveillance. *Science* **2022**, *378*, eabq5358. [CrossRef] [PubMed]
13. Fine, D.H.; Markowitz, K.; Furgang, D.; Fairlie, K.; Ferrandiz, J.; Nasri, C.; McKiernan, M.; Gunsolley, J. *Aggregatibacter actinomycetemcomitans* and its relationship to initiation of localized aggressive periodontitis: Longitudinal cohort study of initially healthy adolescents. *J. Clin. Microbiol.* **2007**, *45*, 3859–3869. [CrossRef] [PubMed]
14. Haubek, D.; Ennibi, O.K.; Poulsen, K.; Poulsen, S.; Benzarti, N.; Kilian, M. Early-onset periodontitis in Morocco is associated with the highly leukotoxic clone of *Actinobacillus actinomycetemcomitans*. *J. Dent. Res.* **2001**, *80*, 1580–1583. [CrossRef] [PubMed]
15. Haubek, D.; Poulsen, K.; Kilian, M. Microevolution and patterns of dissemination of the JP2 clone of *Aggregatibacter (Actinobacillus) actinomycetemcomitans*. *Infect. Immun.* **2007**, *75*, 3080–3088. [CrossRef]
16. Johansson, A.; Claesson, R.; Hoglund Aberg, C.; Haubek, D.; Lindholm, M.; Jasim, S.; Oscarsson, J. Genetic Profiling of *Aggregatibacter actinomycetemcomitans* Serotype B Isolated from Periodontitis Patients Living in Sweden. *Pathogens* **2019**, *8*, 153. [CrossRef]
17. Claesson, R.; Oscarsson, J.; Johansson, A. Carriage of the JP2 Genotype of *Aggregatibacter actinomycetemcomitans* by Periodontitis Patients of Various Geographic Origin, Living in Sweden. *Pathogens* **2022**, *11*, 1233. [CrossRef]
18. Jensen, A.B.; Isidor, F.; Lund, M.; Vaeth, M.; Johansson, A.; Lauritsen, N.N.; Haubek, D. Prevalence of *Aggregatibacter actinomycetemcomitans* and Periodontal Findings among 14 to 15-Year Old Danish Adolescents: A Descriptive Cross-Sectional Study. *Pathogens* **2020**, *9*, 1054. [CrossRef]
19. Meng, H.; Ren, X.; Tian, Y.; Feng, X.; Xu, L.; Zhang, L.; Lu, R.; Shi, D.; Chen, Z. Genetic study of families affected with aggressive periodontitis. *Periodontol. 2000* **2011**, *56*, 87–101. [CrossRef]
20. DiRienzo, J.M.; Slots, J.; Sixou, M.; Sol, M.A.; Harmon, R.; McKay, T.L. Specific genetic variants of *Actinobacillus actinomycetemcomitans* correlate with disease and health in a regional population of families with localized juvenile periodontitis. *Infect. Immun.* **1994**, *62*, 3058–3065. [CrossRef]
21. Kononen, E. Development of oral bacterial flora in young children. *Ann. Med.* **2000**, *32*, 107–112. [CrossRef]
22. Jensen, A.B.; Ennibi, O.K.; Ismaili, Z.; Poulsen, K.; Haubek, D. The JP2 genotype of *Aggregatibacter actinomycetemcomitans* and marginal periodontitis in the mixed dentition. *J. Clin. Periodontol.* **2016**, *43*, 19–25. [CrossRef] [PubMed]
23. Cassini, M.A.; Pilloni, A.; Condo, S.G.; Vitali, L.A.; Pasquantonio, G.; Cerroni, L. Periodontal bacteria in the genital tract: Are they related to adverse pregnancy outcome? *Int. J. Immunopathol. Pharmacol.* **2013**, *26*, 931–939. [CrossRef] [PubMed]
24. Dogan, B.; Kipalev, A.S.; Okte, E.; Sultan, N.; Asikainen, S.E. Consistent intrafamilial transmission of *Actinobacillus actinomycetemcomitans* despite clonal diversity. *J. Periodontol.* **2008**, *79*, 307–315. [CrossRef] [PubMed]
25. Tuite-McDonnell, M.; Griffen, A.L.; Moeschberger, M.L.; Dalton, R.E.; Fuerst, P.A.; Leys, E.J. Concordance of *Porphyromonas gingivalis* colonization in families. *J. Clin. Microbiol.* **1997**, *35*, 455–461. [CrossRef]
26. Lamell, C.W.; Griffen, A.L.; McClellan, D.L.; Leys, E.J. Acquisition and colonization stability of *Actinobacillus actinomycetemcomitans* and *Porphyromonas gingivalis* in children. *J. Clin. Microbiol.* **2000**, *38*, 1196–1199. [CrossRef]
27. Petit, M.D.; van Steenbergen, T.J.; Scholte, L.M.; van der Velden, U.; de Graaff, J. Epidemiology and transmission of *Porphyromonas gingivalis* and *Actinobacillus actinomycetemcomitans* among children and their family members. A report of 4 surveys. *J. Clin. Periodontol.* **1993**, *20*, 641–650. [CrossRef]
28. Monteiro, M.F.; Altabtbaei, K.; Kumar, P.S.; Casati, M.Z.; Ruiz, K.G.S.; Sallum, E.A.; Nociti-Junior, F.H.; Casarin, R.C.V. Parents with periodontitis impact the subgingival colonization of their offspring. *Sci. Rep.* **2021**, *11*, 1357. [CrossRef]
29. Koo, S.S.; Fernandes, J.G.; Li, L.; Huang, H.; Aukhil, I.; Harrison, P.; Diaz, P.I.; Shaddox, L.M. Evaluation of microbiome in primary and permanent dentition in grade C periodontitis in young individuals. *J. Periodontol.* **2024**, *95*, 650–661. [CrossRef]
30. Haffajee, A.D.; Patel, M.; Socransky, S.S. Microbiological changes associated with four different periodontal therapies for the treatment of chronic periodontitis. *Oral Microbiol. Immunol.* **2008**, *23*, 148–157. [CrossRef]
31. Shiloah, J.; Patters, M.R. Repopulation of periodontal pockets by microbial pathogens in the absence of supportive therapy. *J. Periodontol.* **1996**, *67*, 130–139. [CrossRef] [PubMed]

32. Gunsolley, J.C.; Zambon, J.J.; Mellott, C.A.; Brooks, C.N.; Kaugars, C.C. Maintenance therapy in young adults with severe generalized periodontitis. *J. Periodontol.* **1994**, *65*, 274–279. [CrossRef] [PubMed]

33. Kuraji, R.; Sekino, S.; Kapila, Y.; Numabe, Y. Periodontal disease-related nonalcoholic fatty liver disease and nonalcoholic steatohepatitis: An emerging concept of oral-liver axis. *Periodontol. 2000* **2021**, *87*, 204–240. [CrossRef]

34. Ryder, M.I.; Xenoudi, P. Alzheimer disease and the periodontal patient: New insights, connections, and therapies. *Periodontol. 2000* **2021**, *87*, 32–42. [CrossRef] [PubMed]

35. Gualtero, D.F.; Lafaurie, G.I.; Buitrago, D.M.; Castillo, Y.; Vargas-Sanchez, P.K.; Castillo, D.M. Oral microbiome mediated inflammation, a potential inductor of vascular diseases: A comprehensive review. *Front. Cardiovasc. Med.* **2023**, *10*, 1250263. [CrossRef]

36. de Jongh, C.A.; de Vries, T.J.; Bikker, F.J.; Gibbs, S.; Krom, B.P. Mechanisms of *Porphyromonas gingivalis* to translocate over the oral mucosa and other tissue barriers. *J. Oral Microbiol.* **2023**, *15*, 2205291. [CrossRef]

37. Kajiya, M.; Komatsuzawa, H.; Papantonakis, A.; Seki, M.; Makihira, S.; Ouhara, K.; Kusumoto, Y.; Murakami, S.; Taubman, M.A.; Kawai, T. *Aggregatibacter actinomycetemcomitans* Omp29 is associated with bacterial entry to gingival epithelial cells by F-actin rearrangement. *PLoS ONE* **2011**, *6*, e18287. [CrossRef]

38. Yuan, A.; Yang, P.C.; Lee, L.N.; Chang, D.B.; Kuo, S.H.; Luh, K.T. *Actinobacillus actinomycetemcomitans* pneumonia with chest wall involvement and rib destruction. *Chest* **1992**, *101*, 1450–1452. [CrossRef] [PubMed]

39. Kaplan, A.H.; Weber, D.J.; Oddone, E.Z.; Perfect, J.R. Infection due to *Actinobacillus actinomycetemcomitans*: 15 cases and review. *Rev. Infect. Dis.* **1989**, *11*, 46–63. [CrossRef]

40. Paju, S.; Carlson, P.; Jousimies-Somer, H.; Asikainen, S. Heterogeneity of *Actinobacillus actinomycetemcomitans* strains in various human infections and relationships between serotype, genotype, and antimicrobial susceptibility. *J. Clin. Microbiol.* **2000**, *38*, 79–84. [CrossRef]

41. Paturel, L.; Casalta, J.P.; Habib, G.; Nezri, M.; Raoult, D. *Actinobacillus actinomycetemcomitans* endocarditis. *Clin. Microbiol. Infect.* **2004**, *10*, 98–118. [CrossRef] [PubMed]

42. Tang, G.; Kitten, T.; Munro, C.L.; Wellman, G.C.; Mintz, K.P. EmaA, a potential virulence determinant of *Aggregatibacter actinomycetemcomitans* in infective endocarditis. *Infect. Immun.* **2008**, *76*, 2316–2324. [CrossRef] [PubMed]

43. Reyes, L.; Herrera, D.; Kozarov, E.; Rolda, S.; Progulske-Fox, A. Periodontal bacterial invasion and infection: Contribution to atherosclerotic pathology. *J. Periodontol.* **2013**, *84*, S30–S50. [CrossRef]

44. Mark Welch, J.L.; Dewhirst, F.E.; Borisy, G.G. Biogeography of the Oral Microbiome: The Site-Specialist Hypothesis. *Annu. Rev. Microbiol.* **2019**, *73*, 335–358. [CrossRef]

45. Bik, E.M.; Long, C.D.; Armitage, G.C.; Loomer, P.; Emerson, J.; Mongodin, E.F.; Nelson, K.E.; Gill, S.R.; Fraser-Liggett, C.M.; Relman, D.A. Bacterial diversity in the oral cavity of 10 healthy individuals. *ISME J.* **2010**, *4*, 962–974. [CrossRef]

46. Segata, N.; Haake, S.K.; Mannon, P.; Lemon, K.P.; Waldron, L.; Gevers, D.; Huttenhower, C.; Izard, J. Composition of the adult digestive tract bacterial microbiome based on seven mouth surfaces, tonsils, throat and stool samples. *Genome Biol.* **2012**, *13*, R42. [CrossRef]

47. Claesson, R.; Johansson, A.; Belibasakis, G.N. Age-Related Subgingival Colonization of *Aggregatibacter actinomycetemcomitans*, *Porphyromonas gingivalis* and *Parvimonas micra*—A Pragmatic Microbiological Retrospective Report. *Microorganisms* **2023**, *11*, 1434. [CrossRef] [PubMed]

48. Socransky, S.S.; Haffajee, A.D.; Ximenez-Fyvie, L.A.; Feres, M.; Mager, D. Ecological considerations in the treatment of *Actinobacillus actinomycetemcomitans* and *Porphyromonas gingivalis* periodontal infections. *Periodontol. 2000* **1999**, *20*, 341–362. [CrossRef] [PubMed]

49. Zhang, Z.; Liu, D.; Liu, S.; Zhang, S.; Pan, Y. The Role of *Porphyromonas gingivalis* Outer Membrane Vesicles in Periodontal Disease and Related Systemic Diseases. *Front. Cell. Infect. Microbiol.* **2020**, *10*, 585917. [CrossRef]

50. Ha, J.Y.; Seok, J.; Kim, S.J.; Jung, H.J.; Ryu, K.Y.; Nakamura, M.; Jang, I.S.; Hong, S.H.; Lee, Y.; Lee, H.J. Periodontitis promotes bacterial extracellular vesicle-induced neuroinflammation in the brain and trigeminal ganglion. *PLoS Pathog.* **2023**, *19*, e1011743. [CrossRef]

51. Pritchard, A.B.; Fabian, Z.; Lawrence, C.L.; Morton, G.; Crean, S.; Alder, J.E. An Investigation into the Effects of Outer Membrane Vesicles and Lipopolysaccharide of *Porphyromonas gingivalis* on Blood-Brain Barrier Integrity, Permeability, and Disruption of Scaffolding Proteins in a Human in vitro Model. *J. Alzheimer's Dis.* **2022**, *86*, 343–364. [CrossRef] [PubMed]

52. Dominy, S.S.; Lynch, C.; Ermini, F.; Benedyk, M.; Marczyk, A.; Konradi, A.; Nguyen, M.; Haditsch, U.; Raha, D.; Griffin, C.; et al. *Porphyromonas gingivalis* in Alzheimer's disease brains: Evidence for disease causation and treatment with small-molecule inhibitors. *Sci. Adv.* **2019**, *5*, eaau3333. [CrossRef] [PubMed]

53. Slots, J.; Feik, D.; Rams, T.E. *Actinobacillus actinomycetemcomitans* and *Bacteroides intermedius* in human periodontitis: Age relationship and mutual association. *J. Clin. Periodontol.* **1990**, *17*, 659–662. [CrossRef]

54. Haffajee, A.D.; Teles, R.P.; Patel, M.R.; Song, X.; Yaskell, T.; Socransky, S.S. Factors affecting human supragingival biofilm composition. II. Tooth position. *J. Periodontal Res.* **2009**, *44*, 520–528. [CrossRef] [PubMed]

55. Simon-Soro, A.; Tomas, I.; Cabrera-Rubio, R.; Catalan, M.D.; Nyvad, B.; Mira, A. Microbial geography of the oral cavity. *J. Dent. Res.* **2013**, *92*, 616–621. [CrossRef]

56. Haffajee, A.D.; Socransky, S.S.; Smith, C.; Dibart, S.; Goodson, J.M. Subgingival temperature (III). Relation to microbial counts. *J. Clin. Periodontol.* **1992**, *19*, 417–422. [CrossRef]

57. Proctor, D.M.; Fukuyama, J.A.; Loomer, P.M.; Armitage, G.C.; Lee, S.A.; Davis, N.M.; Ryder, M.I.; Holmes, S.P.; Relman, D.A. A spatial gradient of bacterial diversity in the human oral cavity shaped by salivary flow. *Nat. Commun.* **2018**, *9*, 681. [CrossRef]

58. Dawes, C.; Watanabe, S.; Biglow-Lecomte, P.; Dibdin, G.H. Estimation of the velocity of the salivary film at some different locations in the mouth. *J. Dent. Res.* **1989**, *68*, 1479–1482. [CrossRef] [PubMed]

59. Haffajee, A.D.; Teles, R.P.; Patel, M.R.; Song, X.; Veiga, N.; Socransky, S.S. Factors affecting human supragingival biofilm composition. I. Plaque mass. *J. Periodontal Res.* **2009**, *44*, 511–519. [CrossRef]

60. Proctor, D.M.; Shelef, K.M.; Gonzalez, A.; Davis, C.L.; Dethlefsen, L.; Burns, A.R.; Loomer, P.M.; Armitage, G.C.; Ryder, M.I.; Millman, M.E.; et al. Microbial biogeography and ecology of the mouth and implications for periodontal diseases. *Periodontol. 2000* **2020**, *82*, 26–41. [CrossRef]

61. Proctor, D.M.; Relman, D.A. The Landscape Ecology and Microbiota of the Human Nose, Mouth, and Throat. *Cell Host Microbe* **2017**, *21*, 421–432. [CrossRef] [PubMed]

62. Sedghi, L.; DiMassa, V.; Harrington, A.; Lynch, S.V.; Kapila, Y.L. The oral microbiome: Role of key organisms and complex networks in oral health and disease. *Periodontol. 2000* **2021**, *87*, 107–131. [CrossRef] [PubMed]

63. Shaddox, L.M.; Huang, H.; Lin, T.; Hou, W.; Harrison, P.L.; Aukhil, I.; Walker, C.B.; Klepac-Ceraj, V.; Paster, B.J. Microbiological characterization in children with aggressive periodontitis. *J. Dent. Res.* **2012**, *91*, 927–933. [CrossRef]

64. Velsko, I.M.; Harrison, P.; Chalmers, N.; Barb, J.; Huang, H.; Aukhil, I.; Shaddox, L. Grade C molar-incisor pattern periodontitis subgingival microbial profile before and after treatment. *J. Oral Microbiol.* **2020**, *12*, 1814674. [CrossRef] [PubMed]

65. Amado, P.P.P.; Kawamoto, D.; Albuquerque-Souza, E.; Franco, D.C.; Saraiva, L.; Casarin, R.C.V.; Horliana, A.; Mayer, M.P.A. Oral and Fecal Microbiome in Molar-Incisor Pattern Periodontitis. *Front. Cell. Infect. Microbiol.* **2020**, *10*, 583761. [CrossRef]

66. Mombelli, A.; Meier, C. On the symmetry of periodontal disease. *J. Clin. Periodontol.* **2001**, *28*, 741–745. [CrossRef]

67. Haffajee, A.D.; Socransky, S.S.; Smith, C.; Dibart, S. The use of DNA probes to examine the distribution of subgingival species in subjects with different levels of periodontal destruction. *J. Clin. Periodontol.* **1992**, *19*, 84–91. [CrossRef]

68. Clarridge, J.E., 3rd. Impact of 16S rRNA gene sequence analysis for identification of bacteria on clinical microbiology and infectious diseases. *Clin. Microbiol. Rev.* **2004**, *17*, 840–862, table of contents. [CrossRef]

69. Baer, P.N. The case for periodontosis as a clinical entity. *J. Periodontol.* **1971**, *42*, 516–520. [CrossRef]

70. Fine, D.H.; Markowitz, K.; Furgang, D.; Velliyagounder, K. *Aggregatibacter actinomycetemcomitans* as an early colonizer of oral tissues: Epithelium as a reservoir? *J. Clin. Microbiol.* **2010**, *48*, 4464–4473. [CrossRef]

71. Hajishengallis, G.; Lamont, R.J. Dancing with the Stars: How Choreographed Bacterial Interactions Dictate Nososymbiocity and Give Rise to Keystone Pathogens, Accessory Pathogens, and Pathobionts. *Trends Microbiol.* **2016**, *24*, 477–489. [CrossRef] [PubMed]

72. Kolenbrander, P.E.; Palmer, R.J., Jr.; Rickard, A.H.; Jakubovics, N.S.; Chalmers, N.I.; Diaz, P.I. Bacterial interactions and successions during plaque development. *Periodontol. 2000* **2006**, *42*, 47–79. [CrossRef]

73. Moustafa, A.M.; Velusamy, S.K.; Denu, L.; Narechania, A.; Fine, D.H.; Planet, P.J. Adaptation by Ancient Horizontal Acquisition of Butyrate Metabolism Genes in *Aggregatibacter actinomycetemcomitans*. *mBio* **2021**, *12*, 10–1128. [CrossRef] [PubMed]

74. Fine, D.H.; Markowitz, K.; Fairlie, K.; Tischio-Bereski, D.; Ferrendiz, J.; Furgang, D.; Paster, B.J.; Dewhirst, F.E. A consortium of *Aggregatibacter actinomycetemcomitans*, *Streptococcus parasanguinis*, and *Filifactor alocis* is present in sites prior to bone loss in a longitudinal study of localized aggressive periodontitis. *J. Clin. Microbiol.* **2013**, *51*, 2850–2861. [CrossRef]

75. Valm, A.M.; Mark Welch, J.L.; Rieken, C.W.; Hasegawa, Y.; Sogin, M.L.; Oldenbourg, R.; Dewhirst, F.E.; Borisy, G.G. Systems-level analysis of microbial community organization through combinatorial labeling and spectral imaging. *Proc. Natl. Acad. Sci. USA* **2011**, *108*, 4152–4157. [CrossRef]

76. Mark Welch, J.L.; Rossetti, B.J.; Rieken, C.W.; Dewhirst, F.E.; Borisy, G.G. Biogeography of a human oral microbiome at the micron scale. *Proc. Natl. Acad. Sci. USA* **2016**, *113*, E791–E800. [CrossRef] [PubMed]

77. Ramirez-Puebla, S.T.; Mark Welch, J.L.; Borisy, G.G. Improved Visualization of Oral Microbial Consortia. *J. Dent. Res.* **2024**, 220345241251784. [CrossRef] [PubMed]

78. Morillo-Lopez, V.; Sjaarda, A.; Islam, I.; Borisy, G.G.; Mark Welch, J.L. Corncob structures in dental plaque reveal microhabitat taxon specificity. *Microbiome* **2022**, *10*, 145. [CrossRef]

79. Groeger, S.; Zhou, Y.; Ruf, S.; Meyle, J. Pathogenic Mechanisms of *Fusobacterium nucleatum* on Oral Epithelial Cells. *Front. Oral Health* **2022**, *3*, 831607. [CrossRef]

80. Potempa, J.; Banbula, A.; Travis, J. Role of bacterial proteinases in matrix destruction and modulation of host responses. *Periodontol. 2000* **2000**, *24*, 153–192. [CrossRef]

81. Chen, T.; Nakayama, K.; Belliveau, L.; Duncan, M.J. *Porphyromonas gingivalis* gingipains and adhesion to epithelial cells. *Infect. Immun.* **2001**, *69*, 3048–3056. [CrossRef] [PubMed]

82. Haraguchi, A.; Miura, M.; Fujise, O.; Hamachi, T.; Nishimura, F. *Porphyromonas gingivalis* gingipain is involved in the detachment and aggregation of *Aggregatibacter actinomycetemcomitans* biofilm. *Mol. Oral Microbiol.* **2014**, *29*, 131–143. [CrossRef] [PubMed]

83. Takasaki, K.; Fujise, O.; Miura, M.; Hamachi, T.; Maeda, K. *Porphyromonas gingivalis* displays a competitive advantage over *Aggregatibacter actinomycetemcomitans* in co-cultured biofilm. *J. Periodontal Res.* **2013**, *48*, 286–292. [CrossRef]

84. Wright, C.J.; Burns, L.H.; Jack, A.A.; Back, C.R.; Dutton, L.C.; Nobbs, A.H.; Lamont, R.J.; Jenkinson, H.F. Microbial interactions in building of communities. *Mol. Oral Microbiol.* **2013**, *28*, 83–101. [CrossRef] [PubMed]

85. Planet, P.J.; Kachlany, S.C.; Fine, D.H.; DeSalle, R.; Figurski, D.H. The Widespread Colonization Island of *Actinobacillus actinomycetemcomitans*. *Nat. Genet.* **2003**, *34*, 193–198. [CrossRef]
86. Brown, S.A.; Whiteley, M. A novel exclusion mechanism for carbon resource partitioning in *Aggregatibacter actinomycetemcomitans*. *J. Bacteriol.* **2007**, *189*, 6407–6414. [CrossRef]
87. Stacy, A.; Everett, J.; Jorth, P.; Trivedi, U.; Rumbaugh, K.P.; Whiteley, M. Bacterial fight-and-flight responses enhance virulence in a polymicrobial infection. *Proc. Natl. Acad. Sci. USA* **2014**, *111*, 7819–7824. [CrossRef] [PubMed]
88. Ramsey, M.M.; Rumbaugh, K.P.; Whiteley, M. Metabolite cross-feeding enhances virulence in a model polymicrobial infection. *PLoS Pathog.* **2011**, *7*, e1002012. [CrossRef]
89. Razooqi, Z.; Tjellstrom, I.; Hoglund Aberg, C.; Kwamin, F.; Claesson, R.; Haubek, D.; Johansson, A.; Oscarsson, J. Association of *Filifactor alocis* and its RTX toxin gene ftxA with periodontal attachment loss, and in synergy with *Aggregatibacter actinomycetemcomitans*. *Front. Cell. Infect. Microbiol.* **2024**, *14*, 1376358. [CrossRef]
90. Wang, Q.; Wright, C.J.; Dingming, H.; Uriarte, S.M.; Lamont, R.J. Oral community interactions of *Filifactor alocis* in vitro. *PLoS ONE* **2013**, *8*, e76271. [CrossRef]
91. Oscarsson, J.; Claesson, R.; Bao, K.; Brundin, M.; Belibasakis, G.N. Phylogenetic Analysis of *Filifactor alocis* Strains Isolated from Several Oral Infections Identified a Novel RTX Toxin, FtxA. *Toxins* **2020**, *12*, 687. [CrossRef] [PubMed]

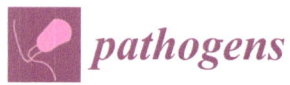

pathogens

MDPI

Article

Dormancy-like Phenotype of *Aggregatibacter actinomycetemcomitans*: Survival during Famine

Natalia O. Tjokro [1], Carolyn B. Marks [2], Ashley Wu [1] and Casey Chen [1,*]

[1] Department of Endodontics and Periodontics, Herman Ostrow School of Dentistry, University of Southern California, 925 W. 34th Street, Los Angeles, CA 90089, USA; ntjokro@ostrow.usc.edu (N.O.T.); ashley99wu@gmail.com (A.W.)

[2] Core Center of Excellence in Nano Imaging, University of Southern California, 1002 Childs Way, Los Angeles, CA 90089, USA; markscar@usc.edu

* Correspondence: cchen@ostrow.usc.edu; Tel.: +1-213-740-7407

Abstract: Microbes frequently experience nutrient deprivations in the natural environment and may enter dormancy. *Aggregatibacter actinomycetemcomitans* is known to establish long-term infections in humans. This study examined the dormancy-like phenotype of an *A. actinomycetemcomitans* strain D7S-1 and its isogenic smooth-colony mutant D7SS. A tissue culture medium RPMI-1640 was nutrient-deficient (ND) and unable to support *A. actinomycetemcomitans* growth. RPMI-1640 amended with bases was nutrient-limited (NL) and supported limited growth of *A. actinomycetemcomitans* less than the nutrient-enriched (NE) laboratory medium did. Strain D7S-1, after an initial 2-log reduction in viability, maintained viability from day 4 to day 15 in the NL medium. Strain D7SS, after 1-log reduction in viability, maintained viability from day 3 to day 5. In contrast, bacteria in the NE medium were either non-recoverable (D7S-1; >6-log reduction) or continued to lose viability (D7SS; 3-log reduction) on day 5 and beyond. Scanning and transmission electron microscopy showed that *A. actinomycetemcomitans* in the NL medium formed robust biofilms similar to those in the NE medium but with evidence of stress. *A. actinomycetemcomitans* in the ND medium revealed scant biofilms and extensive cellular damage. We concluded that *A. actinomycetemcomitans* grown in the NL medium exhibited a dormancy-like phenotype characterized by minimum growth, prolonged viability, and distinct cellular morphology.

Keywords: *Aggregatibacter actinomycetemcomitans*; dormancy; stress response; bacterial physiology

Citation: Tjokro, N.O.; Marks, C.B.; Wu, A.; Chen, C. Dormancy-like Phenotype of *Aggregatibacter actinomycetemcomitans*: Survival during Famine. *Pathogens* **2024**, *13*, 418. https://doi.org/10.3390/pathogens13050418

Academic Editors: Daniel H. Fine and Marat R. Sadykov

Received: 3 March 2024
Revised: 6 May 2024
Accepted: 9 May 2024
Published: 16 May 2024

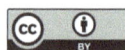
1. Introduction

Most studies on microbial physiology and metabolism have been performed under conditions of nutrient excess. However, microbes are frequently starved for critical growth nutrients in most natural environments [1]. Bacteria may enter a dormancy state in unfavorable environments to ensure long-term survival. Dormancy is a reversible phase in which bacteria are viable but non-replicating and exhibit low levels of metabolic activity with distinct gene expression profiles [1].

Aggregatibacter actinomycetemcomitans is among the best-studied periodontal pathogens. The organism is noted for its association with periodontitis in young individuals and adults with severe periodontitis [2,3]. *A. actinomycetemcomitans* can establish long-term periodontal infections due to persistent subgingival colonization of identical *A. actinomycetemcomitans* clones [4,5]. The mechanism that underpins the organism's persistent colonization remains to be elucidated. Presumably, *A. actinomycetemcomitans* may enter a dormancy phase in vivo when it encounters unfavorable conditions.

We hypothesize that *A. actinomycetemcomitans* may enter dormancy in the in vivo nutrient-limited environment. The in vivo milieu of *A. actinomycetemcomitans* is complex. It involves bacteria- and host-derived factors such as the polymicrobial community and its metabolites, gingival crevicular fluid, various immune cells, cytokines, and chemokines [6–9]. Developing an in vitro model that mimics the in vivo environment is challenging and nearly impossible. Instead, this study examined the potential dormancy phenotype of *A. actinomycetemcomitans* in a relatively simple model by growing bacteria in chemically defined media (CDMs) and characterizing its phenotype. *A. actinomycetemcomitans* in dormancy, in comparison to *A. actinomycetemcomitans* grown in the conventional nutrient-enriched medium, is expected to (i) display no or minimum growth, (ii) remain viable over an extended time, and (iii) demonstrate a distinct cellular morphology. The phenotypes and the mechanism of dormancy will be further tested in animal models in future investigations.

2. Materials and Methods

2.1. Bacterial Strains and Growth Conditions

Bacteria were routinely incubated in an atmosphere supplemented with 5% CO_2 at 37 °C in a humidified incubator. The wildtype rough-colony *A. actinomycetemcomitans* strain D7S-1 and its isogenic smooth-colony mutant D7SS were routinely grown in a modified trypticase soy broth (mTSB) containing 3% trypticase soy broth and 0.6% yeast extract or on mTSB agar (mTSB with 1.5% agar (Becton Dickinson and Company, Franklin Lakes, NJ, USA)).

Three CDMs were tested in the study. A common tissue culture medium, RPMI-1640 (Sigma, St. Louis, MO, USA, Catalog #: R0883), designated as RPMI-1, was used as a CDM base. RPMI-2 was RPMI-1 amended with 10 mg/L uracil and 10 mg/L hypoxanthine. RPMI-3 was RPMI-2 amended with 0.03 mM each of cytidine, guanosine, uridine, adenosine, and thymidine (Sigma, ES-008-D), 10 mM fructose, 2 g/L inosine, 2 mg/L spermidine, 2 mg/L putrescine, 430 mg/L $MgCl_2$, and 2.2 mg/L $CaCl_2$.

Three different protocols were used to prepare *A. actinomycetemcomitans* for electron microscopy: (i) biofilms grown on glass coverslips for SEM, (ii) a bacterial suspension from liquid cultures for SEM, and (iii) bacteria pelleted from liquid cultures for TEM. Briefly, colonies of *A. actinomycetemcomitans* on agar were inoculated into mTSB broth and incubated overnight. Cells were washed with sterile PBS buffer and adjusted to OD_{600} of 0.15 in three test media (i.e., mTSB control, RPMI-1, and RPMI-2). Sterile coverslips were then added to the cultures to support biofilm formation. Cells were collected and prepared for SEM or TEM at designated times.

2.2. Electron Microscopy

Biofilms on coverslips for SEM and the pelleted cells for TEM were fixed by replacing the media with a solution containing 2.5% glutaraldehyde, 2% paraformaldehyde, and 2% sucrose (w/v) in 0.1 M HEPES. The bacterial suspension from cultures was fixed for SEM by adding 100 μL of 25% glutaraldehyde directly to 900 μL of the culture for a final concentration of 2.5% glutaraldehyde. All samples were processed in a Pelco BioWave microwave processor (Ted Pella, Reading, CA, USA) to increase the penetration of samples and decrease processing time, using a Cool Spot to control temperature and reduce standing energy waves. All samples were microwaved for two cycles of 1 min on, 1 min off, and 1 min on at 150 watts, and then this sequence was repeated at 250 w. The samples were stored at 4 °C.

2.3. TEM

Pellets were microwaved with wash buffer (0.1 M HEPES containing 2% sucrose) for 1 min at 250 w. This was repeated three times before quenching with fresh 50 mM ammonium chloride in wash buffer for two cycles of 1 min on, 1 min off, and 1 min at 150 w under vacuum. This was followed by two wash rinses for one minute each at 250 w, then two 18 mΩ water rinses for one minute each at 250 w. Pellets were stained with 1% uranyl acetate in water under vacuum (2 min on, 2 min off, and 2 min on; two cycles at 100 w), followed by two 18 mΩ water rinses before a graded alcohol dehydration series (50%, 70%, 95%, 100%, 100%, and 100%) at 250 w for 1 min at each step.

Before infiltrating the samples with Embed 812 (EMS) epoxy resin, samples were rinsed twice with propylene oxide. BioWave was used for the first two resin dilutions (1:1 and 1:3 of propylene oxide to Embed 812) for 4 min at 250 w. Three pure resin changes followed this before placing the samples into flat molds with paper labels. Blocks were polymerized at 60 °C. Eighty-nanometer sections were cut using a Leica UC6 ultramicrotome (Leica, Wetzlar, Germany) and a Diatome diamond knife. Sections were picked up on 200-mesh thin bar Gilder grids (EMS).

All TEM images were taken using a ThermoFisher (Waltham, MA, USA) Talos FEG TEM at 80 KeV and recorded on a ThermoFisher Ceta16 CMOS camera.

2.4. SEM

Biofilms grown on coverslips were processed the same way as the TEM pellets up to the final dehydration step. After dehydration, the cells adherent to the cover glasses were dried by replacing the 100% ethanol with 100% hexamethyldisilazane (HMDS) three times. With each HMDS change, the samples were microwaved for 45 s at 150 w. Excess HMDS was removed, and samples were dried completely at 37 °C.

The cells in suspension were plated onto poly-l-lysine-coated 12 mm round cover glasses. After a 20-min incubation, samples were processed in terms of the cells grown on cover glass, with the following changes: no Quench step, no UA staining, and Critical Point Dried (Auto-Samdri, Tousimis, Rockland, MD, USA). All SEM samples were mounted to stubs using double-sided carbon sticky tabs and then sputter-coated for 40 s with an 80/20 platinum/palladium target (Cressington 108C Sputter coater, Ted Pella, Reading, CA, USA).

All SEM images were taken on an FEI Nova Nano 50 SEM (Hillsboro, OR, USA) using an Everhart–Thornley detector or a through-the-lens secondary electron detector in immersion mode.

3. Results

3.1. Development of Culture Media That Induce A. actinomycetemcomitans Dormancy-like Phenotype

We hypothesized that specific media may induce an *A. actinomycetemcomitans* dormancy-like phenotype characterized by minimal replication and sustained viability. A common tissue culture medium RPMI-1640, henceforth RPMI-1, was selected as the base of CDMs and further amended to derive RPMI-2 and RPMI-3. We first tested whether the CDMs were nutrient-limited (NL) or nutrient-deficient (ND) for *A. actinomycetemcomitans*. The NL media should possess all essential factors and can sustain the growth of bacteria indefinitely if fresh media are added periodically. In contrast, the ND media lack crucial elements and will not support the growth of bacteria with or without replenishment with fresh media. A modified trypticase soy broth with yeast extract medium (mTSB) was used as the control nutrient-enriched (NE) medium. Both *A. actinomycetemcomitans* D7S-1 and D7SS strains were used in our study to examine their phenotypic differences in different culture media. The comparison between the wildtype biofilm-forming bacteria and the smooth-colony mutant of planktonic bacteria is not the focus of this study.

Figure 1 shows the results of the experiments for strain D7S-1 (A) and D7SS (B) in mTSB, RPMI-1, and RPMI-2. The cultures were diluted 1:1 daily with fresh media for seven days. The dashed reference line represents the CFU/mL if the cultures did not grow or lose viability. Because of the daily dilution of the cultures with fresh media, the CFU of *A. actinomycetemcomitans* is expected to be reduced by 50% every day without gains or losses of cultivable bacteria. Three patterns of growth were observed. As expected, *A. actinomycetemcomitans* grew best in mTSB and was the lowest in RPMI-1. *A. actinomycetemcomitans* in RPMI-2 exhibited less growth than in mTSB. In particular, D7SS in RPMI-2 grew closer to the reference line of no gains and losses. The results suggest that RPMI-1 is an ND medium, and RPMI-2 is an NL medium. The growth of *A. actinomycetemcomitans* in RPMI-3 (RPMI-2 amended with dNTPs) was better than in RPMI-2 but worse than in mTSB (data not shown) and was not further tested.

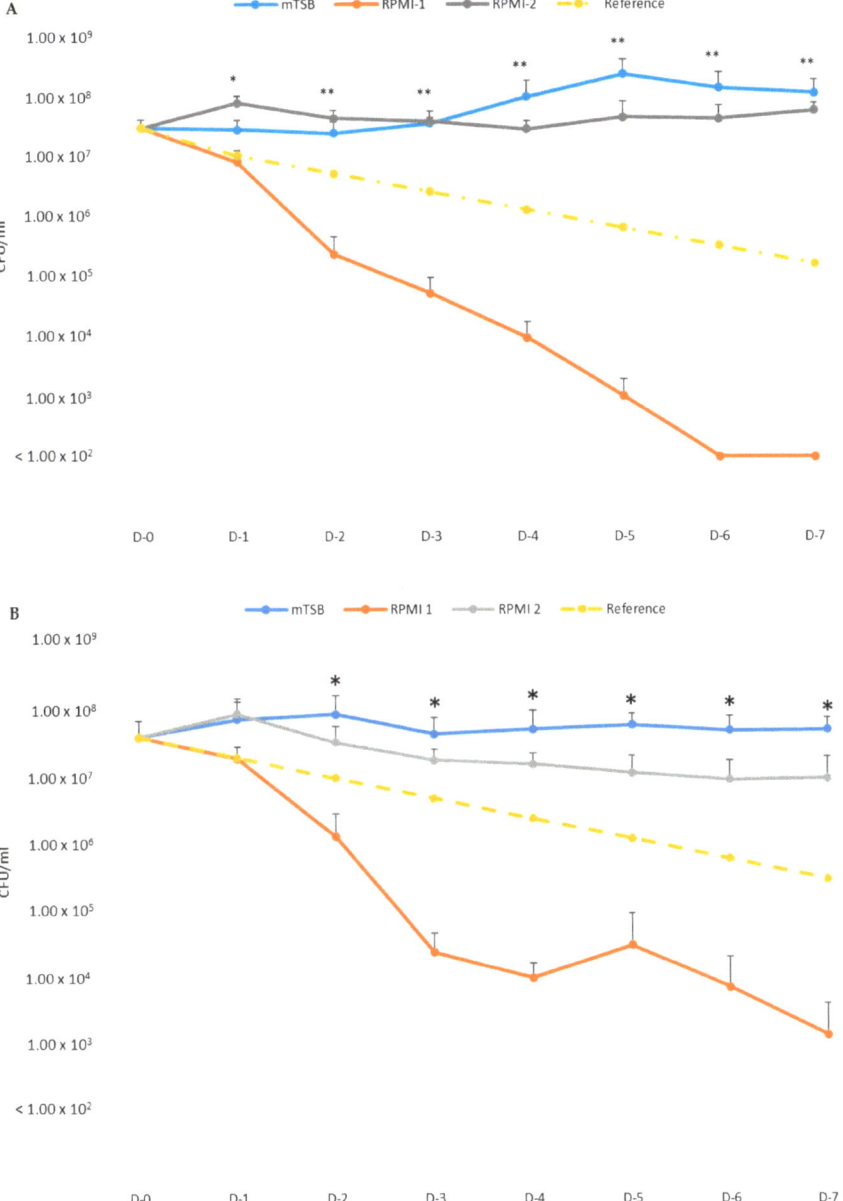

Figure 1. Distinguishing nutrient-deficient and nutrient-limited properties of CDMs. The CFU/mL was determined for *A. actinomycetemcomitans* D7S-1 (**A**) and *A. actinomycetemcomitans* D7SS (**B**) in mTSB, RPMI-1, and RPMI-2, with daily 1:1 dilution with appropriate fresh media. For *A. actinomycetemcomitans* D7S-1: * D-1: ANOVA 0.005419; Tukey HSD Test: RPMI-1 vs. RPMI-2, $p < 0.01$. ** D-2, D-3, D-4, D-5, D-6, and D-7: ANOVA < 0.005; Tukey HSD Test: mTSB vs. RPMI-1, $p < 0.01$; RPMI-1 vs. RPMI-2, $p < 0.01$. For *A. actinomycetemcomitans* D7SS: * D-2, D-3, D-4, D-5, D-6, and D-7: ANOVA < 0.002; Tukey HSD Test: mTSB vs. RPMI-1, $p < 0.01$: RPMI-1 vs. RPMI-2 $p < 0.01$.

We next tested if *A. actinomycetemcomitans* may reflect a dormancy-like phenotype in mTSB, RPMI-1, and RPMI-2 without adding fresh media. Three patterns of growth were also observed (Figure 2). *A. actinomycetemcomitans* D7S-1 cultured in mTSB, following an initial growth, was reduced by more than 2 logs on day 3 and was not cultivable (<100 CFU/mL; >6 logs of reduction) from day 5 to day 15. *A. actinomycetemcomitans* in RPMI-1 showed a continuing decline in viability from day 0 to day 15, when it exhibited about an 800-fold reduction in CFU/mL. Interestingly, *A. actinomycetemcomitans* in RPMI-2, following an initial growth on day 1, showed a decline in viability from day 1 to day 4 (less pronounced than in mTSB) and a period of stable viability from day 5 to day 15 that resembled dormancy. Moreover, the viability of *A. actinomycetemcomitans* in RPMI-2 exceeded 6000-fold greater than in mTSB on day 15. *A. actinomycetemcomitans* D7SS was tested in the three media for five days and showed similar growth trends to those observed for D7S-1. The bacteria exhibited initial growth on day 1 and a rapid decline in viability from day 2 to day 5 in mTSB, and a slower but continuing decrease in viability in RPMI-1 from day 0 to day 5. In contrast, bacteria in RPMI-2 showed initial growth, followed by a slow decline in viability from day 1 to day 3, when it reached a stable period of viability from day 3 to day 5, resembling dormancy. The viability of D7SS in RPMI-2 was 100-fold higher than in mTSB on day 5. The results suggested that *A. actinomycetemcomitans* entered a dormancy-like phase 3 to 4 days after culturing in RPMI-2 and demonstrated sustained viability for up to 15 days.

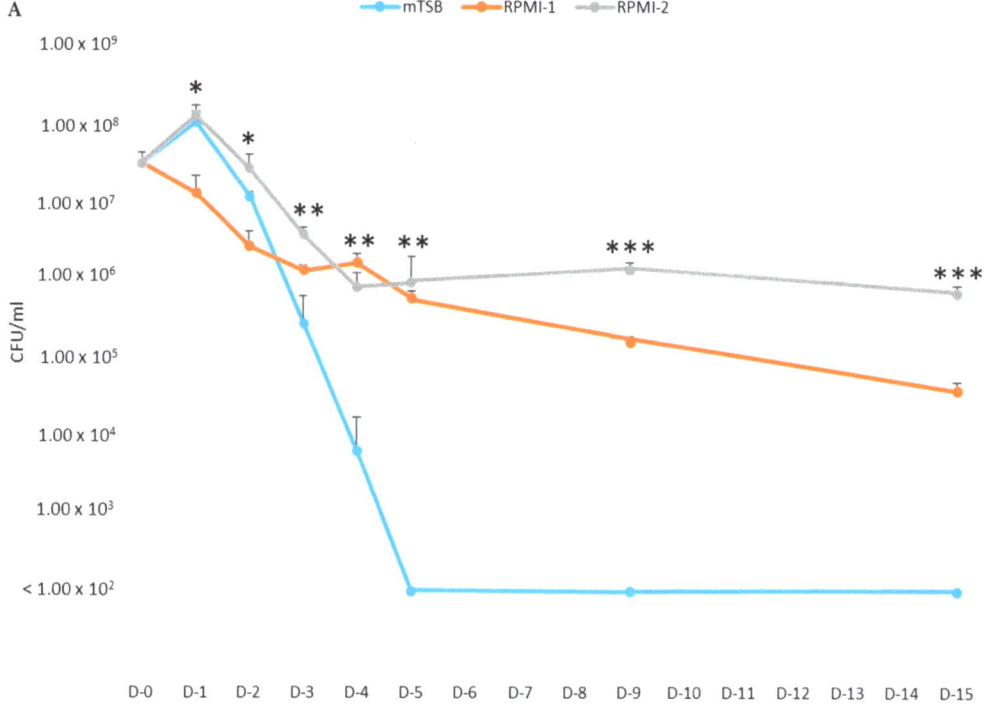

Figure 2. *Cont.*

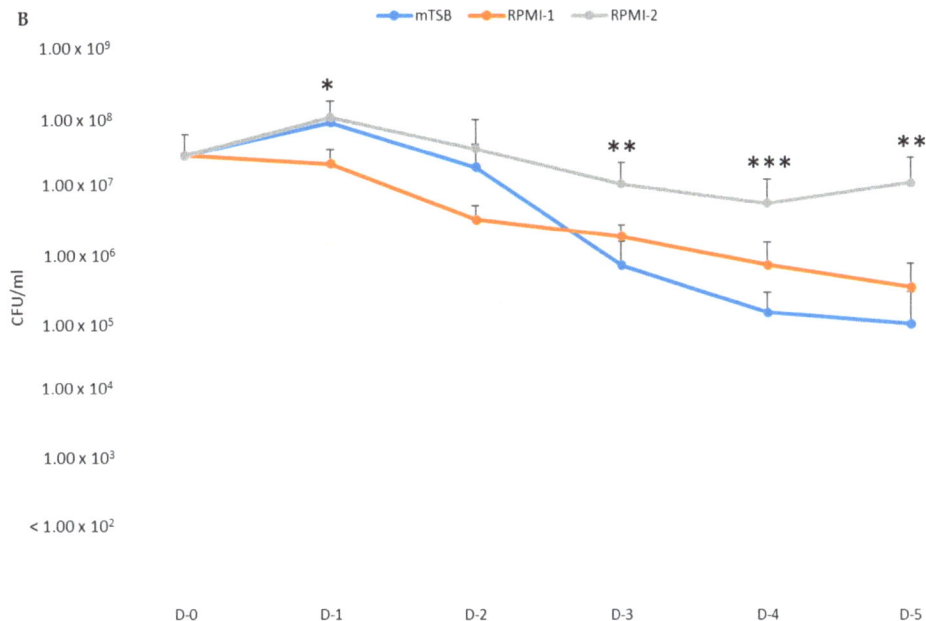

Figure 2. Dormancy-like phenotype of *A. actinomycetemcomitans* in nutrient-limited media. The viability of *A. actinomycetemcomitans* D7S-1 (**A**) and *A. actinomycetemcomitans* D7SS (**B**) in mTSB, RPMI-1, and RPMI-2 without daily addition of fresh media was determined by culturing. For *A. actinomycetemcomitans* D7S-1: * D-1 and D-2: ANOVA < 0.005; Tukey HSD Test: mTSB vs. RPMI-1, $p < 0.01$; RPMI-1 vs. RPMI-2, $p < 0.01$. ** D-3, D-4, and D-5: ANOVA < 0.02; Tukey HSD Test: mTSB vs. RPMI-1, $p < 0.05$; mTSB vs. RPMI-2, $p < 0.01$. *** D-9 and D-15: ANOVA < 0.0001; Tukey HSD Test: mTSB vs. RPMI-1, $p < 0.01$; mTSB vs. RPMI-2, $p < 0.01$; RPMI-1 vs. RPMI-2, $p < 0.01$. For *A. actinomycetemcomitans* D7SS: * D-1: ANOVA $p = 0.034030$; Tukey HSD Test: RPMI-1 vs. RPMI-2, $p < 0.05$. ** D-3 and D-5: ANOVA $p < 0.002$; Tukey HSD Test: mTSB vs. RPMI-2, $p < 0.01$. *** D-4: ANOVA $p = 0.000772$; Tukey HSD Test: mTSB vs. RPMI-2, $p < 0.01$; RPMI-1 vs. RPMI-2, $p < 0.05$.

3.2. Scanning Electron Microscopy (SEM) of A. actinomycetemcomitans

We next examined the cellular morphology of *A. actinomycetemcomitans* cultured in mTSB, RPMI-1, and RPMI-2. The protocol and the list of samples are summarized in Supplementary Figure S1 and Table 1.

Table 1. List of samples for EM.

Strain	Protocol	Timeline
D7S-1 and D7SS	Bacteria cultured in mTSB, RPMI-1, or RPMI-2 media with daily 1:1 dilution with fresh media.	Day 1–Day 4
D7S-1 and D7SS	Bacteria grown in RPMI-2 from Day 1–Day 4 above were transferred to mTSB with daily 1:1 dilution with the fresh medium.	Day 5–Day 7

In mTSB, D7S-1 grew as aggregates of bacteria of 1–2 μm in length (Figure 3A,B). The cells were intact. Numerous fimbria appeared as thin fibrils (orange arrows) or thick bundles (blue arrows) comprised of multiple strands of fimbriae. Moderate amounts of vesicles (~0.1 μm) (red triangles) were noted. In RPMI-1, D7S-1 showed fewer and smaller cell aggregates on the coverslips and fewer fimbriae (Figure 3C,D). Numerous cells appeared either broken or irregularly shaped (yellow arrows). More vesicles of varying sizes were noted. D7S-1 grew less in RPMI-2 than in mTSB but more than in RPMI-1 (Figure 3E,F). The cells also formed aggregates attached to the coverslip, similar to those in mTSB. The cells were intact and demonstrated numerous vesicles of irregular shapes. Both thin and thick fimbriae were noted. A few long cells (3–4 μm) (green arrows) were also found. The cells reverted to the morphology observed in the mTSB control after three days of culturing with the daily dilution of fresh media (Figure 3G,H).

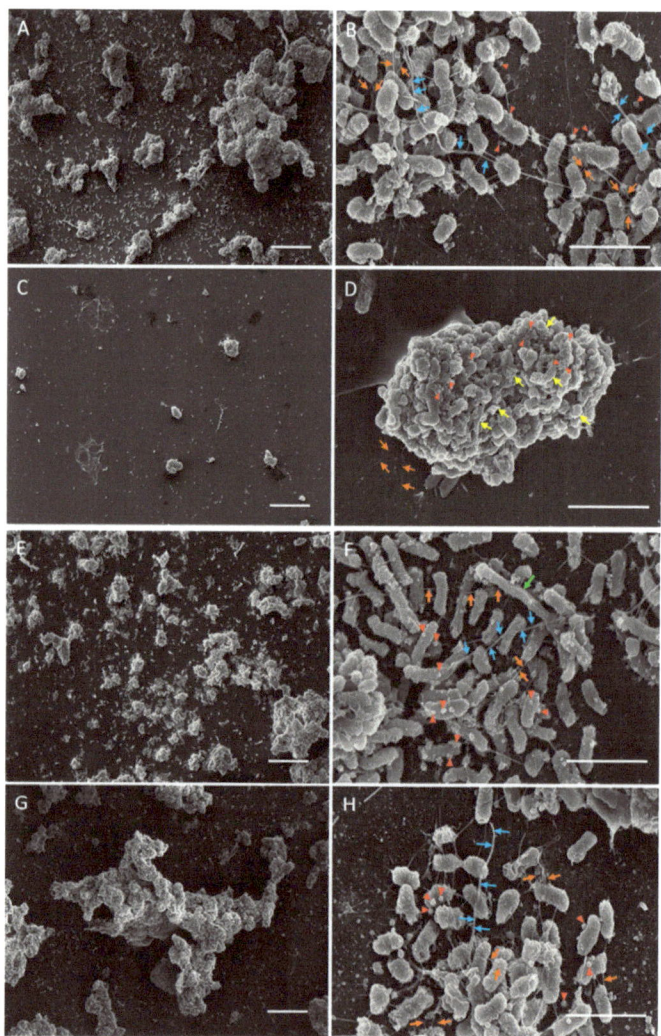

Figure 3. SEM of D7S-1 biofilms formed on the coverslips. The bacteria were cultured with a daily dilution of fresh media for four days in the mTSB control (**A,B**), RPMI-1 (**C,D**), RPMI-2 (**E,F**), or switched from RPMI-2 on day 4 to mTSB and grown with a daily dilution with fresh media until day 7 (**G,H**). Orange arrows indicate thin fibrils of the fimbriae, while blue arrows indicate fimbriae in thick bundles. Vesicles are represented by red triangles, and long cells are represented by green arrows. Yellow arrows indicate broken or irregularly shaped cells. The scale bars on the left and right columns are 20 and 2 μm, respectively.

The morphology of the isogenic smooth-colony mutant D7SS differed from that of D7S-1 in all media tested (Figure 4). In mTSB, D7SS grew as a thick mat of cells. The cells were longer (up to 4 μm) compared to D7S-1 (Figure 4A,B). The cells were intact, with a few vesicles. A few thin fimbriae (orange arrows) (but not the thick bundles of fimbriae) were noted. D7SS in RPMI-1 grew less than in mTSB and exhibited numerous extra-long cells (green arrows) (~10 μm), which may comprise undivided chains of cells (Figure 4C,D). Some of the long cells showed evidence of damage (yellow arrows). A few thin fimbriae (orange arrows) were noted. There were also numerous short and round cells (yellow triangles) not seen in other samples.

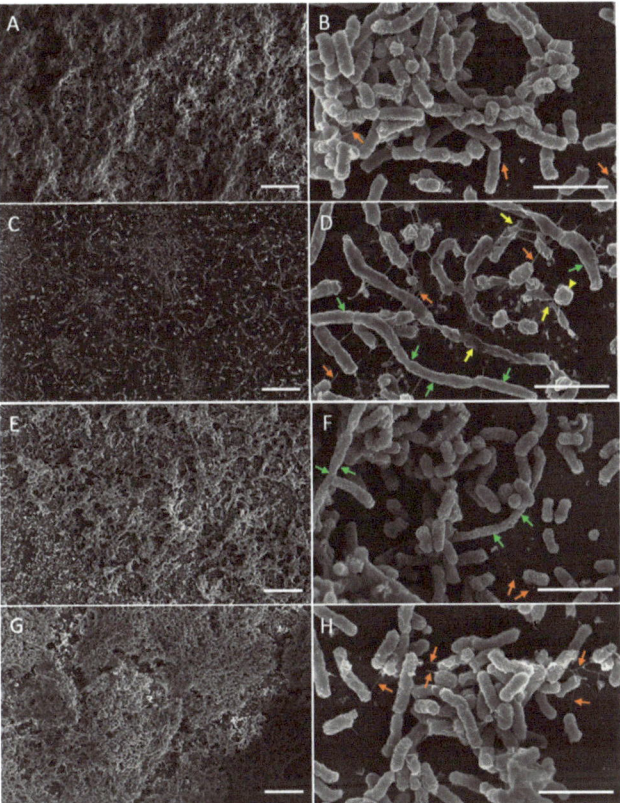

Figure 4. SEM of D7SS. The bacteria were cultured with a daily dilution of fresh media for four days in the mTSB control (**A**,**B**), RPMI-1 (**C**,**D**), RPMI-2 (**E**,**F**), or switched from RPMI-2 on day 4 to mTSB and grown with a daily dilution of fresh media until day 7 (**G**,**H**). Orange arrows represent thin fimbriae, and yellow arrows indicate broken or irregularly shaped cells. Long cells are denoted by green arrows, while yellow triangles indicate short and round cells. The scale bars on the left and right columns are 20 and 2 μm, respectively.

D7SS in RPMI-2 grew as well as in mTSB and was much better than in RPMI-1 (Figure 4E,F). Extra-long cells (green arrows) were found but less numerous than in RPMI-1. Notably, the cells appeared to be largely intact. The small round cells found in RPMI-1 cultures were not present in RPMI-2, and thin fimbriae (orange arrows) were occasionally seen. The morphology of D7SS in RPMI-2 upon culturing in mTSB for three days was indistinguishable from that in mTSB only (Figure 4G,H).

3.3. Transmission Electron Microscopy (TEM) of A. actinomycetemcomitans

The TEM of D7S-1 in the mTSB control showed intact cells (Figure 5A,B) with well-defined cytoplasmic membranes, periplasmic space, and outer membranes (red triangles). The cytoplasm was characterized by a pale-staining area of DNA (yellow arrows) and numerous ribosomes. Thick fimbriae (blue arrows) were also found. We could not find intact D7S-1 in RPMI-1 based on TEM, likely due to the low number of cells in the cultures. D7S-1 in RPMI-2 showed fewer cells than in the mTSB control (Figure 5C,D). However, the cells were largely intact, with well-defined cytoplasmic membranes, periplasmic space, and outer membranes (red triangles). In general, the cytoplasm contained fewer dark-staining ribosomes than in the mTSB control. A few extra-long cells (orange arrows) were noted. D7S-1 in RPMI-2, when cultured in mTSB, reverted to the morphology noted in cells cultured in mTSB only (Figure 5E,F).

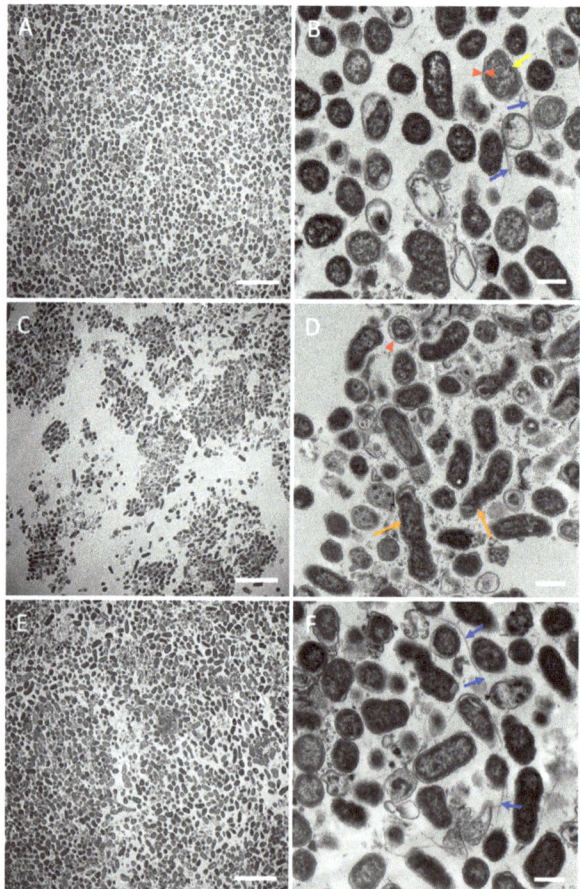

Figure 5. TEM of D7S-1. The bacterial growth conditions are described in Figure 3. The bacteria were pelleted from the cultures and processed for TEM. Intact D7S-1 cells in RPMI-1 could not be found based on TEM, likely due to the low number of cells in the cultures. The samples included D7S-1 in the mTSB control (panels **A,B**) and in RPMI-2 (panels **C,D**), and the bacteria switched from RPMI-2 to mTSB (panels **E,F**). Cellular cytoplasmic membranes, periplasmic space, and outer membranes are indicated by red triangles, while yellow arrows highlight the pale-staining area occupied by genomic DNA. Blue arrows denote thick fimbriae, and extra-long cells are indicated by orange arrows. The scale bars on the left and right columns are 5 μm and 500 nm, respectively.

D7SS in the mTSB control showed intact cells that, on average, were longer than those of D7S-1 (Figure 6A,B). The cells had well-defined cytoplasmic membranes, periplasmic space, and outer membranes (red triangles). The intracellular content was characterized by a pale-staining area of DNA (yellow arrows) and numerous ribosomes. No fimbriae were found. D7SS in RPMI-1 showed very few cells and evidence of damage (Figure 6C,D).

A few intact cells were found, characterized by poorly defined cell wall structures and irregular-shaped outer membranes (red triangles). Relatively few ribosomes were found in the cytoplasm. D7SS in RPMI-2 showed more cells than in RPMI-1 (Figure 6E,F). Occasional extra-long cells (orange arrows) were noted. The cell morphology was similar to that in RPMI-1, with the bacteria displaying irregular-shaped outer membranes. The morphology of the cells in RPMI-2 changed after reversion to the mTSB medium and resembled the cells in mTSB more closely (Figure 6G,H). Notably, the outline of the cells was smoother compared to the bacteria cultured in either RPMI-1 or RPMI-2.

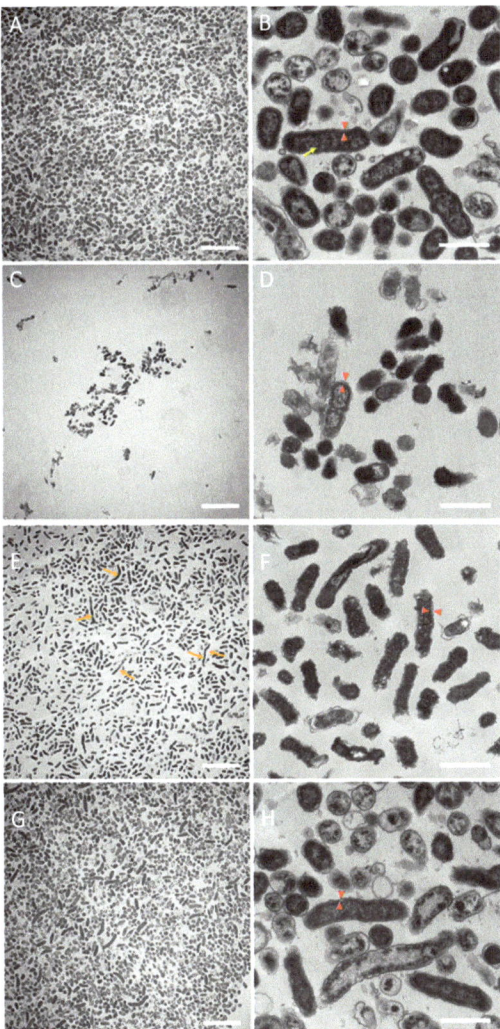

Figure 6. TEM of D7SS. The bacterial growth conditions and sample preparation are described in Figure 3 and include only the bacteria pelleted from cultures. The samples included D7SS in the mTSB control (panels **A,B**), in RPMI-1 (panels **C,D**), and RPMI-2 (panels **E,F**), and bacteria switched from RPMI-2 to mTSB (panels **G,H**). Cytoplasmic membranes, periplasmic space, and outer membranes are represented by red triangles, yellow arrows highlight the pale-staining area occupied by genomic DNA, and extra-long cells are highlighted by orange arrows. The scale bars on the left and right columns are 5 µm and 500 nm, respectively.

4. Discussion

Bacteria cultured in complex media exhibit the typical bacterial lifecycle: a brief lag phase, followed by rapid proliferation during the exponential phase fueled by abundant nutrients. When resources diminish, the rapid growth slows, and bacteria transition into a stationary phase marked by the absence of growth. In a closed culture system, when nutrients are not replenished, bacteria will eventually enter the death phase where, in *Escherichia coli* K12 cultured in Luria Bertani medium, 99% of the viable cells will be lost within three days [10].

In their natural environment, periods of bacterial exponential growth are short as nutrients are typically limited and conditions are generally harsh [11]. Bacteria are often forced to remain in the stationary phase for an extended time [12] until conditions become more favorable. However, when conditions fail to improve, cells may progress into the death phase. The mechanisms underlying the transition from the stationary phase to the death phase are poorly understood [10]. One theory hypothesizes that whenever the bacterial load exceeds the support potential of the culture, cells begin to die as there are no sufficient resources to continue their metabolism and carry out the repair and maintenance functions. This death then releases cell contents, including amino acids from proteins, carbohydrates from the cell walls, lipids from cell membrane materials, and DNA, that can be utilized by the surviving siblings [10,13]. Another theory proposed that in a high-density culture, cells can sense that resources are becoming limited, and a proportion of cells will automatically go through altruistic suicide so that others can continue to grow utilizing the remaining nutrients and survive [10,11,13].

Despite the death of the majority of the population during the transition from the stationary to death phase, some proportions of cells may survive [11] and enter into dormancy instead. They are viable but non-replicating in this state and exhibit low metabolic rates with distinct gene expression profiles [14]. Metabolic activities slow down to a minimum to conserve energy and increase their likelihood of survival. This group of surviving cells makes up what is known as the seed bank, and it serves to ensure that at least some cells can be resuscitated when conditions improve in the future [14].

Dormancy, however, is an energetically expensive process [14]. Although energy production slows to the bare minimum, bacteria must still allocate resources to maintain cellular structures and machinery [14]. They still need to spend energy maintaining surveillance of their environment to detect the appropriate time to exit dormancy and resume normal metabolism [14]. Yet, this energy investment will almost guarantee their survival.

In this study, we attempted to generate an in vitro dormancy model for *A. actinomycetemcomitans*. Most in vitro bacterial studies have relied on the use of complex media, and this strategy has significant drawbacks in microbial research. First, the undefined nature of the complex medium components frequently impedes hypothesis testing. Additionally, complex media do not accurately simulate the nutrient constraints of the in vivo environment where bacteria often experience starvation. Therefore, we chose CDMs to test our hypothesis. The precise formulations of CDMs allow us to make specific modifications to develop different media with distinct growth support properties. RPMI-1640 was selected as the base of our CDMs because our previous study showed that this medium (i.e., RPMI-1 in this study) supported the viability of *A. actinomycetemcomitans* for 24 h, with no apparent growth, and induced a distinct gene expression profile [15]. RPMI-1 was further amended to derive RPMI-2 and RPMI-3, and these amendments were tailored to *A. actinomycetemcomitans* based on its genome analysis [16] and growth requirements of *Haemophilus influenzae* [17–19]. *H. influenzae* and *A. actinomycetemcomitans* are genetically related and may share similar growth requirements.

We first determined whether the media were nutrient-deficient or nutrient-limited using the conventional enriched medium mTSB as a control (Figure 1). The critical finding was the difference between the growth phenotypes of *A. actinomycetemcomitans* in RPMI-1 and RPMI-2. The exhaustion of essential growth factors cannot explain the difference. A key finding to the formulation of the media is the requirement of nucleotide synthesis via salvage pathways for *A actinomycetemcomitans*. RPMI-1640, amended with uracil and hypoxanthine, provided all necessary components for the growth of *A. actinomycetemcomitans*. The results suggested that RPMI-1 is an ND medium, while RPMI-2 is an NL medium. Our results for RPMI-1 differed from the observation by Sreenivasan et al. [20], which suggested that RPMI-1 could sustain *A. actinomycetemcomitans'* growth. However, in their study, the growth of *A. actinomycetemcomitans* was monitored for 24 h only, which did not allow for sufficient time to demonstrate the decline in viability over time.

The growth differences in D7S-1 between mTSB and RPMI-2 were statistically significantly different. However, the differences were less than those in D7SS in the same media. It appears that D7S-1 was more resistant to nutrient limitations, which was more evident in the experiment in Figure 2. *A. actinomycetemcomitans* exhibited distinct cellular morphology when cultured in mTSB, RPMI-1, and RPMI-2. While there were differences in the cellular morphology of D7S-1 and D7SS, and the growth conditions were not the same as those tested in growth studies, the results suggested that *A. actinomycetemcomitans* in RPMI-2 was largely intact, remained relatively healthy, and exhibited a morphology distinct from that in mTSB. Perhaps not surprisingly, *A. actinomycetemcomitans* grown in RPMI-1 was significantly stressed, with numerous cells showing extensive damage, and was not considered dormant as defined by our study. In RPMI-2, the morphology of *A. actinomycetemcomitans* showed characteristics that were somewhat between the morphology in mTSB and RPMI-1, and the phenotype was reversible if the bacteria were transferred back to complex mTSB medium; they became indistinguishable from those with no exposure to the nutrient-limited medium.

We noted the presence of thin fimbriae but never thick bundles of fimbriae in the smooth-colony D7SS in liquid cultures. The strain D7SS has a point mutation in the promoter region of the fimbria biogenesis operon [21]. The results suggested that the point mutation's effect on fimbria expression is leaky, leading to the expression of thin fimbriae but not the thick bundles of fimbriae noted in the wildtype D7S-1. A similar observation that smooth-colony mutants expressed a lower abundance of and shorter fimbriae has been reported previously [22]. The role of the thin fimbriae in adherence and aggregation for *A. actinomycetemcomitans* remains to be elucidated.

Our lab routinely cultured *A. actinomycetemcomitans* in NE media for growth study and consistently observed a death phase typically after two days of incubation, when the bacteria were not recoverable. Therefore, the result of the sustained viability of D7S-1 in RPMI-2 was striking. Notably, the bacteria appeared to enter a phase of sustained viability starting from day 4, and the viability remained unchanged until the end of the experimentation. It is unknown how long the viability can last if we continue the experiment.

A. actinomycetemcomitans in RPMI-1 also exhibited a sustained but declining viability. This phenotype cannot be explained by the exhaustion of essential growth nutrients in the media because of the typical death phase encountered by *A. actinomycetemcomitans* grown in NE medium in 2–3 days. We hypothesize that the induction of *A. actinomycetemcomitans* dormancy requires both a specific formulation of the media and the presence of essential components to maintain dormancy.

There are several limitations and caveats to this study. The proportions of live and dead cells in EM studies were unknown. Future studies should include live/dead staining of both planktonic and biofilms in different culture conditions. The cellular morphology achieved by using EM was descriptive, and there is a need for quantitative analysis of the cells (e.g., cell size). Also, the pathogenesis of *A. actinomycetemcomitans* in periodontitis is complex. The simple model of this study does not simulate the complex in vivo growth condition, but will be useful for further investigation into the survival mechanism of *A. actinomycetemcomitans* in vivo.

Our study has not resolved when and how to distinguish dormancy and starvation and whether these conditions have overlapping phenotypes and mechanisms. These are the issues that require additional experiments for clarification. In the current study, we chose to avoid starvation by replenishing the media in the experiments to examine the cellular morphology by EM. We are currently investigating the genes involved in the phenotypes observed in this study by employing transcriptomics and Tn-seq. Once a list of candidate genes is identified, we will begin sorting out the genes involved in dormancy, starvation, or both. To the best of our knowledge, this is the first study to identify a growth phenotype of *A. actinomycetemcomitans* that resembles dormancy. Experiments are underway to investigate the essential genes and the transcriptomes of the putative *A. actinomycetemcomitans* dormancy. The information may provide insight into the pathogenesis of *A. actinomycetemcomitans* in periodontitis. Moreover, RPMI-1640 may be amended as a CDM for experiments that require specific information on each ingredient in the media. RPMI-1640 may also be tailored to other oral species based on genome analysis. We plan to test the CDMs developed in this study as growth media for in vitro polymicrobial models. These CDMs may be useful in investigating the complex bacteria-to-bacteria relationships in dental biofilms.

5. Conclusions

RPMI-1640 and its amendments are CDMs that can be used to test hypotheses related to the growth of *A. actinomycetemcomitans*. Specifically, we discovered *A. actinomycetemcomitans'* dormancy-like phenotype when the bacteria were cultured in a nutrient-limited RPMI-1640 amended with bases. The *A. actinomycetemcomitans* dormancy-like phenotype is characterized by a reduced but stable viability without the death phase, in contrast to the bacteria grown in enriched laboratory media. The *A. actinomycetemcomitans* dormancy-like phenotype exhibits distinct cellular morphology examined by SEM and TEM. The dormancy-like phenotype is reversible upon culturing in enriched laboratory media. The in vitro dormancy model may be useful for investigating the mechanisms of the survival of *A. actinomycetemcomitans* in nutrient-limited conditions.

Supplementary Materials: The following supporting information can be downloaded at: https://www.mdpi.com/article/10.3390/pathogens13050418/s1, Figure S1: Summary of protocols used to prepare *A. actinomycetemcomitans* samples for electron microscopy.

Author Contributions: Conception and study design, C.C. and N.O.T.; performing experiments and data analysis, C.C., N.O.T., C.B.M. and A.W.; writing—original draft preparation, C.C., N.O.T. and C.B.M.; writing—review and editing, C.C. and N.O.T. All authors have read and agreed to the published version of the manuscript.

Funding: This research was funded by NIH R01 DE012212 (CC).

Institutional Review Board Statement: Not applicable.

Informed Consent Statement: Not applicable.

Data Availability Statement: Data are contained within the article.

Conflicts of Interest: The authors declare no conflicts of interest.

References

1. McDonald, M.D.; Owusu-Ansah, C.; Ellenbogen, J.B.; Malone, Z.D.; Ricketts, M.P.; Frolking, S.E.; Ernakovich, J.G.; Ibba, M.; Bagby, S.C.; Weissman, J.L. What Is Microbial Dormancy? *Trends Microbiol.* **2024**, 32, 142–150. [CrossRef] [PubMed]
2. Fine, D.H.; Kaplan, J.B.; Kachlany, S.C.; Schreiner, H.C. How We Got Attached to *Actinobacillus actinomycetemcomitans*: A Model for Infectious Diseases. *Periodontol. 2000* **2006**, 42, 114–157. [CrossRef] [PubMed]
3. Kittichotirat, W.; Bumgarner, R.E.; Chen, C. Evolutionary Divergence of *Aggregatibacter actinomycetemcomitans*. *J. Dent. Res.* **2016**, 95, 94–101. [CrossRef] [PubMed]
4. Sun, R.; Kittichotirat, W.; Wang, J.; Jan, M.; Chen, W.; Asikainen, S.; Bumgarner, R.; Chen, C. Genomic Stability of *Aggregatibacter actinomycetemcomitans* during Persistent Oral Infection in Human. *PLoS ONE* **2013**, 8, e66472. [CrossRef] [PubMed]
5. Saarela, M.; Asikainen, S.; Alaluusua, S.; Pyhälä, L.; Lai, C.-H.; Jousimies-Somer, H. Frequency and Stability of Mono-or Poly-Infection by *Actinobacillus actinomycetemcomitans* Serotypes a, b, c, d or e. *Oral Microbiol. Immunol.* **1992**, 7, 277–279. [CrossRef] [PubMed]

6. Fine, D.H.; Schreiner, H.; Velusamy, S.K. Aggregatibacter, a Low Abundance Pathobiont That Influences Biogeography, Microbial Dysbiosis, and Host Defense Capabilities in Periodontitis: The History of a Bug, and Localization of Disease. *Pathogens* **2020**, *9*, 179. [CrossRef]
7. Nakamura, Y.; Watanabe, K.; Yoshioka, Y.; Ariyoshi, W.; Yamasaki, R. Persister Cell Formation and Elevated lsrA and lsrC Gene Expression upon Hydrogen Peroxide Exposure in a Periodontal Pathogen *Aggregatibacter actinomycetemcomitans*. *Microorganisms* **2023**, *11*, 1402. [CrossRef] [PubMed]
8. Vahvelainen, N.; Bozkurt, E.; Maula, T.; Johansson, A.; Pöllänen, M.T.; Ihalin, R. Pilus PilA of the Naturally Competent HACEK Group Pathogen *Aggregatibacter actinomycetemcomitans* Stimulates Human Leukocytes and Interacts with Both DNA and Proinflammatory Cytokines. *Microb. Pathog.* **2022**, *173*, 105843. [CrossRef] [PubMed]
9. Kelk, P.; Moghbel, N.S.; Hirschfeld, J.; Johansson, A. *Aggregatibacter actinomycetemcomitans* Leukotoxin Activates the NLRP3 Inflammasome and Cell-to-Cell Communication. *Pathogens* **2022**, *11*, 159. [CrossRef]
10. Finkel, S.E. Long-Term Survival during Stationary Phase: Evolution and the GASP Phenotype. *Nat. Rev. Microbiol.* **2006**, *4*, 113–120. [CrossRef]
11. Pletnev, P.; Osterman, I.; Sergiev, P.; Bogdanov, A.; Dontsova, O. Survival Guide: Escherichia Coli in the Stationary Phase. *Acta Naturae* **2015**, *7*, 22–33. [CrossRef] [PubMed]
12. Kolter, R.; Siegele, D.A.; Tormo, A. The Stationary Phase of the Bacterial Life Cycle. *Annu. Rev. Microbiol.* **1993**, *47*, 855–874. [CrossRef] [PubMed]
13. Navarro Llorens, J.M.; Tormo, A.; Martínez-García, E. Stationary Phase in Gram-Negative Bacteria. *FEMS Microbiol. Rev.* **2010**, *34*, 476–495. [CrossRef] [PubMed]
14. Lennon, J.T.; Jones, S.E. Microbial Seed Banks: The Ecological and Evolutionary Implications of Dormancy. *Nat. Rev. Microbiol.* **2011**, *9*, 119–130. [CrossRef] [PubMed]
15. Tjokro, N.O.; Kittichotirat, W.; Torittu, A.; Ihalin, R.; Bumgarner, R.E.; Chen, C. Transcriptomic Analysis of *Aggregatibacter actinomycetemcomitans* Core and Accessory Genes in Different Growth Conditions. *Pathogens* **2019**, *8*, 282. [CrossRef] [PubMed]
16. Najar, F. Sequence and Analysis of *Actinobacillus actinomycetemcomitans*. Ph.D. Thesis, University of Oklahoma, Norman, OK, USA, 2002.
17. Klein, R.; Luginbuhl, G. Simplified Media for the Growth of Haemophilus Influenzae from Clinical and Normal Flora Sources. *Microbiology* **1979**, *113*, 409–411. [CrossRef] [PubMed]
18. Schilling, C.H.; Palsson, B.Ø. Assessment of the Metabolic Capabilities of *Haemophilus influenzae* Rd through a Genome-Scale Pathway Analysis. *J. Theor. Biol.* **2000**, *203*, 249–283. [CrossRef]
19. Coleman, H.N.; Daines, D.A.; Jarisch, J.; Smith, A.L. Chemically Defined Media for Growth of Haemophilus Influenzae Strains. *J. Clin. Microbiol.* **2003**, *41*, 4408–4410. [CrossRef]
20. Sreenivasan, P.K.; Meyer, D.H.; Fives-Taylor, P.M. Factors Influencing the Growth and Viability of *Actinobacillus actinomycetemcomitans*. *Oral Microbiol. Immunol.* **1993**, *8*, 361–369. [CrossRef]
21. Wang, Y.; Liu, A.; Chen, C. Genetic Basis for Conversion of Rough-to-Smooth Colony Morphology in *Actinobacillus actinomycetemcomitans*. *Infect. Immun.* **2005**, *73*, 3749–3753. [CrossRef]
22. Fu, Y.; Maaβ, S.; du Teil Espina, M.; Wolters, A.H.G.; Gong, Y.; de Jong, A.; Raangs, E.; Buist, G.; Westra, J.; Becher, D.; et al. Connections between Exoproteome Heterogeneity and Virulence in the Oral Pathogen *Aggregatibacter actinomycetemcomitans*. *mSystems* **2022**, *7*, e00254-22. [CrossRef] [PubMed]

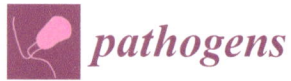

Article

Leukotoxin A Production and Release by JP2 and Non-JP2 Genotype *Aggregatibacter actinomycetemcomitans* in Relation to Culture Conditions

Sotirios Kalfas [1], Zahra Khayyat Pour [2], Rolf Claesson [2] and Anders Johansson [2,*]

[1] Department of Preventive Dentistry, Periodontology and Implant Biology, Aristotle University of Thessaloniki, 54124 Thessaloniki, Greece; kalfas@dent.auth.gr
[2] Department of Odontology, Umeå University, 90187 Umeå, Sweden; z.khayyatpour@allt1.se (Z.K.P.); rlkc1952@gmail.com (R.C.)
* Correspondence: anders.p.johansson@umu.se; Tel.: +46-90-7856291

Abstract: Aggressive forms of periodontitis, especially in young patients, are often associated with an increased proportion of the Gram-negative bacterium *Aggregatibacter actinomycetemcomitans* of the microbiota of the affected periodontal sites. One of the virulence factors of *A. actinomycetemcomitans* is a leukotoxin (LtxA) that induces a pro-inflammatory cell death process in leukocytes. *A. actinomycetemcomitans* exhibits a large genetic diversity and different genotypes vary in LtxA production capacity. The genotype JP2 is a heavy LtxA producer due to a 530-base pair deletion in the promoter for the toxin genes, and this trait has been associated with an increased pathogenic potential. The present study focused on the production and release of LtxA by different *A. actinomycetemcomitans* genotypes and serotypes under various growth conditions. Four different strains of this bacterium were cultured in two different culture broths, and the amount of LtxA bound to the bacterial surface or released into the broths was determined. The cultures were examined during the logarithmic and the early stationary phases of growth. The JP2 genotype exhibited the highest LtxA production among the strains tested, and production was not affected by the growth phase. The opposite was observed with the other strains. The composition of the culture broth had no effect on the growth pattern of the tested strains. However, the abundant release of LtxA from the bacterial surface into the culture broth was found in the presence of horse serum. Besides confirming the enhanced leucotoxicity of the JP2 genotype, the study provides new data on LtxA production in the logarithmic and stationary phases of growth and the effect of media composition on the release of the toxin from the bacterial membrane.

Keywords: *Aggregatibacter actinomycetemcomitans*; leukotoxin release; JP2-genotype; culture conditions

Citation: Kalfas, S.; Pour, Z.K.; Claesson, R.; Johansson, A. Leukotoxin A Production and Release by JP2 and Non-JP2 Genotype *Aggregatibacter actinomycetemcomitans* in Relation to Culture Conditions. *Pathogens* **2024**, *13*, 569. https://doi.org/10.3390/pathogens13070569

Academic Editor: Daniel H. Fine

Received: 7 May 2024
Revised: 19 June 2024
Accepted: 4 July 2024
Published: 6 July 2024

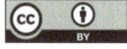
1. Introduction

The Gram-negative facultative anaerobic bacterial species *Aggregatibacter actinomycetemcomitans* is associated with periodontitis in young individuals [1,2]. A leukotoxin (LtxA) produced by this bacterium is closely linked to the initiation of degenerative processes involved in the disease [3,4]. LtxA is a large pore-forming protein internalized by the β_2 integrin LFA-1 (CD11a/CD18) expressed by human immune cells [5]. The interaction of LtxA with leukocytes activates the release of interleukin (IL)-1β from human macrophages and of proteolytic enzymes from neutrophils [6] and ultimately causes cell death. LtxA-induced macrophage death involves the activation of the NLRP3 inflammasome in a process defined as pyroptosis [7]. The NLRP3 inflammasome plays a central role in many degenerative diseases and is a possible target for future strategies in periodontal therapy [8]. *A. actinomycetemcomitans* shows a substantial genetic diversity and seven serotypes (a–g) have been described till now [9,10]. A specific variant of serotype b, the JP2 genotype, produces large amounts of LtxA and is characterized by the absence of a 530-base pair (bp) sequence within the *ltxCABD* promoter region [11].

The JP2 genotype was initially detected in individuals with origins in the Mediterranean part of Africa, following a dissemination route through West Africa, and further to North and South America via the transatlantic slave trade [12]. Today, there are several reports on the carriage of the JP2 genotype by individuals outside the North and West African regions [13]. Young carriers of the JP2 genotype of *A. actinomycetemcomitans* are at high risk of developing periodontitis [14]. In addition to the JP2 genotype, an additional marker for highly leukotoxic genotypes of *A. actinomycetemcomitans* has been discovered [15]. This genotype contains an intact *cagE* gene and includes JP2, as well as a subgroup of non-JP2 isolates with genetic similarities to JP2 [16].

LtxA production substantially varies among different genotypes, being highest in strains of the JP2 genotype [17]. The role of the 530 bp deletion in the promoter region of the leukotoxin operon for the regulation of LtxA expression is not fully understood [18]. The deletion of a specific 100 bp region within the 530 bp promoter deletion region was shown to be a leukotoxin repressor, thus enhancing LtxA production [19]. As a supplement to this finding another recently discovered leukotoxin promoter deletion outside this 100 bp deletion also resulted in enhanced LtxA production in the JP2 genotype, further illustrating the complexity of leukotoxin production [20]. These discrepancies in the role of the promoter deletion for LtxA production indicate a complex regulation with alternative signaling pathways. Environmental factors and growth conditions have also been described as interfering with LtxA production [21–23].

LtxA is a 1055 amino acid protein post-translationally activated through acylation before being secreted by a Type I secretion system [24]. The secreted LtxA may either be released into the culture media or stay bound to the bacterial outer membrane [25,26]. The presence of serum proteins induces the release of LtxA from the bacterial outer membrane [27]. The ionic strength of the environment also affects this release [28]. Serum protease inhibitors protect LtxA from proteolytic degradation, which, in turn, promotes increased leukotoxic activity [29].

The aim of the present study was to examine LtxA production by the JP2 and non-JP2 genotypes of *A. actinomycetemcomitans* in relation to certain culture conditions, such as the culture medium and the phase of growth.

2. Materials and Methods

2.1. Culture Media and Bacterial Strains

Two sterile-filtered culture broths, peptone yeast extract glucose (PYG) [4] and Bacteroides medium (BM) [30] were used. Their composition is shown in Table 1. All chemicals were obtained from Sigma-Aldrich (St. Louis, MA, USA).

Table 1. Composition of the two culture broths.

PYG Medium	BM Medium
Bacto peptone 0.5%	Trypticase (BBL) 1%
Trypticase peptone 0.5%	Proteose peptone (Oxoid) 1%
Glucose 1%	Glucose 0.5%
Yeast extract 1%,	Yeast extract 0.5%
NaCl 1.36 mM	NaCl 1.13 mM
$MgSO_4$ 0.03 mM	Sterile horse serum 2%
K_2HPO_4 0.22 mM	Hemin 5 mg/L
KH_2PO_4 0.29 mM	Vitamin K 10 mg/L
$CaCl_2$ 0.05 mM	
$NaHCO_3$ 4.7 mM	

The growth of four *A. actinomycetemcomitans* strains, NCTC 9710, HK 1519 (JP2 geno-type), SUNY ab75, and Y4, isolated from human plaque, was initially examined in the two broths (Table 2). A total of 1 mL of an overnight culture was inoculated into 50 mL of fresh broth and incubated at 37 °C in air with 5% CO_2. The bacterial growth was followed by measuring the optical density at 600 nm (OD_{600}) of the culture at certain time points. The growth was followed for 24 h.

Table 2. Generation time in minutes of various strains of *A. actinomycetemcomitans* in two different culture media. Mean ± standard deviation of 3 experiments with each strain.

A. actinomycetemcomitans Strains	PYG Broth	BM Broth
NCTC 9710 (serotype c)	92 ± 9	96 ± 6
HK 1519 (serotype b, JP2 genotype)	108 ± 6	96 ± 27
SUNY ab75 (serotype a)	116 ± 12	94 ± 24
Y4 (serotype b, non-JP2 genotype)	92 ± 9	92 ± 18

For the analysis of LtxA production, half of the culture was harvested in the late logarithmic phase of growth after about 8 h of incubation and the rest of the culture after an additional 12 h incubation, i.e., in the stationary phase of growth.

2.2. Extraction of LtxA from Bacterial Cells

Each culture sample was immediately centrifuged at 10,000× *g* and 4 °C for 30 min, and the bacterial pellet was re-suspended in 50 mM phosphate buffer containing 0.45 M NaCl, pH 7.0, and the density was adjusted to 3×10^{11} cells/mL. The suspension was incubated under gentle rocking at 4 °C for 1 h to release LtxA and other outer membrane proteins from the bacterial cells [28]. At the end of the incubation, the cells were removed by centrifugation (10,000× *g* at 4 °C for 20 min), and the supernatant was stored at −80 °C until analyzed.

2.3. Precipitation of LtxA Released into the Culture Medium

LtxA and other proteins released from the bacteria into the broth were precipitated by the addition of trichloroacetic acid to the culture supernatant to a final concentration of 5% and incubated overnight at 4 °C. The precipitate was harvested by centrifugation (3000× *g* at 4 °C for 15 min) and resuspended in 0.1 M NaOH to a final volume that corresponded to protein extraction from 3×10^{11} bacteria/mL, this concentration being comparable with the one in LtxA extracts from the bacterial cells. The solution was stored at −80 °C until analyzed.

2.4. Detection of LtxA in Electrophoresis Gel

The proteins in the precipitates of culture broths and in cell extracts were separated by sodium dodecyl sulphate polyacrylamide gel electrophoresis (SDS-PAGE, 8%). Each sample was mixed with an equal volume of buffer (50 μL 50 mM Tris-buffer, pH 7.4, containing 2% SDS, 0.03% bromophenol blue, 20% sucrose, and 5% mercaptothion) and heated at 100 °C for 5 min. The protein bands in the gel were stained with Coomassie brilliant blue R-250 (Bio-Rad Laboratories, Hercules, CA, USA) and the amount of protein in the 116 kDa band that corresponds to leukotoxin was coarsely determined with the Model Gs-700 Imaging Densitometer and the Molecular Analyst™ software version 1.4 (Bio-Rad Laboratories).

2.5. Detection of LtxA by Western Blot Analysis and Amino Acid Sequencing

The proteins in the SDS-PAGE were transferred from the gel to a Polyscreen™ transfer membrane (NEN Life Science Products, Mechelen, Belgium) as previously described [28]. The membrane was incubated in a TBS buffer (20 mM Tris and 500 mM NaCl, pH 7.5) containing rabbit anti-leukotoxin serum (diluted 1:1000) for 1–2 h. As a secondary antibody, goat anti-rabbit HRP (DAKO A/S. Glostrup, Denmark) was used (diluted 1:1000 in TBS-buffer) for 1 h. The immunoreactive bands were visualized on film (Kodak) with ECL development solution according to the manufacturer's instructions (PIERCE, Rockford, IL, USA).

The N-terminal amino acid sequence analysis of the 116 kDa protein band, transferred from the gel to a Polyscreen™ membrane, was performed with the Procise™ 494 (Applied Biosystems, Foster City, CA, USA) protein sequencing system, using programs and chemicals recommended by the manufacturer [28].

2.6. Isolation of PMN from Peripheral Blood

Human polymorphonuclear leukocytes (PMNs) were prepared from peripheral blood collected in sodium heparin-containing vacuum tubes from two healthy donors (co-authors RC and AJ). After sedimentation in Macrodex (Pharmacia, Uppsala, Sweden), the upper phase was centrifuged ($150\times$ *g* at 4 °C for 12 min) and the cell pellet was resuspended in distilled water for 30 s to lyse remaining red blood cells. Thereafter, NaCl was added to make the solution isotonic, and the cells were washed twice with PBS before being resuspended in RPMI medium with 20% fetal calf serum. The cell concentration in the suspension was determined in a Bürker chamber under $400\times$ magnification and adjusted to 4×10^6 cells/mL. The final preparation contained 90–95% PMN cells.

2.7. Assay of Leukotoxic Activity

The leukotoxicity of the various samples was determined by the activity of lactate dehydrogenase [28] released from injured PMN cells upon exposure to the samples. A volume of 75 µL of PMN suspensions (2×10^6 cells/mL) was mixed with an equal volume of bacterial cell suspensions in RPMI with 20% FCS. Mixtures with a bacterial/PMN ratio of 3, 6, 12, 25, 50, 100, and 200 were prepared and incubated at 37 °C in air with 5% CO_2 for 2 h. The leukocytes were pelleted by centrifugation ($250\times$ *g* for 5 min), and the activity of lactate dehydrogenase released in the supernatant was determined [31]. The positive and negative controls were PMN lysed with 0.1% Triton X-100 and PMN only in RPMI, respectively.

A leukotoxicity assay was run in triplicate in a 96-well flat-bottomed microtiter plate. The reaction mixture contained 20 µL sample (supernatant from the centrifuged mixtures) and 180 µL LDH-buffer (0.1 M sodium phosphate buffer pH 7.0, with 2 mM Na-pyruvate and 0.154 mM NADH-Na). The activity of LDH was monitored at room temperature in a spectrophotometer (Multiscan MCC/340, Labsystems Diagnostic Oy, Vantaa, Finland) by continuously measuring the change in absorbance at 340 nm, indicative of NADH oxidation, for 2–5 min. The LDH activity of each sample was recorded as the decrease in absorbance/minute (DA) and the relative leukotoxicity (RL) of each sample was expressed in percent (%) and calculated by the formula:

$$\text{RL (\%)} = 100 \times (\text{DA}_{\text{sample}} - \text{DA}_{\text{neg.control}})/(\text{DA}_{\text{pos.control}} - \text{DA}_{\text{neg.control}}) \tag{1}$$

3. Results

3.1. Bacterial Growth

The estimation of bacterial growth in two different culture media did not show any substantial differences among the four tested bacterial strains (Figure 1). All strains reached the stationary phase of growth after 9–11 h of incubation at 37 °C.

The generation time for each bacterial strain in both culture media was calculated and presented in Table 2.

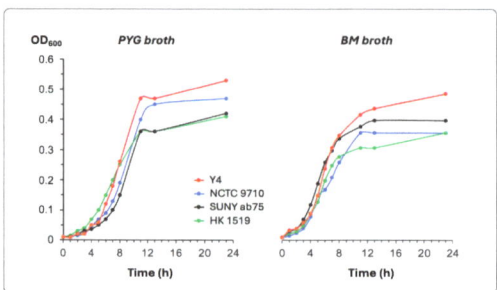

Figure 1. Growth curves in PYG and BM broths of the four bacterial strains. The growth was determined by the change in the optical density of the culture at 600 nm (OD_{600}).

3.2. Cell Surface-Associated LtxA

The extraction of leukotoxin from bacterial cells showed that strains HK 1519 and Y4 produced high amounts of LtxA during the log phase. The LtxA production by the NCTC 9710 and SUNY ab75 strains was very low or undetectable. During the stationary phase, the HK 1519 strain exhibited more LtxA per bacterial cell than during the log phase, while Y4 showed no change in its content of leukotoxin.

In the log phase, both HK 1519 and Y4 had more leukotoxin associated with the bacterial cells in PYG than in BM. On the other hand, during the stationary phase, strain HK 1519 released more leukotoxin in PYG than in BM, while Y4 had more leukotoxin in BM media compared with PYG (Figure 2 and Table 3). Within the quantitative limitations of the method, the JP2 genotype (strain HK 1519) appeared to continue producing high amounts of LtxA also in the stationary phase of growth, while a more variable LtxA production was observed in the other non-JP2 strains (Table 3). This phenomenon seemed most pronounced in PYG broth.

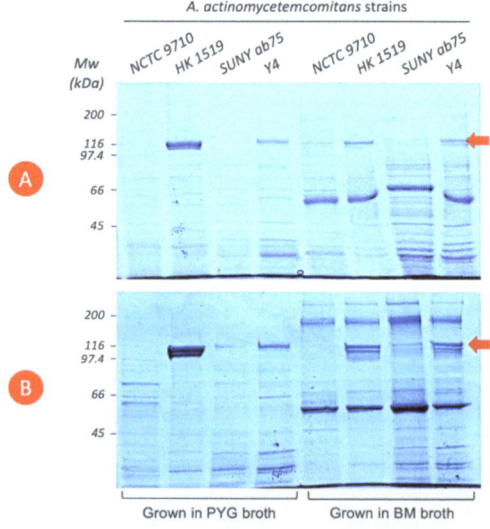

Figure 2. Cell surface-associated LtxA extracted from *A. actinomycetemcomitans* strains cultured in PYG or BM broth. The cells were harvested during the logarithmic (**A**) or stationary (**B**) phases of growth. The leukotoxin appears as a protein band at the 116 kDa position (arrow) in SDS-PAGE (8%). Data from representative experiments are shown.

Table 3. Leukotoxin content of extracts from bacteria cultured in two different media and harvested during the logarithmic or stationary phases of growth. The amount of leukotoxin was determined by densitometric analysis (OD × mm^2) of the LtxA band in the SDS-PAGE of the extracts. Data from two experiments (Exp. 1 and Exp. 2) with each strain are presented.

Strain	PYG Broth				BM Broth			
	Logarithmic		Stationary		Logarithmic		Stationary	
	Exp. 1	Exp. 2	Exp. 1	Exp. 2	Exp. 1	Exp. 2	Exp. 1	Exp. 2
NCTC 9710	0.14	0.68	0.73	0.67	−0.02	0.94	1.33	0.81
HK1519	2.85	4.72	19.7	8.75	2.54	1.62	7.65	7.10
SUNY ab75	0.25	0.17	0.71	0.68	0.74	0.64	0.91	1.51
Y4	3.81	1.52	1.24	1.61	1.66	1.87	3.08	2.79

An abundance of LtxA compared with the other proteins in the cell extracts from the JP2 genotype was observed (Figure 2). The analysis of leukotoxin precipitated from the supernatants of the different bacterial cultures showed very low or no detectable amount of leukotoxin in SDS-PAGE gels.

The immunoblotting of gels with the SDS-PAGE separated extracts showed a high specificity of the polyclonal leukotoxin antiserum for the 116 kDa protein band (Figure 3). The amino acid sequence analyses of this protein band showed a complete sequence homology with *A. actinomycetemcomitans* LtxA, (accession number P16462, https://www.uniprot.org/uniprotkb/P16462/entry, accessed on 7 January 2015).

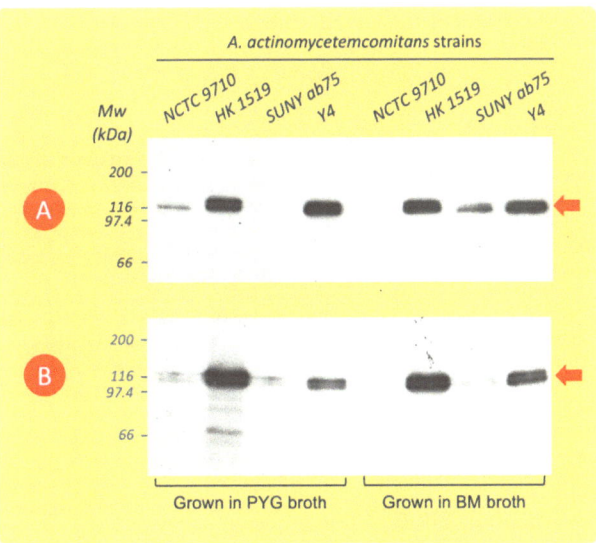

Figure 3. Western blot analysis (with polyclonal rabbit LtxA antiserum) of cell surface-associated LtxA extracted from *A. actinomycetemcomitans* strains cultured in PYG or BM broth. The cells were harvested during the logarithmic (**A**) or stationary (**B**) phases of growth. Data from representative experiments are shown. The leukotoxin appears at the 116 kDa position (arrow).

3.3. LtxA Released in the Culture Broth

The detection of LtxA released into the growth broth was accomplished by the immunoblotting of the proteins precipitated from the culture supernatants and separated by SDS-PAGE, as described above.

The immunoblot revealed antiserum reactivity with proteins precipitated only from BM culture supernatants (Figure 4). The antibodies bound to the protein band with the molecular weight of leukotoxin and to protein bands at positions of lower or higher molecular weights ranging between 70 and >200 kDa.

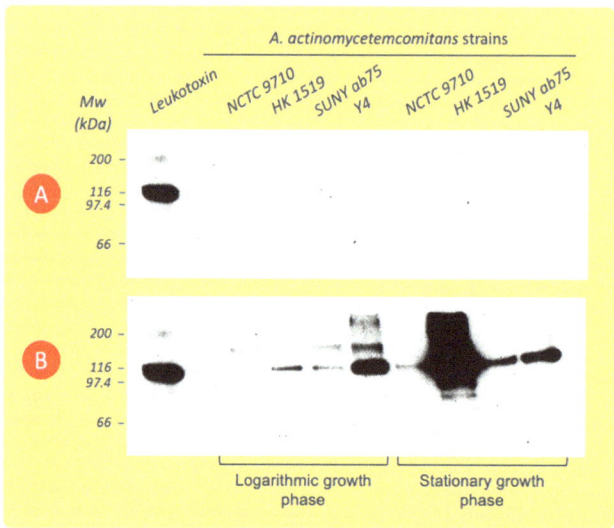

Figure 4. Western blots of proteins precipitated from culture supernatants of various *A. actinomycetemcomitans* strains and separated by SDS-PAGE before being exposed to polyclonal rabbit LtxA antiserum. The supernatants were collected during the logarithmic or stationary phases of growth in PYG (**A**) or BM (**B**) broth. Data from representative experiments are shown.

3.4. Screening of Leukotoxicity by the Cytolytic Assay

The LtxA-induced lysis of human PMNs showed that the JP2 genotype (strain HK1519) exhibited the highest activity irrespective of the culture condition (Figure 5). Strain Y4 also showed leukotoxic activity; however, it was lower than that of the JP2 genotype.

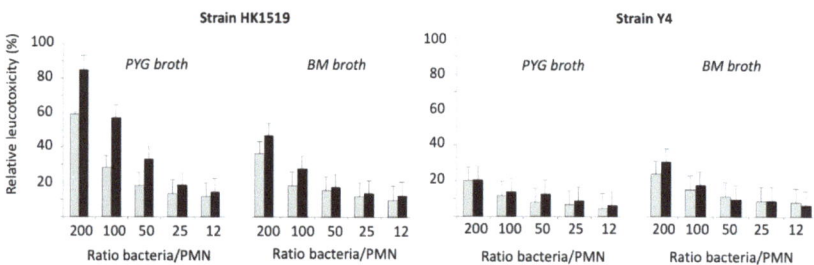

Figure 5. Relative leukotoxicity of *A. actinomycetemcomitans* HK1519 and Y4 grown in PYG or BM broth and harvested during the logarithmic (grey bars) or stationary (black bars) phases of growth. The leukotoxic activity was examined at various ratios of bacteria/PMN.

At a ratio of 200 bacteria/PMN, the RLs of HK1519 cells from the logarithmic and stationary growth phases were 60% and 85%, respectively. The corresponding RLs of strain Y4 were lower, ranging from about 20 to 30% (Figure 5).

In all experiments, the leukotoxicity of strains NCTC 9710 and Suny ab75 was somewhat lower compared to the one of strain Y4, and it reached detectable levels under the conditions displayed in Figure 6.

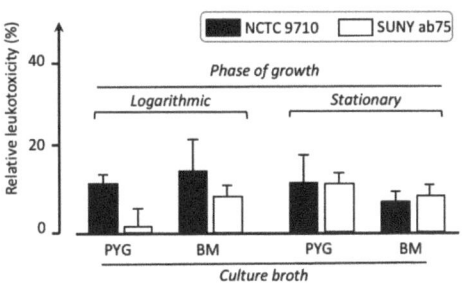

Figure 6. Leukotoxicity of *A. actinomycetemcomitans* strains NCTC 9710 and SUNY ab75 under different growth conditions. Mean ± SD of three replicates.

4. Discussion

It is evident from the present findings that the growth conditions may affect the leukotoxicity of *A. actinomycetemcomitans*, which may partly explain the discrepancies in leukotoxin production and leukotoxicity observed for the same strains by various researchers. Both the composition of the culture medium and the phase of growth at which the bacteria were harvested influenced the relative leukotoxicity; however, strain-dependent patterns were found. Although the leukotoxicity of the non-JP2 genotype strains showed a tendency to be slightly increased in cultures from BM broth, the highest leukotoxic activity is to be expected with all strains when grown in the absence of blood or serum proteins, such as in PYG broth, due to the minimal loss of the toxin from the bacterial surface into the culture medium. Except for the JP2 genotype, which continued its high LtxA production during the stationary phase of growth, the other strains exhibited higher or equally high leukotoxic activity during the logarithmic phase than during the stationary phase of growth. It is worth noting that in the studies mentioned above, *A. actinomycetemcomitans* was cultured on agar media supplemented with blood or serum, usually for 48 h, before assaying the leukotoxicity. These conditions probably had a considerable impact on the outcome of these studies.

The culture broths studied have a chemically non-defined composition and are widely used for the cultivation of oral bacteria. The two broths supported the growth of all strains tested, and no significant difference was found in either the generation time, the duration of the lag phase, or the final cell density when the cultures reached the stationary phase of growth. Thus, the variation in leukotoxicity cannot be attributed to differences in the growth pattern.

The main difference between PYG and BM broth is the presence of hemin, vitamin K, and horse serum in the latter. Judging from the equally good growth of all strains in both media, it may be suggested that these supplements do not cover the nutritional demands of *A. actinomycetemcomitans*, as also shown elsewhere [32]. Serum was thought to support growth and was used in selective media to secure good growth upon primary cultivation; however, the opposite effect was observed [33]. Supplementing BM with these compounds was originally suggested to support the growth of fastidious anaerobes such as *Prevotella* and *Porphyromonas* species, formerly classified as *Bacteroides* species [30,34,35].

Despite the similar growth in the two broths, a consistent difference in the release of LtxA from the bacterial cells appears to occur with all strains, with the release being more extensive in BM cultures. The release of membrane-bound active LtxA, both as free molecules and incorporated in outer membrane vesicles, was previously shown to occur upon a 1 h incubation of the bacteria with human serum or serum albumin at 4 °C, with the release being concentration-dependent [27]. Possibly, the horse serum in BM has a similar effect on the release of the toxin.

In the previous study [27], the leukotoxic activity of the JP2 genotype was also examined with cultures in PYG supplemented with various concentrations of human serum. Intact LtxA and other protein bands of smaller molecular weight that reacted with LtxA-antiserum were detected both in the samples of culture supernatants and the cell extracts. However, the preparations lacked leukotoxic activity even from cultures with low serum concentrations (5%), which could possibly depend on the degradation and inactivation of LtxA by the components of the human serum. This was not observed in this study, which may indicate important differences between the inactivated horse serum used in BM and the human serum previously studied.

The Y4 strain seems to produce more LtxA, either released in the medium or kept bound to the bacterial cells, when grown in BM than in PYG. As mentioned, a strain-dependent pattern appears to exist in LtxA production, with the pattern being influenced by the medium composition. Possibly, these strains may respond to small molecules and nutritional cues of their environment with an altered virulence expression, as also observed with other periodontopathogens [36].

In accordance with previous observations, the JP2 genotype (strain HK1519) of *A. actinomycetemcomitans* exhibited a much higher LtxA production than the non-JP2 genotypes [17]. Moreover, the present results indicate that the enhanced LtxA production by the JP2 genotype is more pronounced during the stationary phase of growth. This strain continued to accumulate LtxA bound to the outer membrane, while the non-JP2 genotype (strain Y4) already reached maximal LtxA content in the late logarithmic growth phase. This is opposite to the large previously reported reduction in LtxA expression in the JP2 genotype when approaching the stationary phase of growth [37]. Differences in the culture conditions may be responsible for the discrepant results, as already mentioned above.

Some authors suggested an enhanced pathogenic potential of *A. actinomycetemcomitans* strains belonging to serotype b due to their increased LtxA production [4,38]. LtxA induces a substantial pro-inflammatory response in macrophages by targeting the NLRP3 inflammasome [7,39]. The genotyping of serotype b isolates revealed a subgroup with high virulence [40]. More recently, a genetic marker, the *cagE* gene, was identified for this subgroup [15], which includes the JP2 genotype and about one-third of the non-JP2 serotype b isolates with shared properties of high LtxA production and pathogenicity [16]. The serotype b strain Y4 lacks the *cagE* gene [16]. This genetic difference between the two serotype b strains HK1519 and Y4 agrees with the large difference in their LtxA production as presently found. It remains to be discovered whether the *cagE* gene has a role in the enhanced *LtxA* production and virulence associated with this genotype [15,16].

Extrapolating these in vitro findings to the clinical situation, it seems plausible to expect that the nutritional environment of the inflamed periodontal pocket favors the production and release of LtxA by *A. actinomycetemcomitans*. Especially, strains characterized as heavy LtxA producers, such as those of the JP2 genotype, might stably express this virulence factor at maximum capacity, irrespective of their growth phase. The high pathogenic potential ascribed to the JP2 genotype [41,42] and to other strains of the *cagE* subgroup is probably potentiated by the enhanced release of the toxin from the bacterial surface, due to the presence of serum compounds. Depending on the proteolytic activity of the environment, the free LtxA may be degraded and lose its toxicity [28,29] or remain intact. The higher the production and release of LtxA, the higher the amount of intact toxin molecules that may diffuse into the neighboring soft tissue and trigger inflammatory reactions or kill defense cells [6,43]. The present study supports this hypothesis of the pathogenic potential of specific *A. actinomycetemcomitans* strains and the possible mechanisms.

Author Contributions: Conceptualization, A.J., S.K. and R.C.; methodology, A.J., Z.K.P. and R.C.; software, A.J.; validation, A.J., S.K. and R.C.; formal analysis, A.J., R.C. and Z.K.P.; investigation, R.C. and A.J.; resources, A.J., S.K. and R.C.; data curation, A.J., S.K. and Z.K.P.; writing—original draft preparation, A.J.; writing—review and editing, A.J., S.K., Z.K.P. and R.C.; funding acquisition, A.J. and S.K. All authors have read and agreed to the published version of the manuscript.

Funding: This research was funded by TUA grants from the County Council of Västerbotten, Sweden (A.J.; 7003193).

Institutional Review Board Statement: Not applicable.

Informed Consent Statement: Not applicable.

Data Availability Statement: Data are available from the corresponding author, Department of Odontology, Umeå University.

Acknowledgments: *A. actinomycetemcomitans* strain HK 1519 (serotype b, JP2 genotype) was kindly provided by M. Kilian, Aarhus, Denmark.

Conflicts of Interest: The authors declare no conflicts of interest.

References

1. Fine, D.H.; Patil, A.G.; Velusamy, S.K. *Aggregatibacter actinomycetemcomitans* (Aa) Under the Radar: Myths and Misunderstandings of Aa and Its Role in Aggressive Periodontitis. *Front. Immunol.* **2019**, *10*, 728. [CrossRef] [PubMed]
2. Hbibi, A.; Bouziane, A.; Lyoussi, B.; Zouhdi, M.; Benazza, D. *Aggregatibacter actinomycetemcomitans*: From Basic to Advanced Research. In *Periodontitis: Advances in Experimental Research*; Springer International Publishing: Cham, Switzerland, 2022; Volume 1373, pp. 45–67.
3. Kelk, P.; Claesson, R.; Chen, C.; Sjöstedt, A.; Johansson, A. IL-1beta secretion induced by *Aggregatibacter* (*Actinobacillus*) *actinomycetemcomitans* is mainly caused by the leukotoxin. *Int. J. Med. Microbiol.* **2008**, *298*, 529–541. [CrossRef] [PubMed]
4. Åberg, C.H.; Haubek, D.; Kwamin, F.; Johansson, A.; Claesson, R. Leukotoxic activity of *Aggregatibacter actinomycetemcomitans* and periodontal attachment loss. *PLoS ONE* **2014**, *9*, e104095. [CrossRef]
5. Lally, E.T.; Kieba, I.R.; Sato, A.; Green, C.L.; Rosenbloom, J.; Korostoff, J.; Wang, J.F.; Shenker, B.J.; Ortlepp, S.; Robinson, M.K.; et al. RTX toxins recognize a beta2 integrin on the surface of human target cells. *J. Biol. Chem.* **1997**, *272*, 30463–30469. [CrossRef]
6. Johansson, A. *Aggregatibacter actinomycetemcomitans* leukotoxin: A powerful tool with capacity to cause imbalance in the host inflammatory response. *Toxins* **2011**, *3*, 242–259. [CrossRef] [PubMed]
7. Kelk, P.; Moghbel, N.S.; Hirschfeld, J.; Johansson, A. *Aggregatibacter actinomycetemcomitans* Leukotoxin Activates the NLRP3 Inflammasome and Cell-to-Cell Communication. *Pathogens* **2022**, *11*, 159. [CrossRef] [PubMed]
8. Zhao, Y.; Quan, Y.; Lei, T.; Fan, L.; Ge, X.; Hu, S. The Role of Inflammasome NLPR3 in the Development and Therapy of Periodontitis. *Int. J. Med. Sci.* **2022**, *19*, 1603–1614. [CrossRef] [PubMed]
9. Kaplan, J.B.; Perry, M.B.; MacLean, L.L.; Furgang, D.; Wilson, M.E.; Fine, D.H. Structural and genetic analyses of O polysaccharide from *Actinobacillus actinomycetemcomitans* serotype f. *Infect. Immun.* **2001**, *69*, 5375–5384. [CrossRef] [PubMed]
10. Kittichotirat, W.; Bumgarner, R.; Chen, C. Evolutionary Divergence of *Aggregatibacter actinomycetemcomitans*. *J. Dent. Res.* **2016**, *95*, 94–101. [CrossRef]
11. Brogan, J.M.; Lally, E.T.; Poulsen, K.; Kilian, M.; Demuth, D.R. Regulation of *Actinobacillus actinomycetemcomitans* leukotoxin expression: Analysis of the promoter regions of leukotoxic and minimally leukotoxic strains. *Infect. Immun.* **1994**, *62*, 501–508. [CrossRef]
12. Haubek, D.; Poulsen, K.; Kilian, M. Microevolution and Patterns of Dissemination of the JP2 Clone of *Aggregatibacter* (*Actinobacillus*) *actinomycetemcomitans*. *Infect. Immun.* **2007**, *75*, 3080–3088. [CrossRef] [PubMed]
13. Khzam, N.; Miranda, L.A.; Kujan, O.; Shearston, K.; Haubek, D. Prevalence of the JP2 genotype of *Aggregatibacter actinomycetemcomitans* in the world population: A systematic review. *Clin. Oral Investig.* **2022**, *26*, 2317–2334. [CrossRef] [PubMed]
14. Mehta, J.; Eaton, C.; AlAmri, M.; Lin, G.; Nibali, L. The association between *Aggregatibacter actinomycetemcomitans* JP2 clone and periodontitis: A systematic review and meta-analysis. *J. Periodontal Res.* **2023**, *58*, 465–482. [CrossRef]
15. Johansson, A.; Claesson, R.; Åberg, C.H.; Haubek, D.; Oscarsson, J. The *cagE* gene sequence as a diagnostic marker to identify JP2 and non-JP2 highly leukotoxic *Aggregatibacter actinomycetemcomitans* serotype b strains. *J. Periodontal Res.* **2017**, *52*, 903–912. [CrossRef] [PubMed]
16. Johansson, A.; Claesson, R.; Åberg, C.H.; Haubek, D.; Lindholm, M.; Jasim, S.; Oscarsson, J. Genetic Profiling of *Aggregatibacter actinomycetemcomitans* Serotype B Isolated from Periodontitis Patients Living in Sweden. *Pathogens* **2019**, *8*, 153. [CrossRef] [PubMed]
17. Jensen, A.B.; Lund, M.; Nørskov-Lauritsen, N.; Johansson, A.; Claesson, R.; Reinholdt, J.; Haubek, D. Differential Cell Lysis Among Periodontal Strains of JP2 and Non-JP2 Genotype of *Aggregatibacter actinomycetemcomitans* Serotype B Is Not Reflected in Dissimilar Expression and Production of Leukotoxin. *Pathogens* **2019**, *8*, 211. [CrossRef] [PubMed]
18. Hritz, M.; Fisher, E.; Demuth, D.R. Differential regulation of the leukotoxin operon in highly leukotoxic and minimally leukotoxic strains of Actinobacillus actinomycetemcomitans. *Infect. Immun.* **1996**, *64*, 2724–2729. [CrossRef]
19. Sampathkumar, V.; Velusamy, S.K.; Godboley, D.; Fine, D.H. Increased leukotoxin production: Characterization of 100 base pairs within the 530 base pair leukotoxin promoter region of *Aggregatibacter actinomycetemcomitans*. *Sci. Rep.* **2017**, *7*, 1887. [CrossRef]

20. Claesson, R.; Chiang, H.M.; Lindholm, M.; Höglund Åberg, C.; Haubek, D.; Johansson, A.; Oscarsson, J. Characterization of *Aggregatibacter actinomycetemcomitans* Serotype b Strains with Five Different, Including Two Novel, Leukotoxin Promoter Structures. *Vaccines* **2020**, *8*, 398. [CrossRef]

21. Kolodrubetz, D.; Spitznagel, J.; Wang, B.; Phillips, L.H.; Jacobs, C.; Kraig, E. cis Elements and trans factors are both important in strain-specific regulation of the leukotoxin gene in Actinobacillus actinomycetemcomitans. *Infect. Immun.* **1996**, *64*, 3451–3460. [CrossRef]

22. Childress, C.; Feuerbacher, L.A.; Phillips, L.; Burgum, A.; Kolodrubetz, D. Mlc is a transcriptional activator with a key role in integrating cyclic AMP receptor protein and integration host factor regulation of leukotoxin RNA synthesis in *Aggregatibacter actinomycetemcomitans*. *J. Bacteriol.* **2013**, *195*, 2284–2297. [CrossRef]

23. Shakya, S.; Danshiitsoodol, N.; Noda, M.; Inoue, Y.; Sugiyama, M. 3-Phenyllactic acid generated in medicinal plant extracts fermented with plant-derived lactic acid bacteria inhibits the biofilm synthesis of *Aggregatibacter actinomycetemcomitans*. *Front. Microbiol.* **2022**, *13*, 991144. [CrossRef] [PubMed]

24. Fong, K.; Tang, H.; Brown, A.; Kieba, I.; Speicher, D.; Boesze-Battaglia, K.; Lally, E. *Aggregatibacter actinomycetemcomitans* leukotoxin is post-translationally modified by addition of either saturated or hydroxylated fatty acyl chains. *Mol. Oral Microbiol.* **2011**, *26*, 262–276. [CrossRef] [PubMed]

25. Balashova, N.V.; Diaz, R.; Balashov, S.V.; Crosby, J.A.; Kachlany, S.C. Regulation of *Aggregatibacter* (*Actinobacillus*) *actinomycetemcomitans* leukotoxin secretion by iron. *J. Bacteriol.* **2006**, *188*, 8658–8661. [CrossRef] [PubMed]

26. Tang, G.; Kawai, T.; Komatsuzawa, H.; Mintz, K.P. Lipopolysaccharides mediate leukotoxin secretion in *Aggregatibacter actino-mycetem-comitans*. *Mol. Oral Microbiol.* **2012**, *27*, 70–82. [CrossRef]

27. Johansson, A.; Claesson, R.; Hänström, L.; Kalfas, S. Serum-mediated release of leukotoxin from the cell surface of the periodontal pathogen *Actinobacillus actinomycetemcomitans*. *Eur. J. Oral Sci.* **2003**, *111*, 209–215. [CrossRef] [PubMed]

28. Johansson, A.; Hänström, L.; Kalfas, S. Inhibition of *Actinobacillus actinomycetemcomitans* leukotoxicity by bacteria from the subgingival flora. *Oral Microbiol. Immunol.* **2000**, *15*, 218–225. [CrossRef] [PubMed]

29. Johansson, A.; Claesson, R.; Belibasakis, G.; Makoveichuk, E.; Hänström, L.; Olivecrona, G.; Sandström, G.; Kalfas, S. Protease inhibitors, the responsible components for the serum-dependent enhancement of *Actinobacillus actinomycetemcomitans* leukotoxicity. *Eur. J. Oral. Sci.* **2001**, *109*, 335–341. [CrossRef]

30. Shah, H.N.; Bowden, G.H.; Hardie, J.M.; Williams, R.A.D. Comparison of the biochemical properties of *Bacteroides melaninogenicus* from human dental plaque and other sites. *J. Appl. Bacteriol.* **1976**, *41*, 473–492. [CrossRef]

31. Johansson, A.; Kalfas, S. Characterization of the proteinase-dependent cytotoxicity of *Porphyromonas gingivalis*. *Eur. J. Oral Sci.* **1998**, *106*, 863–871. [CrossRef]

32. Nørskov-Lauritsen, N.; Kilian, M. Reclassification of *Actinobacillus actinomycetemcomitans, Haemophilus aphrophilus, Haemophilus paraphrophilus* and *Haemophilus segnis* as *Aggregatibacter actinomycetemcomitans* gen. nov., comb. nov., Aggregatibacter aphrophilus comb. nov. and Aggregatibacter segnis comb. nov., and emended description of *Aggregatibacter aphrophilus* to include V factor-dependent and V factor-independent isolates. *Int. J. Syst. Evol. Microbiol.* **2006**, *56 Pt 9*, 2135–2146. [PubMed]

33. Tsuzukibashi, O.; Takada, K.; Saito, M.; Kimura, C.; Yoshikawa, T.; Makimura, M.; Hirasawa, M. A novel selective medium for isolation of *Aggregatibacter* (*Actinobacillus*) *actinomycetemcomitans*. *J. Periodontal Res.* **2008**, *43*, 544–548. [CrossRef] [PubMed]

34. Hunt, D.E.; Jones, J.V.; Dowell, V.R. Selective medium for the isolation of *Bacteroides gingivalis*. *J. Clin. Microbiol.* **1986**, *23*, 441–445. [CrossRef]

35. Gibbons, R.J.; Macdonald, J.B. Hemin and vitamin K compounds as required factors for the cultivation of certain strains of *Bacteroides melaninogenicus*. *J. Bacteriol.* **1960**, *80*, 164–170. [CrossRef] [PubMed]

36. Lamont, R.J.; Kuboniwa, M. The polymicrobial pathogenicity of *Porphyromonas gingivalis*. *Front. Oral Health* **2024**, *5*, 1404917. [CrossRef] [PubMed]

37. Spitznagel, J., Jr.; Kraig, E.; Kolodrubetz, D. Regulation of leukotoxin in leukotoxic and nonleukotoxic strains of *Actinobacillus actinomycetemcomitans*. *Infect. Immun.* **1991**, *59*, 1394–1401. [CrossRef]

38. Yang, H.W.; Asikainen, S.; Doğan, B.; Suda, R.; Lai, C.H. Relationship of *Actinobacillus actinomycetemcomitans* serotype b to aggressive periodontitis: Frequency in pure cultured isolates. *J. Periodontol.* **2004**, *75*, 592–599. [CrossRef]

39. Kelk, P.; Johansson, A.; Claesson, R.; Hanstrom, L.; Kalfas, S. Caspase 1 involvement in human monocyte lysis induced by *Actinobacillus actino-mycetemcomitans* leukotoxin. *Infect. Immun.* **2003**, *71*, 4448–4455. [CrossRef] [PubMed]

40. Asikainen, S.; Chen, C.; Slots, J. *Actinobacillus actinomycetemcomitans* genotypes in relation to serotypes and periodontal status. *Oral Microbiol. Immunol.* **1995**, *10*, 65–68. [CrossRef] [PubMed]

41. Haubek, D.; Ennibi, O.-K.; Poulsen, K.; Væth, M.; Poulsen, S.; Kilian, M. Risk of aggressive periodontitis in adolescent carriers of the JP2 clone of *Aggregatibacter* (*Actinobacillus*) *actinomycetemcomitans* in Morocco: A prospective longitudinal cohort study. *Lancet* **2008**, *371*, 237–242. [CrossRef]

42. Krueger, E.; Brown, A.C. *Aggregatibacter actinomycetemcomitans* leukotoxin: From mechanism to targeted anti-toxin therapeutics. *Mol. Oral Microbiol.* **2020**, *35*, 85–105. [CrossRef] [PubMed]

43. Johansson, A.; Kalfas, S. Virulence mechanisms of leukotoxin from *Aggregatibacter actinomycetem-comitans*. In *Oral Health Care, Prosthodontics, Periodontology, Biology, Research and Systemic Conditions*; IntechOpen: London, UK, 2012; Volume 2, pp. 165–192.

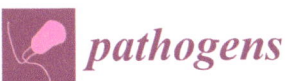

Review

The Trimeric Autotransporter Adhesin EmaA and Infective Endocarditis [†]

Keith P. Mintz [1,*], David R. Danforth [1] and Teresa Ruiz [2]

[1] Department of Microbiology and Molecular Genetics, University of Vermont, Burlington, VT 05405, USA; david.danforth@cuanschutz.edu

[2] Department of Molecular Physiology and Biophysics, University of Vermont, Burlington, VT 05405, USA; teresa.ruiz@uvm.edu

[*] Correspondence: keith.mintz@uvm.edu

[†] Dedicated to the memory of Javier Ruiz Rejas.

Abstract: Infective endocarditis (IE), a disease of the endocardial surface of the heart, is usually of bacterial origin and disproportionally affects individuals with underlying structural heart disease. Although IE is typically associated with Gram-positive bacteria, a minority of cases are caused by a group of Gram-negative species referred to as the HACEK group. These species, classically associated with the oral cavity, consist of bacteria from the genera *Haemophilus* (excluding *Haemophilus influenzae*), *Aggregatibacter*, *Cardiobacterium*, *Eikenella*, and *Kingella*. *Aggregatibacter actinomycetemcomitans*, a bacterium of the Pasteurellaceae family, is classically associated with Aggressive Periodontitis and is also concomitant with the chronic form of the disease. Bacterial colonization of the oral cavity serves as a reservoir for infection at distal body sites via hematological spreading. *A. actinomycetemcomitans* adheres to and causes disease at multiple physiologic niches using a diverse array of bacterial cell surface structures, which include both fimbrial and nonfimbrial adhesins. The nonfimbrial adhesin EmaA (extracellular matrix binding protein adhesin A), which displays sequence heterogeneity dependent on the serotype of the bacterium, has been identified as a virulence determinant in the initiation of IE. In this chapter, we will discuss the known biochemical, molecular, and structural aspects of this protein, including its interactions with extracellular matrix components and how this multifunctional adhesin may contribute to the pathogenicity of A. actinomycetemcomitans.

Keywords: bacterial adhesin; collagen interactions; electron tomography; 3D structure; biofilm

Citation: Mintz, K.P.; Danforth, D.R.; Ruiz, T. The Trimeric Autotransporter Adhesin EmaA and Infective Endocarditis. *Pathogens* **2024**, *13*, 99. https://doi.org/10.3390/pathogens13020099

Academic Editor: Daniel H. Fine

Received: 11 December 2023
Revised: 18 January 2024
Accepted: 22 January 2024
Published: 23 January 2024

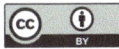
1. Infectious Endocarditis

Infective endocarditis (IE) is initiated by the exposure of the underlying extracellular matrix of the cardiac valve surface due to physiological perturbation of the valve. Damage to the endothelium and exposure of the matrix leads to the binding and activation of circulating platelets, resulting in fibrin deposition, the product of blood coagulation. In the presence of transient bacteremia, bacteria can bind to the underlying matrix proteins or platelets to ultimately form an infective mass or "vegetation" composed of serum components and bacteria, which disrupts the normal flow of the blood through the heart [1].

The majority of bacterial IE cases are attributable to Gram-positive Streptococci, Staphylococci, and Enterococci species [1]. However, in up to 6% of the cases, the HACEK group of bacteria has been identified as the causative agents [2]. These species, classically associated with the oral cavity, consist of bacteria from the genera *Haemophilus* (excluding *Haemophilus* influenzae), *Aggregatibacter*, *Cardiobacterium*, *Eikenella*, and *Kingella* [3,4]. IE caused by the HACEK group of bacteria affects younger individuals and is more likely to be community-acquired than nosocomial [2,5]. These microorganisms can be detected using modern blood culture methods [6], although they may also cause "culture-negative" endocarditis, an infection from which no organisms can be isolated [5]. Among these

Gram-negative organisms, *Haemophilus* and *Aggregatibacter* were the predominant genera in causing IE [7,8].

2. *A. actinomycetemcomitans* Physiology

A. actinomycetemcomitans are coccobacillus with shapes ranging from nearly cocci (0.5 μm × 0.6 μm) to bacilli (0.5 μm × 1.5 μm), depending on the culture conditions and bacterial growth phases. In contrast to most Gram-negative bacteria, which display smooth or flat outer membrane surfaces (e.g., Enterobacteriaceae), the outer membrane of the Pasteurellaceae and Moraxellaceae families displays a convoluted or corrugated morphology [9–11] (Figure 1A). The topography of the outer membrane of *A. actinomycetemcomitans* was described by utilizing 3D electron tomography of negatively stained bacterial preparations and using atomic force microscopy [9]. Analysis of the section profiles provided detailed information about the dimensions of the bacterial cell surface convolutions: the grooves were 12.4 ± 1.3 nm in depth and approximately 100–150 nm in diameter with a distance between grooves ranging from 65 to 165 nm. The outer membrane convolutions of *A. actinomycetemcomitans*, however, do not mirror the topography of the inner membrane, which presented a flat appearance, lacking convolutions (Figure 1B,C). The greater outer membrane surface area afforded by the convolutions may represent a selective advantage in nutrient acquisition for *A. actinomycetemcomitans* in the oral cavity. Furthermore, the dissimilarity between the inner and outer membranes may impose restrictions in the secretion and presentation of outer membrane proteins on the bacterial cell surface.

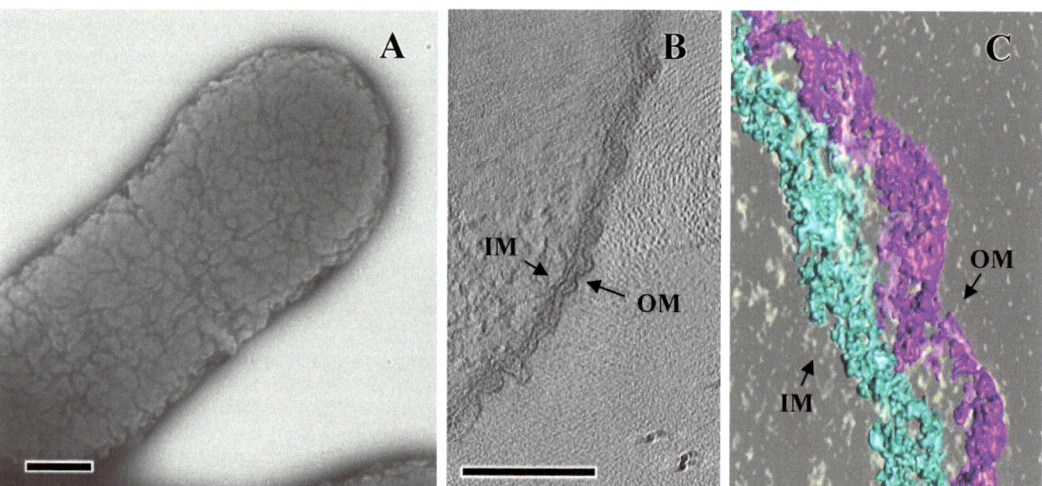

Figure 1. Bacterial cell surface of *A. actinomycetemcomitans*: (**A**) transmission electron micrograph of whole-mount preparations. (**B**) Central slice of a tomogram of ultrathin sections after high-pressure freezing and freeze substitution. (**C**) Segmentation of a small area of the inner (IM) and outer (OM) membranes from the tomogram. Bar, 100 nm. Adapted from [9].

The rugose morphology is attributed to the presence of a large (141 kDa) inner membrane protein, Morphogenesis protein C (MorC), that was first identified in *A. actinomycetemcomitans* and named for its effect on the outer membrane morphology, as visualized using transmission electron microscopy [10]. The absence of MorC in the cell membrane of *A. actinomycetemcomitans* results in a bacterium with a smooth outer membrane appearance when visualized using 2D electron microscopy [9,10]. The wild-type bacterial cell exhibits a higher curvature of the outer membrane and a periplasmic space with a two-fold larger volume/area ratio when compared to the MorC mutant, as revealed using 3D electron tomography and atomic force microscopy [9]. In addition to changes in the outer membrane morphology, the inactivation of *morC* also resulted in a reduction in leukotoxin secretion in *A. actinomycetemcomitans* [10,12]. Concomitant with a reduction in leukotoxin is a reduction in cell size, an increase in autoaggregation, [10] and an increased sensitivity to membrane-destabilizing agents [13]. These pleiotropic effects are associated with changes in the abundance of multiple proteins in the membrane, including chaperones, oxidative stress response proteins, and components of the fimbrial secretion system [14]. A reduction in fimbrial subunit secretion results in a decreased number of fimbriae observed on the surface of the mutant strain and in an altered biofilm microcolony architecture [13].

In other organisms, the MorC homologs are involved in autotransporter protein incorporation into the outer membrane. However, in *A. actinomycetemcomitans*, there appears to be no impact on the autotransporter abundance in the *morC* mutant strains [12].

3. *A. actinomycetemcomitans* Interactions with Collagen

Bacterial colonization of the oral cavity serves as a reservoir for infection at distal body sites via hematological spreading, and poor dental health is a known risk factor for IE [15]. As stated above, IE is initiated due to the exposure of the extracellular matrix underlying the endothelium of the cardiac valve. The major component of the extracellular matrix is collagen, present in 28 different types. All collagens are composed of three polypeptide chains coiled around each other into a triple helical conformation [16]. The most abundant types of collagens include types I-III, V, and XI, which are categorized as banded or fiber-forming collagens [16]. Type IV collagen, which differs in structure from the fiber-forming collagens, is the major component of the basement membrane [16]. Less abundant non-collagenous proteins include the highly glycosylated proteins laminin and fibronectin, proteoglycans containing protein-bound glycosaminoglycan chains, and unique proteins found associated with specific tissues [17].

A common theme among both Gram-positive and Gram-negative pathogens is the ability to bind to proteins of the extracellular matrix [18]. *A. actinomycetemcomitans* has been found in the deep connective tissue, in contact with the collagen fibers of the periodontium of individuals afflicted with the aggressive form of the disease [19,20], which suggests that this bacterium interacts with collagen fibers. Studies indicate that *A. actinomycetemcomitans* binds to multiple types of immobilized, acid-solubilized collagen (types I–III and V) but not basement membrane type IV [21]. Furthermore, this organism also binds to fibronectin and laminin [21,22], additional components of the ECM.

4. Extracellular Matrix Protein Adhesin A (EmaA)

Bacterial outer membrane proteins were found to be essential to the interactions with the extracellular matrix [21], and several genes associated with binding to ECM proteins were identified following the screening of a transposon mutant library [21]. Disruption of a novel 5895 base pair open reading frame was identified in mutants that demonstrated a significant decrease in type V collagen binding, the collagen type found in abundance in cardiac tissue [23]. The gene product was deduced to code for a 1965 amino acid protein (202 kDa). Antibodies specific to the protein confirmed the presence of a protein of this mass associated with the outer membrane of *A. actinomycetemcomitans* [24]. The gene was designated as <u>e</u>xtracellular <u>m</u>atrix protein <u>a</u>dhesin A (*emaA*).

The EmaA protein is unique to *A. actinomycetemcomitans* [24]. However, sequence analysis suggested that EmaA belongs to a class of nonfimbrial oligomeric coiled-coil adhesins [25] or trimeric autotransporter adhesins [26], a subclass of type V secreted proteins [27] of which YadA of the *Yersinia* species is the prototypic protein. The monomer molecular mass of 202 kDa makes EmaA one of the larger members of this family of proteins, compared with YadA (42 kDa), UspA1 (83 kDa), UspA2 (60 kDa), Hia (114 kDa), and BadA (340 kDa) [28–31]. In contrast to YadA, UspA1/UspA2, and BadA, which are expressed at high densities on the bacterial surface [32], EmaA is sparsely distributed on the surface and can be more easily found at the apical end of the bacterium [33–36] (Figure 2A).

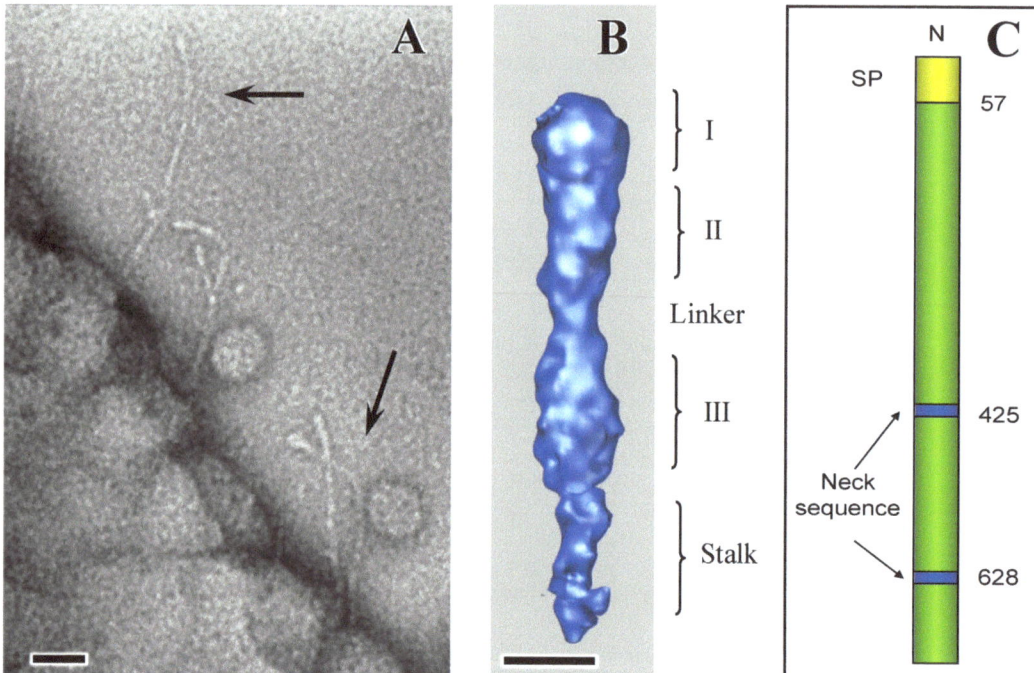

Figure 2. EmaA structure: (**A**) transmission electron micrograph of EmaA appendages acquired from a whole-mount preparation of a nonfimbriated bacterium showing the typical bends of the adhesin. Bar, 20 nm. Black arrows point to the most characteristic bend. (**B**) Surface representation of the 3D structure of the functional domain of EmaA obtained using electron tomography and subvolume averaging. (**C**) Cartoon with the corresponding amino acids. Only the head (57–627) and portion of the stalk domains are presented in (**B**) and (**C**). I, II and III represent subdomains SI-SIII; N: NH₂-terminus of the polypeptide; SP: signal peptide; 57 is the start of the polypeptide after cleavage of the signal peptide; 425 and 628 represent the start amino acids of the neck sequences. Bar, 5 nm. Adapted from [35].

The prototypical EmaA structure consists of three identical subunits, assembled on the bacterial outer membrane, which form antenna-like structures of 3–5 nm in diameter, projecting at least 150 nm away from the bacterial surface (Figure 2A) [34]. These structures are absent in strains following the disruption of the gene sequence [34]. Three-dimensional structures of the canonical serotype b EmaA, using by 3D electron tomography and image processing, indicated that the antenna-like structure is composed of multiple domains, including an ellipsoidal-shaped head domain at the distal end of the structure, and a long stalk, which is connected to a flexible neck region [34]. The collagen-binding activity is attributed to the head domain, which corresponds to amino acids 57–627 of the monomer and encompasses the most apical 30 nm of the antennae-like structures [33,35,36]. The head domain is composed of three subdomains: a globular subdomain I (amino acids 57–225) with a diameter of ~5 nm; a cylindrical subdomain II (~4.4 × 5.8 nm, amino acids 225–433); a narrow linker with a diameter of ~3 nm; followed by another cylindrical subdomain III (~4.6 × 6.6 nm, amino acids 433–627) [33,36] (Figure 2B,C). Adjacent to the head domain is a rod-like stalk that adopts either a straight or a bent conformation at various positions along the length of the stalk structure [34,35]. The flexibility in the angular orientation of the stalk relative to the head domain is suggested to be required for optimal positioning of the functional domain to interact with collagen fibers [35].

5. *EmaA* Interactions with Collagen

The collagen-binding properties of EmaA were investigated utilizing acid-solubilized collagen either bound to plastic wells or embedded into an artificial basement membrane extracellular environment [37]. Since these preparations do not adequately represent the native collagen of animal tissue, isolated mouse heart valves were utilized as a representative of the in vivo conditions. The extracellular matrix (ECM) protein composition and stratification of the heart valves are conserved between humans and rabbits [38]. In this model system, both the wild-type and an isogenic *emaA* mutant bacteria had similar affinity for the tissue when the endothelium was left intact. However, following enzymatic removal of the endothelium, the mutant showed a 5–10-fold reduction in binding to the exposed underlying ECM, as compared with the wild-type bacteria. This finding indicates that EmaA plays a major role in the interaction of *A. actinomycetemcomitans* with native collagen.

The association of EmaA binding to native collagen and potentially binding to the heart valves in vivo was investigated using a well-established rabbit model for endocarditis [39]. In this model, a catheter is introduced from the carotid artery to past the aortic valve to induce minor damage in the valve tissue, resulting in the formation of sterile vegetation composed mostly of platelets and fibrin, in the absence of bacteria. Bacteria are typically injected into the animal 48 h post catheterization. Visible vegetation was formed in all three rabbits 72 h after inoculation with 1.5 or 15×10^7 CFU of the bacterium. However, few, if any, bacteria were recovered from the vegetation. This is in sharp contrast to the high recovery rate typically obtained for Streptococci [40] and Staphylococci [41,42]. Taken together, these observations suggested that *A. actinomycetemcomitans* directly attaches to the damaged valve tissue rather than to the vegetation. In subsequent experiments, the rabbits were either singly or repeatedly inoculated with the bacterium at different time points either immediately or/and 48 h after catheterization [38]. The animals were euthanized ~3 h after the second inoculation and the entire aortic valves, as well as any visible vegetation, were isolated for bacterial recovery. The vegetation appeared smaller than in the prior experiment and *A. actinomycetemcomitans* was recovered, supporting the higher affinity of the bacterium for ECM molecules over the proteins composing the vegetation (e.g., fibrin).

In vivo competition studies were conducted using equal inoculum of wild-type and *emaA* isogenic mutants utilizing the modified time of inoculation in the rabbit model system. The rabbits were euthanized, and the aortic valve leaflets and any visible vegetation were removed, homogenized, and cultured onto growth media with and without the presence of antibiotics [38]. The competition index (CI) was calculated, and the value was determined to an order of magnitude less than 1 (1 indicating no difference in competitiveness between the mutant and wild-type strains). The data suggest that the *emaA* mutant colonized the traumatized heart valve approximately 10-fold less effectively than the wild-type strain, suggesting that this adhesin is a virulence determinant of *A. actinomycetemcomitans* involved in the initiation of infective endocarditis.

The fine structural details of the interaction of EmaA and collagen were analyzed using 3D electron tomography and image processing techniques and using reconstituted bacterial adhesin/small collagen fiber complexes (Figure 3A) [43]. Analysis of the extracted subvolumes containing the EmaA functional domain interacting with collagen (Figure 3B) indicated that although all three subdomains (SI, SII, and SIII) of EmaA mediate the interaction, SII and SIII are more often found bound to collagen. Subdomain SII showed stronger interactions with the collagen fiber than subdomain SIII, and occasionally the tip of the apical domain SI was involved in the interactions [43]. The number of EmaA adhesins exhibiting a bend between subdomains SII and SIII (the linker region) in the bound state is higher than for the unliganded adhesin [36,43]. This bend is evocative of the one observed in the G162S EmaA substitution mutant (Subdomain SI) that could not bind collagen efficiently [33,35], which indicates that the G162S mutant adhesin is locked into a bound conformation. Furthermore, EmaA binds to collagen fibrils in a different manner than Gram-positive bacteria following either the dock, lock, and latch model [44] or the collagen hug model [45]. The EmaA/collagen interaction agrees more closely with the model proposed for the binding of YadA to collagen [46]. In this model, the interaction is governed by the electrostatic forces between the collagen fibrils and the charged residues of the trimeric YadA surface.

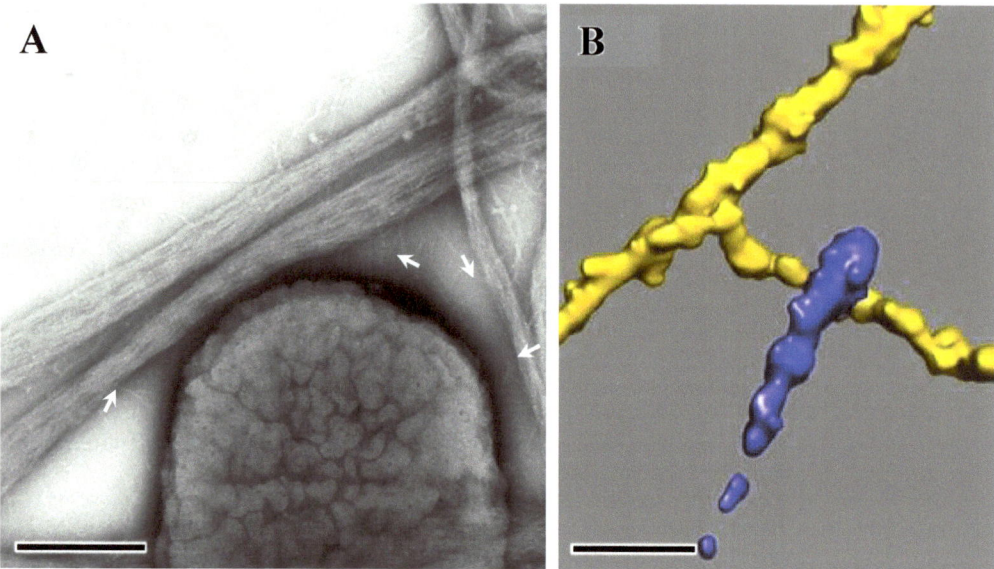

Figure 3. Interactions of *A. actinomycetemcomitans* with collagen visualized using electron microscopy. (**A**) Low-magnification micrograph. Arrows point to the EmaA adhesin. Bar, 0.25 nm. (**B**) Segmentation of the 3D reconstructions of the functional domain of EmaA bound to collagen. Collagen (yellow) and EmaA (blue). Bar, 10 nm. Adapted from [43].

6. Secretion of EmaA and Cell Surface Expression

Proteins either targeted to the membrane or secreted into the environment are transported from the site of synthesis in the cytoplasm (by ribosomes) through the inner membrane and the periplasm and toward the outer membrane or the extracellular space. Therefore, Gram-negative bacteria utilize multiple protein secretion machineries, termed secretion systems, for transport [27,47,48]. Secretion systems are composed of protein complexes responsible for facilitating the transport of polypeptides across membranes and the periplasmic space. In the general secretory pathway, proteins are transported across the inner membrane by the Sec translocon and contain a signal peptide that indicates the protein is to be released into the periplasmic space [48]. Concomitant with translocation to the periplasm, the signal peptide is cleaved by a signal peptidase [49]. Periplasmic chaperones protect the protein from degradation on its way to the outer membrane [50].

Proteins secreted via the type V secretion system, which is dependent on the Sec translocon, encode all of the information necessary to catalyze transport across the outer membrane, giving them the name "autotransporters" [27]. This is accomplished by two main domains: the translocator domain (also known as the beta domain) and the passenger domain. The translocator domain may be composed of a single polypeptide (as is the case for monomeric autotransporters, type V_a) or three polypeptides in the case of trimeric autotransporters, type V_c [51]. In both cases, the translocator domain inserts into the outer membrane and catalyzes the transport of the passenger domain through the outer membrane with assistance from the beta-barrel assembly module (BAM) complex [27,52,53]. After transport through the pore, the passenger domain is exposed to the extracellular environment. This process requires no energy and is independent of other protein factors [27].

The signal peptide of the majority of secreted proteins is found in the amino terminus of the protein. These peptides exhibit limited sequence similarity but are composed of clusters of charged or hydrophobic amino acids that are required for interaction with the protein secretory machinery in the cytoplasm [54]. Typical signal peptides are divided into three regions, containing a variable number of amino acids. An uncommon number of charged amino acids, located following the start methionine, constitute the N region, followed by a region of hydrophobic amino acids (H region) adjacent to a sequence containing the cleavage site for the inner-membrane-bound signal peptidase (C region). The later region contains small, slightly polar amino acids at the -1 and -3 positions of the signal peptide cleavage site [55].

A typical signal peptide contains between 15 and 25 amino acids [54]. However, algorithms predicted a signal peptidase cleavage site between amino acids 56 and 57 of the EmaA sequence [56]. Studies utilizing signal peptide fusion constructs with alkaline phosphatase lacking a functional signal peptide demonstrated that the first 56 amino acids acted as a signal to target the protein for translocation across the inner membrane [56] (Figure 4). Proteins containing long signal peptides are usually found in eukaryotes; however, they have also been observed in viral and other bacterial autotransporter proteins [57,58]. The individual EmaA monomers are transported to the Sec translocon via a chaperone-dependent pathway, and a specific sequence within the extended signal peptide is required for the proper secretion of EmaA at elevated temperatures that mimic the physiological temperatures the bacterium encounters during inflammation [56,59]. Following translocation and cleavage of the signal peptide, the carboxyl termini of the three EmaA monomers interact with the inner leaflet of the outer membrane and form a transmembrane pore for the presentation of an intact structure on the surface of the bacteria (Figure 4).

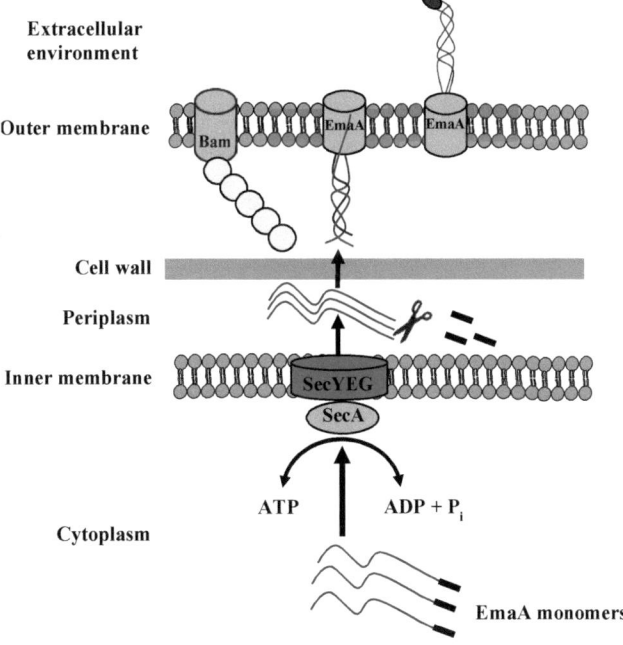

Figure 4. Type V secretion system of a trimeric autotransporter. Bam: β-barrel assembly machinery; EmaA: extracellular matrix protein adhesin A; SecYEG: complex of the general secretion system; SecA: ATPase motor protein associated with SecYEG.

7. *A. actinomycetemcomitans* Serotypes and the Molecular Heterogeneity of EmaA

Bacterial serotypes are dependent on the composition of the lipopolysaccharide (LPS) expressed on the surface of the bacterium. Seven serotypes (a–f) have been identified for *A. actinomycetemcomitans* [60]. Phylogenetic analysis of the *emaA* DNA sequences revealed that *A. actinomycetemcomitans* strains can be segregated cleanly into two clusters based upon serotype [61]: one cluster comprises serotypes b and c, while the remaining serotypes comprise the other [37]. Perhaps not coincidentally, EmaA is expressed as two isoforms, which are correlated with the serotype of the bacterium (Figure 5). Serotypes b and c express the cognate full-length isoform (b-EmaA, 202 kDa monomers), whereas serotypes a and d express an intermediate isoform, which is a shorter variant of EmaA containing a 279-amino-acid deletion (a-EmaA, 173 kDa monomers) [37]. Moreover, in some strains, point mutations in the DNA sequence result in truncated proteins, which are not expressed on the surface of the bacterium [37]. Both molecular isoforms of the protein (full-length and intermediate) bind to collagen [62].

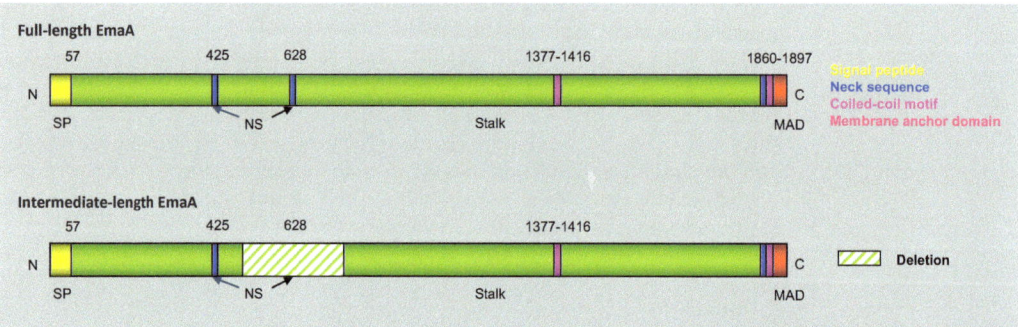

Figure 5. Molecular forms of EmaA proteins. Two forms of EmaA are shown: full-length and intermediate, which lacks 279 amino acids after the first neck sequence at amino acid 425. The full-length EmaA was found mainly in serotypes b and c while the intermediate EmaA was only present in serotypes d and a. Numbers correspond to amino acid number of the predicted protein. N: NH$_2$-terminus of the polypeptide; SP: signal peptide; MAD: membrane anchor domain; C: COOH-terminus of the polypeptide. The whole polypeptide is represented as green with specific motifs colored as indicated in the legend.

LPS is synthesized utilizing a well-defined sequence of enzymatic reactions, which include enzymes associated with sugar synthesis, an ABC sugar transport protein (wzt), and an O-antigen ligase (waaL) [63] (Figure 6). The enzymes in this pathway have been identified in *A. actinomycetemcomitans* [64–66]. Interestingly, genetic and pharmacological studies disrupting O-PS synthesis in both the serotype a and b strains revealed changes in the mass of the protein monomers (as visualized by a change in the electrophoretic mobility of the monomers) and a reduction in the amount of EmaA associated with the membrane [64]. In addition, a lectin specific to one of the serotype b O-PS sugars was demonstrated to bind to the protein [64]. These experiments suggest that: (1) EmaA is a glycoprotein modified with the sugars associated with the O-antigen and (2) EmaA utilizes the same enzymatic mechanism for post translational modification as the O-antigen does for conjugation to the LPS core oligosaccharide.

Additional experiments [67] have clearly demonstrated that *A. actinomycetemcomitans waaL* is required for the collagen-binding activity associated with EmaA and suggests that the ligase activity is important for conferring changes in the structure of this adhesin important for collagen binding.

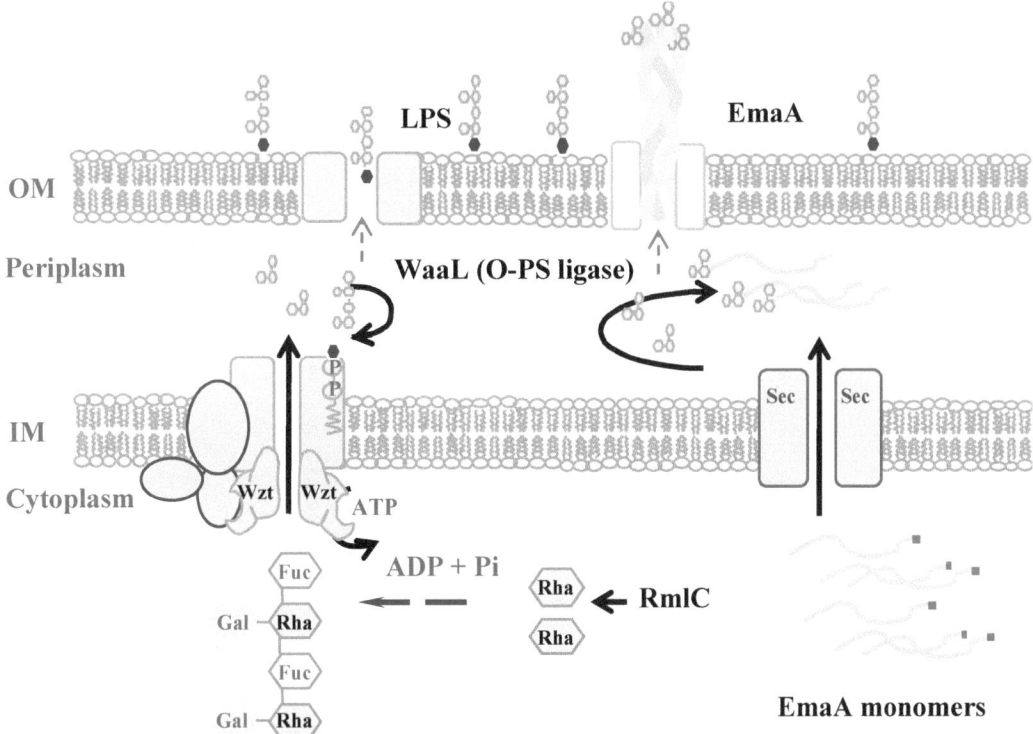

Figure 6. Model for the hypothetical glycosylation pathway for the trimeric autotransporter adhesin EmaA. IM: inner membrane; OM: outer membrane; LPS: lipopolysaccharide; Fuc: fucose, Rha: rhamnose; Gal: galactose; Wzt: ABC sugar transport protein; RmlC: rhamnose epimerase; WaaL: O-antigen ligase.

Genetic and biochemical studies suggest that glycosylation is required for collagen binding and the stability of the protein [64,68]. A structural analysis using 3D electron tomography, iterative multireference alignment algorithms and 3D classification [62,69–72] of glycosylation-deficient mutants enables the determination of the structural role of this modification in collagen binding. The 3D structures of the functional domain of EmaA from mutant strains with glycosylation disrupted at two different stages—the *rmlc* mutant, which does not express the rhamnose epimerase, and the *waaL* mutant, which lacks the O-antigen ligase—were analyzed [70,73,74]. The structural studies of the EmaA adhesins expressed in the mutant strains suggest that glycosylation is important to maintaining the overall structural stability of the adhesin and, specifically, the proper conformation of the functional domain. Glycosylation-deficient mutant strains exhibit far fewer EmaA adhesins on the bacterial surface than the wild-type strain, which is consistent with previous protein immunoblot and mRNA expression analysis results [64,75]. In addition, the adhesins seem to "hug" the cell surface, which might ensue from modifications to the electrostatic properties of both surfaces, thus supporting YadA-like interactions with collagen. The averages from all the groups demonstrate that the mutant strain adhesins lack the three-fold symmetry characteristic of the wild-type strain and manifest a high degree of flexibility. An apparent difference between the mutant and wild-type adhesins is the overall reduced density in the structures expressed in the glycosylation mutant strains.

Subtomograms encompassing the EmaA functional domain of the *rmlc* mutant strain were separated into eight subgroups (G1–G8), with memberships ranging from 18% to 6% [70,74]. The EmaAs from this glycosylation-deficient strain exhibit reduced structural stability and clearly differ from the wild-type strain (Figure 7). Groups G4, G6, and G8 exhibit extremely low density in subdomain SIII and the stalk region, while in groups G1 and G3, the stalk is the main affected region. Only groups G2, G5, and G7 present complete functional domains comparable to those observed in wild-type EmaA [33,36,69]. However, all groups manifest a certain degree of curvature and/or bends (kinks) localized close to the linker region, either between subdomain SII and the linker or between the linker and subdomain SIII. In addition, when the structures present a complete functional domain, subdomain SIII consistently has a smaller diameter size, which can be interpreted as a reduction in either the mass or stability of the protein conformation. Similar overall characteristics were observed when analyzing subtomograms containing the EmaA functional domain of the *waaL* mutant strain, which were separated into eight subgroups (G1–G8), with memberships ranging from 25% to 6% [73,74]. With the exception of G7, all other subgroups have a strong curvature along the whole length of the functional domain (Figure 8). In most of the subgroups, subdomain SI has a larger diameter than in the wild-type strain, while the density of subdomain SIII appears weaker. In addition, a large percentage of the mutant adhesins display a strong curvature along the whole length of the functional domain and exhibit bends in places beyond the characteristic bend of the wild-type strain at the linker region [74]. The observed subtle bend between subdomains SI and SII (noticeable in G3 and G8) is reminiscent of the structural changes observed in a different G162S substitution mutant strain that exhibits greatly reduced collagen-binding activity [33,35,36,74]. Thus, the observed structural differences indicate that the lack of glycans reduces the stability of EmaA and prevents it from adopting the proper fold necessary to correctly express a functional structure capable of binding collagen. Moreover, the partial glycosylation in the *rmlC* mutant adhesins (presence of fucose) [68] has a greater impact on the structural integrity of the functional domain than the absence of ligase in the *waaL* mutant adhesins [74].

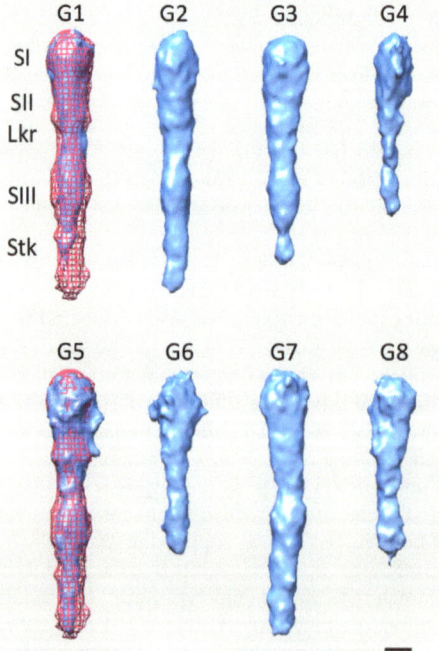

Figure 7. Surface representations of the EmaA averages of subgroups G1–G8 from *rmlC* mutant strains [70,74]. Mesh: wild-type EmaA structure; EmaA subdomains: SI–SIII; Lkr: linker region; Stk: stalk region. Bar, 3 nm.

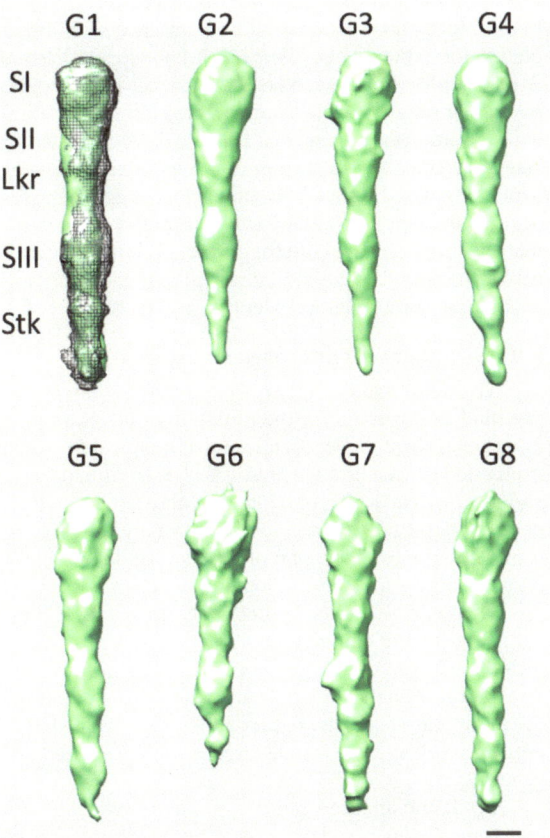

Figure 8. Surface representations of the EmaA averages of subgroups G1–G8 from *waaL* mutant strains [73,74]. Mesh: wild-type EmaA structure; EmaA subdomains: SI–SIII; Lkr: linker region; Stk: stalk region. Bar, 3 nm.

8. EmaA and Biofilm Formation

EmaA, originally identified as a collagen-binding adhesin, has been recently implicated in biofilm biogenesis. The absence of the protein results in strains with reduced biofilm potential, as shown in multiple fimbriated and nonfimbriated strains [76]. The lack of EmaA leads to changes in the cell density of the microcolonies formed during biofilm biogenesis, which suggests that EmaA plays an important role in mediating cell-to-cell interactions. EmaA-mediated biofilm formation is independent of the glycosylation state and the precise 3D structure of the protein, which differs from the requirements demonstrated for the collagen-binding activity of the cognate full-length isoform but more closely resembles the requirements of the shorter a-EmaA isoform [33,35,36,43]. This implies that the mechanisms governing the role of EmaA in biofilm formation and collagen binding differ [76].

Cells formed a diminished biofilm in strains lacking both fimbriae and EmaA [76]. It was hypothesized that a functional overlap or redundancy with either Aae or ApiA/Omp100 may explain these results. Epithelial cell adhesin (Aae) is a monomeric autotransporter with a mass of 130 kDa [77,78]. Whereas, ApiA/Omp100, a trimeric autotransporter with a monomeric molecular mass of 37 kDa, is a multifunctional adhesin associated with collagen binding, epithelial cell invasion, and resistance to serum killing [79,80].

The validity of the hypothesis was addressed by generating single and double mutant strains to investigate the contribution of ApiA/Omp100 and Aae to biofilm formation [81].

In the strains expressing fimbriae, the absence of ApiA/Omp100 and/or Aae did not impact biofilm formation. However, in the absence of fimbriae and EmaA, only Aae mediated biofilm formation. ApiA/Omp100 did not appear to contribute to the biofilm formation in *A. actinomycetemcomitans*. Nonetheless, when *aae* and *apiA/omp100* were expressed in *E. coli*, both strains demonstrated comparable biofilm formation but to a lesser degree compared with the strain expressing *emaA*. These data suggested that the contribution of EmaA and Aae to biofilm formation is highly dependent on the genetic background of the strains expressing the adhesins. The data further suggest the existence of a hierarchical functional order of these protein adhesins in biofilm formation: fimbriae (the longest of the adhesins) make primary contact with the surface, followed by the increased aggregation of bacterial cells as mediated by EmaA, culminating in more efficient adherence to the surface on the part of Aae and to a lesser extent (if any) on the part of ApiA/Omp100.

9. Transcriptional Control of *emaA* Expression

The adaptation of organisms to varying environmental or physiological niches is essential to survival. For the initiation of infection under the specific conditions inside a particular host niche, bacteria must adapt to the environment by reprogramming the expression of specific gene products. The environmental changes experienced by *A. actinomycetemcomitans* during oral infection and dissemination in the blood initiate the induction or repression of the expression of EmaA and other surface proteins. This modulation of expression is most likely part of a global regulatory reprogramming that leads to enhanced bacterial fitness for colonization of these disparate tissues.

The DNA sequence immediately upstream of the translational start site of *emaA* is sufficient for the complementation of *emaA* mutants [35,76]. This region of the DNA includes a 339 bp of the 3′ end of the CoA ligase gene based on sequence homology [24,76]. Truncation of the CoA ligase sequence, which resulted in a sequence containing only the intergenic sequence, reduced the promoter activity. This finding suggested that the regulatory elements for *emaA* expression are located within the 3′ end of the CoA ligase gene [82].

CpxR and an ArcA-binding sequence were identified using in silico analysis of the intergenic region, based on *E. coli* consensus sequences [82]. CpxR represents the response regulator for the *E. coli*/CpxAR two-component signaling system. Under stress conditions, misfolded envelope proteins accumulate, leading to the autophosphorylation of CpxA, a histidine kinase, that transfers the phosphate group to CpxR, resulting in the upregulation of a series of chaperonins and proteases that either degrade or refold the misfolded proteins, lessening envelope stress [83,84]. Furthermore, CpxR, in concert with the σ^E envelope stress response, contributes to the regulation of the periplasmic chaperone system [83–86]. In *E. coli*, this stress response is coupled with surface sensing and is demonstrated to control genes involved in adhesion and biofilm formation [83,87–91]. Thus, these systems may assist in the folding and secretion of the EmaA adhesin [82]. Over-expression of *cpxR* (in the absence of the CpxA kinase) reduces the amount of EmaA synthesized, which suggested that, at relatively high concentrations, *cpxR* downregulates EmaA expression [82]. Therefore, *cpxR* may act as a repressor instead of an activator under the growth conditions used in this study.

ArcA is the DNA-binding response regulator of the two-component regulatory system ArcAB, which regulates the adaptation of the organism to respiratory growth conditions and oxygen tension [92–95]. Under anaerobic or microaerobic respiratory conditions, ArcB, a transmembrane sensor kinase, undergoes autophosphorylation and coordinates changes in gene expression in response to changes in the respiratory and fermentative state of the cell [93,96]. The environmental niches occupied by *A. actinomycetemcomitans* during disease within or outside of the oral cavity, where EmaA is important to tissue colonization [38], reflect conditions that most likely regulate gene expression. In experiments resulting in the over-expression of the protein or genetic inactivation of *arcA*, a significant reduction in the amount of EmaA synthesized and the mass of the biofilm formed was observed [82]. Dual activation and repression by ArcA have also been reported in other bacterial species [97].

An *emaA* mutant strain, against the same fimbriated background, was observed to have a lesser effect on biofilm formation than the *arcA* mutant strain [76]. This suggests that the inactivation of *arcA* may impact other adhesins involved in biofilm formation. ArcA has been shown to regulate biofilm formation in several other species of bacteria [97–99]. The data suggest that ArcA acts primarily as a positive regulator of *emaA* transcription. This regulation may be mediated by either the binding of ArcA directly to the DNA or indirectly by competing with a negative regulator in response to changes in the environment.

Over-expression of two other transcriptional regulators (OxyR and DeoR) also reduced the expression of EmaA; however, little effect was detected when the same plasmids were expressed in *E. coli*. OxyR, the hydrogen peroxide stress response regulator, activates genes in the oxidative stress response system in *E. coli* [100], which regulates the surface proteins associated with an altered colony morphology and auto-aggregation [101]. OxyR is suggested to be involved in the regulation of the fimbrial secretion apparatus [102] and the autotransporter adhesin ApiA in *A. actinomycetemcomitans* [103]. DeoR regulates nucleotide catabolism and toxin production in *E. coli* [104]. The changes in *emaA* synthesis, based on excess production of specific transcription factors, do not necessarily correlate with a direct regulation by any of the proposed trans-acting regulatory elements [105]. The *A. actinomycetemcomitans* regulons are still unknown, and these proteins may interact with a large array of genes, including genes of other transcription factors, forming a network regulatory cascade that can indirectly change the expression level of a myriad of different target genes.

The minimal sequence necessary from which transcription can be initiated has been elucidated, and potential binding sites for trans-acting regulatory factors, such as CpxR and ArcA, have been deduced [82]. Interestingly, the *emaA* promoter region resembles the promoters of other major virulence adhesins of *A. actinomycetemcomitans*, including *flp*, *aae*, and *apiA* [82]. Based on these observations, it is suggested that these transcriptional regulators are involved in coordinate regulation of the adhesins required for *A. actinomycetemcomitans* colonization and pathogenesis.

10. Summary and Conclusions

Adhesion and tissue colonization are crucial phases during the infective process. Bacterial adhesion to extracellular matrix (ECM) proteins is a paradigm used by many pathogens for colonization and the tropism of infections. *A. actinomycetemcomitans* is typically found within the connective tissue of the periodontium in contact with collagen fibers in individuals with periodontitis [19,20,106]. The presence of bacteria in the connective tissue suggests that this organism establishes a reservoir for the continuous release of bacteria for re-infection of the gingival pocket or for the transient bacteremia responsible for systemic infections. This hypothesis is supported by the observations that the bacterium binds to the exposed underlying connective tissue of damaged heart valves and forms vegetation that alters the blood flow around the valve, leading to the development of endocarditis [5,107].

A. actinomycetemcomitans expresses multiple proteins associated with adhesion that are vital for colonization and contribute to its virulence [14,21,35,77,108,109]. These adhesins function hierarchically in biofilm formation: fimbriae (the longest of the adhesins) make primary contact with the surface, followed by enhanced binding and increased aggregation of the bacterial cells, as mediated by the extracellular matrix protein adhesin A (EmaA), and culminating in more specific adherence to targeted surfaces on the part of Aae and ApiA/Omp100 [76,81,110].

EmaA, the largest autotransporter protein of *A. actinomycetemcomitans*, is required for collagen binding, biofilm formation, and cell-to-cell interaction [24,36,38,76]. Three identical EmaA monomers form visible antenna-like appendages that extend 150 nm away from the bacterial surface [34,35]. The functional domain, subdivided into three subdomains (SI-SIII), is located at the distal end of the adhesin and mediates the adhesin/collagen interaction [33,35,36,43]. Moreover, EmaA is modified by a novel glycosylation mechanism involving the sugars and enzymes associated with the O-polysaccharide region of the lipopolysaccharide [64,67,68]. This post translational modification increases the stability of the adhesin and promotes a structural conformation required for collagen binding [70,73,74]. However, it does not affect other known functions [76].

11. Future Directions

A. actinomycetemcomitans expresses adhesins with molecular masses almost 20 times larger than the mass of typical bacterial proteins, suggesting that synthesis of these adhesins is regulated coordinately to manage cellular resources when their functions are not needed. Our work suggests that these adhesins are coordinately regulated by shared transcription factors [82]. To date, only a limited number of genes have been studied at the transcriptional level [111], and these studies have nearly uniformly been undertaken in highly manipulated and passaged laboratory strains that lose responsiveness during culture adaptation. A minimally manipulated strain isolated from an individual with *A. actinomycetemcomitans*-related infective endocarditis (IE) demonstrated differential regulation of *emaA* and other adhesins when grown on blood versus laboratory media, thus retaining manipulable adhesin expression). Passage of the IE strain on laboratory media reduces the surface adhesin expression, leading to an altered state, a process we refer to as transcriptional "senescence", in which specific regulons are no longer responsive to external or intracellular signaling. This dysfunctional regulatory state has broad implications when studying gene regulation using culture-adapted laboratory strains.

This fully documented provenance and limited manipulation under well-defined environmental conditions will allow for the unique opportunity to investigate the transcriptional control of *emaA* and other virulence-related adhesins, opening up new avenues of investigation into the gene regulation and pathogenicity of this organism. Furthermore, comparison of the colonization of vastly different tissue environments by this bacterium may provide insight into the physiological changes required for this strain to transition from the oral cavity in the bloodstream into the heart.

Funding: This research was funded by multiple awards from NIH/NIDCR and NSF.

Institutional Review Board Statement: This study did not require ethical approval.

Informed Consent Statement: Not applicable.

Data Availability Statement: No new data were created or analyzed in this study. Data sharing is not applicable to this article.

Conflicts of Interest: The authors declare no conflict of interest.

References

1. Holland, T.L.; Baddour, L.M.; Bayer, A.S.; Hoen, B.; Miro, J.M.; Fowler, V.G., Jr. Infective endocarditis. *Nat. Rev. Dis. Primers* **2016**, *2*, 16059. [CrossRef] [PubMed]
2. Chambers, S.T.; Murdoch, D.; Morris, A.; Holland, D.; Pappas, P.; Almela, M.; Fernandez-Hidalgo, N.; Almirante, B.; Bouza, E.; Forno, D.; et al. HACEK infective endocarditis: Characteristics and outcomes from a large, multi-national cohort. *PLoS ONE* **2013**, *8*, e63181. [CrossRef]
3. Cahill, T.J.; Prendergast, B.D. Infective endocarditis. *Lancet* **2016**, *387*, 882–893. [CrossRef] [PubMed]
4. Akifusa, S.; Poole, S.; Lewthwaite, J.; Henderson, B.; Nair, S.P. Recombinant *Actinobacillus actinomycetemcomitans* cytolethal distending toxin proteins are required to interact to inhibit human cell cycle progression and to stimulate human leukocyte cytokine synthesis. *Infect. Immun.* **2001**, *69*, 5925–5930. [CrossRef] [PubMed]
5. Paturel, L.; Casalta, J.P.; Habib, G.; Nezri, M.; Raoult, D. *Actinobacillus actinomycetemcomitans* endocarditis. *Clin. Microbiol. Infect. Off. Publ. Eur. Soc. Clin. Microbiol. Infect. Dis.* **2004**, *10*, 98–118. [CrossRef] [PubMed]
6. Petti, C.A.; Bhally, H.S.; Weinstein, M.P.; Joho, K.; Wakefield, T.; Reller, L.B.; Carroll, K.C. Utility of extended blood culture incubation for isolation of *Haemophilus, Actinobacillus, Cardiobacterium, Eikenella,* and *Kingella* organisms: A retrospective multicenter evaluation. *J. Clin. Microbiol.* **2006**, *44*, 257–259. [CrossRef] [PubMed]
7. Blackberg, A.; Morenius, C.; Olaison, L.; Berge, A.; Rasmussen, M. Infective endocarditis caused by HACEK group bacteria—A registry-based comparative study. *Eur. J. Clin. Microbiol. Infect. Dis.* **2021**, *40*, 1919–1924. [CrossRef]

8. Yew, H.S.; Chambers, S.T.; Roberts, S.A.; Holland, D.J.; Julian, K.A.; Raymond, N.J.; Beardsley, J.; Read, K.M.; Murdoch, D.R. Association between HACEK bacteraemia and endocarditis. *J. Med. Microbiol.* **2014**, *63*, 892–895. [CrossRef]
9. Azari, F.; Nyland, L.; Yu, C.; Radermacher, M.; Mintz, K.P.; Ruiz, T. Ultrastructural analysis of the rugose cell envelope of a member of the *Pasteurellaceae* family. *J. Bacteriol.* **2013**, *195*, 1680–1688. [CrossRef]
10. Gallant, C.V.; Sedic, M.; Chicoine, E.A.; Ruiz, T.; Mintz, K.P. Membrane morphology and leukotoxin secretion are associated with a novel membrane protein of *Aggregatibacter actinomycetemcomitans*. *J. Bacteriol.* **2008**, *190*, 5972–5980. [CrossRef]
11. Smith, K.P.; Voogt, R.D.; Ruiz, T.; Mintz, K.P. The conserved carboxyl domain of MorC, an inner membrane protein of *Aggregatibacter actinomycetemcomitans*, is essential for membrane function. *Mol. Oral. Microbiol.* **2016**, *31*, 43–58. [CrossRef] [PubMed]
12. Smith, K.P.; Fields, J.G.; Voogt, R.D.; Deng, B.; Lam, Y.W.; Mintz, K.P. Alteration in abundance of specific membrane proteins of *Aggregatibacter actinomycetemcomitans* is attributed to deletion of the inner membrane protein MorC. *Proteomics* **2015**, *15*, 1859–1867. [CrossRef] [PubMed]
13. Smith, K.P.; Ruiz, T.; Mintz, K.P. Inner-membrane protein MorC is involved in fimbriae production and biofilm formation in *Aggregatibacter actinomycetemcomitans*. *Microbiology* **2016**, *162*, 513–525. [CrossRef] [PubMed]
14. Smith, K.P.; Fields, J.G.; Voogt, R.D.; Deng, B.; Lam, Y.W.; Mintz, K.P. The cell envelope proteome of *Aggregatibacter actinomycetemcomitans*. *Mol. Oral. Microbiol.* **2015**, *30*, 97–110. [CrossRef] [PubMed]
15. Lockhart, P.B.; Brennan, M.T.; Thornhill, M.; Michalowicz, B.S.; Noll, J.; Bahrani-Mougeot, F.K.; Sasser, H.C. Poor oral hygiene as a risk factor for infective endocarditis-related bacteremia. *J. Am. Dent. Assoc.* **2009**, *140*, 1238–1244. [CrossRef]
16. Shoulders, M.D.; Raines, R.T. Collagen structure and stability. *Annu. Rev. Biochem.* **2009**, *78*, 929–958. [CrossRef]
17. Halper, J. Basic components of connective tissues and extracellular matrix: Fibronectin, fibrinogen, laminin, elastin, fibrillins, fibulins, matrilins, tenascins and thrombospondins. *Adv. Exp. Med. Biol.* **2021**, *1348*, 105–126. [CrossRef]
18. Westerlund, B.; Korhonen, T.K. Bacterial proteins binding to the mammalian extracellular matrix. *Mol. Microbiol.* **1993**, *9*, 687–694. [CrossRef]
19. Carranza, F.A., Jr.; Saglie, R.; Newman, M.G.; Valentin, P.L. Scanning and transmission electron microscopic study of tissue-invading microorganisms in localized juvenile periodontitis. *J. Periodontol.* **1983**, *54*, 598–617. [CrossRef]
20. Gillett, R.; Johnson, N.W. Bacterial invasion of the periodontium in a case of juvenile periodontitis. *J. Clin. Periodontol.* **1982**, *9*, 93–100. [CrossRef]
21. Mintz, K.P.; Fives-Taylor, P.M. Binding of the periodontal pathogen *Actinobacillus actinomycetemcomitans* to extracellular matrix proteins. *Oral. Microbiol. Immunol.* **1999**, *14*, 109–116. [CrossRef]
22. Alugupalli, K.R.; Kalfas, S.; Forsgren, A. Laminin binding to a heat-modifiable outer membrane protein of *Actinobacillus actinomycetemcomitans*. *Oral. Microbiol. Immunol.* **1996**, *11*, 326–331. [CrossRef] [PubMed]
23. Cole, W.G.; Chan, D.; Hickey, A.J.; Wilcken, D.E. Collagen composition of normal and myxomatous human mitral heart valves. *Biochem. J.* **1984**, *219*, 451–460. [CrossRef] [PubMed]
24. Mintz, K.P. Identification of an extracellular matrix protein adhesin, EmaA, which mediates the adhesion of *Actinobacillus actinomycetemcomitans* to collagen. *Microbiology* **2004**, *150*, 2677–2688. [CrossRef] [PubMed]
25. Ackermann, N.; Tiller, M.; Anding, G.; Roggenkamp, A.; Heesemann, J.; Akifusa, S.; Poole, S.; Lewthwaite, J.; Henderson, B.; Nair, S.P. Contribution of trimeric autotransporter C-terminal domains of oligomeric coiled-coil adhesin (Oca) family members YadA, UspA1, EibA, and Hia to translocation of the YadA passenger domain and virulence of *Yersinia enterocolitica*. *J. Bacteriol.* **2008**, *190*, 5031–5043. [CrossRef]
26. Chauhan, N.; Hatlem, D.; Orwick-Rydmark, M.; Schneider, K.; Floetenmeyer, M.; van Rossum, B.; Leo, J.C.; Linke, D. Insights into the autotransport process of a trimeric autotransporter, Yersinia Adhesin A (YadA). *Mol. Microbiol.* **2019**, *111*, 844–862. [CrossRef]
27. Leo, J.C.; Grin, I.; Linke, D. Type V secretion: Mechanism(s) of autotransport through the bacterial outer membrane. *Philos. Trans. R. Soc. Lond. B Biol. Sci.* **2012**, *367*, 1088–1101. [CrossRef]
28. Hoiczyk, E.; Roggenkamp, A.; Reichenbecher, M.; Lupas, A.; Heesemann, J. Structure and sequence analysis of *Yersinia* YadA and *Moraxella* UspAs reveal a novel class of adhesins. *EMBO J.* **2000**, *19*, 5989–5999. [CrossRef]
29. Laarmann, S.; Cutter, D.; Juehne, T.; Barenkamp, S.J.; St Geme, J.W. The *Haemophilus influenzae* Hia autotransporter harbours two adhesive pockets that reside in the passenger domain and recognize the same host cell receptor. *Mol. Microbiol.* **2002**, *46*, 731–743. [CrossRef]
30. Lafontaine, E.R.; Cope, L.D.; Aebi, C.; Latimer, J.L.; McCracken, G.H., Jr.; Hansen, E.J. The UspA1 protein and a second type of UspA2 protein mediate adherence of *Moraxella catarrhalis* to human epithelial cells in vitro. *J. Bacteriol.* **2000**, *182*, 1364–1373. [CrossRef]
31. Riess, T.; Andersson, S.G.; Lupas, A.; Schaller, M.; Schafer, A.; Kyme, P.; Martin, J.; Walzlein, J.H.; Ehehalt, U.; Lindroos, H.; et al. Bartonella adhesin A mediates a proangiogenic host cell response. *J. Exp. Med.* **2004**, *200*, 1267–1278. [CrossRef] [PubMed]
32. Tahir, Y.E.; Kuusela, P.; Skurnik, M. Functional mapping of the *Yersinia enterocolitica* adhesin YadA. Identification Of eight NSVAIG—S motifs in the amino-terminal half of the protein involved in collagen binding. *Mol. Microbiol.* **2000**, *37*, 192–206. [CrossRef] [PubMed]
33. Azari, F.; Radermacher, M.; Mintz, K.P.; Ruiz, T. Correlation of the amino-acid sequence and the 3D structure of the functional domain of EmaA from *Aggregatibacter actinomycetemcomitans*. *J. Struct. Biol.* **2012**, *177*, 439–446. [CrossRef] [PubMed]

34. Ruiz, T.; Lenox, C.; Radermacher, M.; Mintz, K.P. Novel surface structures are associated with the adhesion of *Actinobacillus actinomycetemcomitans* to collagen. *Infect. Immun.* **2006**, *74*, 6163–6170. [CrossRef]

35. Yu, C.; Ruiz, T.; Lenox, C.; Mintz, K.P. Functional mapping of an oligomeric autotransporter adhesin of *Aggregatibacter actinomycetemcomitans*. *J. Bacteriol.* **2008**, *190*, 3098–3109. [CrossRef]

36. Yu, C.; Mintz, K.P.; Ruiz, T. Investigation of the three-dimensional architecture of the collagen adhesin EmaA of *Aggregatibacter actinomycetemcomitans* by electron tomography. *J. Bacteriol.* **2009**, *191*, 6253–6261. [CrossRef]

37. Tang, G.; Ruiz, T.; Barrantes-Reynolds, R.; Mintz, K.P. Molecular heterogeneity of EmaA, an oligomeric autotransporter adhesin of *Aggregatibacter* (*Actinobacillus*) *actinomycetemcomitans*. *Microbiology* **2007**, *153*, 2447–2457. [CrossRef]

38. Tang, G.; Kitten, T.; Munro, C.L.; Wellman, G.C.; Mintz, K.P. EmaA, a potential virulence determinant of *Aggregatibacter actinomycetemcomitans* in infective endocarditis. *Infect. Immun.* **2008**, *76*, 2316–2324. [CrossRef]

39. Paik, S.; Senty, L.; Das, S.; Noe, J.C.; Munro, C.L.; Kitten, T. Identification of virulence determinants for endocarditis in *Streptococcus sanguinis* by signature-tagged mutagenesis. *Infect. Immun.* **2005**, *73*, 6064–6074. [CrossRef]

40. Hook, E.W., 3rd; Sande, M.A. Role of the vegetation in experimental *Streptococcus viridans* endocarditis. *Infect. Immun.* **1974**, *10*, 1433–1438. [CrossRef]

41. Bayer, A.S.; Coulter, S.N.; Stover, C.K.; Schwan, W.R. Impact of the high-affinity proline permease gene (putP) on the virulence of *Staphylococcus aureus* in experimental endocarditis. *Infect. Immun.* **1999**, *67*, 740–744. [CrossRef] [PubMed]

42. Veltrop, M.H.; Bancsi, M.J.; Bertina, R.M.; Thompson, J. Role of monocytes in experimental *Staphylococcus aureus* endocarditis. *Infect. Immun.* **2000**, *68*, 4818–4821. [CrossRef]

43. Azari, F.; Radermacher, M.; Mintz, K.P.; Ruiz, T. Interactions between the trimeric autotransporter adhesin EmaA and collagen revealed by three-dimensional electron tomography. *J. Bacteriol.* **2019**, *201*, e00297-19. [CrossRef] [PubMed]

44. Ponnuraj, K.; Bowden, M.G.; Davis, S.; Gurusiddappa, S.; Moore, D.; Choe, D.; Xu, Y.; Hook, M.; Narayana, S.V. A "dock, lock, and latch" structural model for a staphylococcal adhesin binding to fibrinogen. *Cell* **2003**, *115*, 217–228. [CrossRef] [PubMed]

45. Zong, Y.; Xu, Y.; Liang, X.; Keene, D.R.; Hook, A.; Gurusiddappa, S.; Hook, M.; Narayana, S.V. A 'Collagen Hug' model for *Staphylococcus aureus* CNA binding to collagen. *EMBO J.* **2005**, *24*, 4224–4236. [CrossRef]

46. Nummelin, H.; Merckel, M.C.; Leo, J.C.; Lankinen, H.; Skurnik, M.; Goldman, A. The *Yersinia* adhesin YadA collagen-binding domain structure is a novel left-handed parallel beta-roll. *EMBO J.* **2004**, *23*, 701–711. [CrossRef] [PubMed]

47. Delepelaire, P. Type I secretion in gram-negative bacteria. *Biochim. Biophys. Acta* **2004**, *1694*, 149–161. [CrossRef]

48. Pugsley, A.P. The complete general secretory pathway in gram-negative bacteria. *Microbiol. Rev.* **1993**, *57*, 50–108. [CrossRef]

49. Zwizinski, C.; Wickner, W. Purification and characterization of leader (signal) peptidase from *Escherichia coli*. *J. Biol. Chem.* **1980**, *255*, 7973–7977. [CrossRef]

50. Silhavy, T.J.; Kahne, D.; Walker, S. The bacterial cell envelope. *Cold Spring Harb. Perspect. Biol.* **2010**, *2*, a000414. [CrossRef]

51. Leyton, D.L.; Rossiter, A.E.; Henderson, I.R. From self sufficiency to dependence: Mechanisms and factors important for autotransporter biogenesis. *Nat. Rev. Microbiol.* **2012**, *10*, 213–225. [CrossRef] [PubMed]

52. Bernstein, H.D. Looks can be deceiving: Recent insights into the mechanism of protein secretion by the autotransporter pathway. *Mol. Microbiol.* **2015**, *97*, 205–215. [CrossRef] [PubMed]

53. Rossiter, A.E.; Leyton, D.L.; Tveen-Jensen, K.; Browning, D.F.; Sevastsyanovich, Y.; Knowles, T.J.; Nichols, K.B.; Cunningham, A.F.; Overduin, M.; Schembri, M.A.; et al. The essential beta-barrel assembly machinery complex components BamD and BamA are required for autotransporter biogenesis. *J. Bacteriol.* **2011**, *193*, 4250–4253. [CrossRef] [PubMed]

54. Owji, H.; Nezafat, N.; Negahdaripour, M.; Hajiebrahimi, A.; Ghasemi, Y. A comprehensive review of signal peptides: Structure, roles, and applications. *Eur. J. Cell Biol.* **2018**, *97*, 422–441. [CrossRef] [PubMed]

55. von Heijne, G. The signal peptide. *J. Membr. Biol.* **1990**, *115*, 195–201. [CrossRef] [PubMed]

56. Jiang, X.; Ruiz, T.; Mintz, K.P. The extended signal peptide of the trimeric autotransporter EmaA of *Aggregatibacter actinomycetemcomitans* modulates secretion. *J. Bacteriol.* **2011**, *193*, 6983–6994. [CrossRef]

57. Hiss, J.A.; Schneider, G. Domain organization of long autotransporter signal sequences. *Bioinform. Biol. Insights* **2009**, *3*, 189–204. [CrossRef]

58. Szabady, R.L.; Peterson, J.H.; Skillman, K.M.; Bernstein, H.D. An unusual signal peptide facilitates late steps in the biogenesis of a bacterial autotransporter. *Proc. Natl. Acad. Sci. USA* **2005**, *102*, 221–226. [CrossRef]

59. Jiang, X.; Ruiz, T.; Mintz, K.P. Characterization of the secretion pathway of the collagen adhesin EmaA of *Aggregatibacter actinomycetemcomitans*. *Mol. Oral. Microbiol.* **2012**, *27*, 382–396. [CrossRef]

60. Takada, K.; Saito, M.; Tsuzukibashi, O.; Kawashima, Y.; Ishida, S.; Hirasawa, M. Characterization of a new serotype g isolate of *Aggregatibacter actinomycetemcomitans*. *Mol. Oral. Microbiol.* **2010**, *25*, 200–206. [CrossRef]

61. Kittichotirat, W.; Bumgarner, R.E.; Chen, C. Evolutionary divergence of *Aggregatibacter actinomycetemcomitans*. *J. Dent. Res.* **2016**, *95*, 94–101. [CrossRef] [PubMed]

62. Tang-Siegel, G.G.; Danforth, D.R.; Tristano, J.; Ruiz, T.; Mintz, K.P. The serotype a-EmaA adhesin of *Aggregatibacter actinomycetemcomitans* does not require O-PS synthesis for collagen binding activity. *Microbiology* **2022**, *168*, 001191. [CrossRef] [PubMed]

63. Bertani, B.; Ruiz, N. Function and biogenesis of lipopolysaccharides. *EcoSal Plus* **2018**, *8*. [CrossRef] [PubMed]

64. Tang, G.; Mintz, K.P. Glycosylation of the collagen adhesin EmaA of *Aggregatibacter actinomycetemcomitans* is dependent upon the lipopolysaccharide biosynthetic pathway. *J. Bacteriol.* **2010**, *192*, 1395–1404. [CrossRef] [PubMed]

65. Yoshida, Y.; Nakano, Y.; Nezu, T.; Yamashita, Y.; Koga, T. A novel NDP-6-deoxyhexosyl-4-ulose reductase in the pathway for the synthesis of thymidine diphosphate-D-fucose. *J. Biol. Chem.* **1999**, *274*, 16933–16939. [CrossRef]
66. Yoshida, Y.; Nakano, Y.; Yamashita, Y.; Koga, T. Identification of a genetic locus essential for serotype b-specific antigen synthesis in *Actinobacillus actinomycetemcomitans*. *Infect. Immun.* **1998**, *66*, 107–114. [CrossRef] [PubMed]
67. Danforth, D.R.; Melloni, M.; Thorpe, R.; Cohen, A.; Voogt, R.; Tristano, J.; Mintz, K.P. Dual function of the O-antigen WaaL ligase of *Aggregatibacter actinomycetemcomitans*. *Mol. Oral. Microbiol.* **2023**, *38*, 471–488. [CrossRef]
68. Tang, G.; Ruiz, T.; Mintz, K.P. O-polysaccharide glycosylation is required for stability and function of the collagen adhesin EmaA of *Aggregatibacter actinomycetemcomitans*. *Infect. Immun.* **2012**, *80*, 2868–2877. [CrossRef]
69. Brooks, C.J.; Mintz, K.P.; Radermacher, M.; Ruiz, T. 3D structural analysis and classification of EmaA, a collagen binding adhesin. *Microsc. Microanal.* **2017**, *23*, 1260–1261. [CrossRef]
70. Brooks, C.J.; Ruiz, T.; Radermacher, M. The alignment and classification of 3D reconstructions of rod-like molecules obtained by electron tomography. *Microsc. Microanal.* **2017**, *23*, 1118–1119. [CrossRef]
71. Radermacher, M. A new environment for modular image reconstruction and data analysis. *Microsc. Microanal.* **2013**, *19*, 762–763. [CrossRef]
72. Yu, L.; Snapp, R.R.; Ruiz, T.; Radermacher, M. Probabilistic principal component analysis with expectation maximization (PPCA-EM) facilitates volume classification and estimates the missing data. *J. Struct. Biol.* **2010**, *171*, 18–30. [CrossRef]
73. Watson, A.; Naughton, H.; Radermacher, M.; Mintz, K.P.; Ruiz, T. Tomographic analysis of EmaA adhesin glycosylation in *Aggregatibacter actinomycetemcomitans*. *Microsc. Microanal.* **2015**, *21*, 899–900. [CrossRef]
74. Watson, A.; Tang-Siegel, G.; Brooks, C.J.; Radermacher, M.; Mintz, K.P.; Ruiz, T. Structural significance of EmaA glycosylation in *A. actinomycetemcomitans*. *Microsc. Microanal.* **2016**, *22*, 1132–1133. [CrossRef]
75. Tang, G.; Kawai, T.; Komatsuzawa, H.; Mintz, K.P. Lipopolysaccharides mediate leukotoxin secretion in *Aggregatibacter actinomycetemcomitans*. *Mol. Oral. Microbiol.* **2012**, *27*, 70–82. [CrossRef]
76. Danforth, D.R.; Tang-Siegel, G.; Ruiz, T.; Mintz, K.P. A non-fimbrial adhesin of *Aggregatibacter actinomycetemcomitans* mediates biofilm biogenesis. *Infect. Immun.* **2018**, *87*, 70–82. [CrossRef]
77. Fine, D.H.; Velliyagounder, K.; Furgang, D.; Kaplan, J.B. The *Actinobacillus actinomycetemcomitans* autotransporter adhesin Aae exhibits specificity for buccal epithelial cells from humans and old world primates. *Infect. Immun.* **2005**, *73*, 1947–1953. [CrossRef]
78. Rose, J.E.; Meyer, D.H.; Fives-Taylor, P.M. Aae, an autotransporter involved in adhesion of *Actinobacillus actinomycetemcomitans* to epithelial cells. *Infect. Immun.* **2003**, *71*, 2384–2393. [CrossRef]
79. Asakawa, R.; Komatsuzawa, H.; Kawai, T.; Yamada, S.; Goncalves, R.B.; Izumi, S.; Fujiwara, T.; Nakano, Y.; Suzuki, N.; Uchida, Y.; et al. Outer membrane protein 100, a versatile virulence factor of *Actinobacillus actinomycetemcomitans*. *Mol. Microbiol.* **2003**, *50*, 1125–1139. [CrossRef]
80. Yue, G.; Kaplan, J.B.; Furgang, D.; Mansfield, K.G.; Fine, D.H. A second *Aggregatibacter actinomycetemcomitans* autotransporter adhesin exhibits specificity for buccal epithelial cells in humans and Old World primates. *Infect. Immun.* **2007**, *75*, 4440–4448. [CrossRef]
81. Danforth, D.R.; Melloni, M.; Tristano, J.; Mintz, K.P. Contribution of adhesion proteins to *Aggregatibacter actinomycetemcomitans* biofilm formation. *Mol. Oral. Microbiol.* **2021**, *36*, 243–253. [CrossRef]
82. Tristano, J.; Danforth, D.R.; Wargo, M.J.; Mintz, K.P. Regulation of adhesin synthesis in *Aggregatibacter actinomycetemcomitans*. *Mol. Oral. Microbiol.* **2023**, *38*, 237–250. [CrossRef]
83. Price, N.L.; Raivio, T.L. Characterization of the Cpx regulon in *Escherichia coli* strain MC4100. *J. Bacteriol.* **2009**, *191*, 1798–1815. [CrossRef]
84. Raivio, T.L.; Silhavy, T.J. Periplasmic stress and ECF sigma factors. *Annu. Rev. Microbiol.* **2001**, *55*, 591–624. [CrossRef]
85. Danese, P.N.; Silhavy, T.J. The sigma(E) and the Cpx signal transduction systems control the synthesis of periplasmic protein-folding enzymes in *Escherichia coli*. *Genes. Dev.* **1997**, *11*, 1183–1193. [CrossRef]
86. Danese, P.N.; Snyder, W.B.; Cosma, C.L.; Davis, L.J.; Silhavy, T.J. The Cpx two-component signal transduction pathway of *Escherichia coli* regulates transcription of the gene specifying the stress-inducible periplasmic protease, DegP. *Genes. Dev.* **1995**, *9*, 387–398. [CrossRef]
87. Dorel, C.; Lejeune, P.; Rodrigue, A. The Cpx system of *Escherichia coli*, a strategic signaling pathway for confronting adverse conditions and for settling biofilm communities? *Res. Microbiol.* **2006**, *157*, 306–314. [CrossRef]
88. Dorel, C.; Vidal, O.; Prigent-Combaret, C.; Vallet, I.; Lejeune, P. Involvement of the Cpx signal transduction pathway of *E. coli* in biofilm formation. *FEMS Microbiol. Lett.* **1999**, *178*, 169–175. [CrossRef]
89. Jubelin, G.; Vianney, A.; Beloin, C.; Ghigo, J.M.; Lazzaroni, J.C.; Lejeune, P.; Dorel, C. CpxR/OmpR interplay regulates curli gene expression in response to osmolarity in *Escherichia coli*. *J. Bacteriol.* **2005**, *187*, 2038–2049. [CrossRef]
90. Kershaw, C.J.; Brown, N.L.; Constantinidou, C.; Patel, M.D.; Hobman, J.L. The expression profile of *Escherichia coli* K-12 in response to minimal, optimal and excess copper concentrations. *Microbiology* **2005**, *151*, 1187–1198. [CrossRef] [PubMed]
91. Nevesinjac, A.Z.; Raivio, T.L. The Cpx envelope stress response affects expression of the type IV bundle-forming pili of enteropathogenic *Escherichia coli*. *J. Bacteriol.* **2005**, *187*, 672–686. [CrossRef] [PubMed]
92. Alvarez, A.F.; Georgellis, D.; Brown, A.N.; Anderson, M.T.; Bachman, M.A.; Mobley, H.L.T. In vitro and in vivo analysis of the ArcB/A redox signaling pathway. *Methods Enzymol.* **2010**, *471*, 205–228. [CrossRef]

93. Brown, A.N.; Anderson, M.T.; Bachman, M.A.; Mobley, H.L.T. The ArcAB two-component system: Function in metabolism, redox control, and infection. *Microbiol. Mol. Biol. Rev.* **2022**, *86*, e0011021. [CrossRef]
94. Longo, P.; Ota-Tsuzuki, C.; Nunes, A.; Fernandes, B.; Mintz, K.; Fives-Taylor, P.; Mayer, M. *Aggregatibacter actinomycetemcomitans* arcB influences hydrophobic properties, biofilm formation and adhesion to hydroxyapatite. *Braz. J. Microbiol.* **2009**, *40*, 550–562. [CrossRef]
95. Shalel-Levanon, S.; San, K.Y.; Bennett, G.N. Effect of ArcA and FNR on the expression of genes related to the oxygen regulation and the glycolysis pathway in *Escherichia coli* under microaerobic growth conditions. *Biotechnol. Bioeng.* **2005**, *92*, 147–159. [CrossRef]
96. Pena-Sandoval, G.R.; Georgellis, D. The ArcB sensor kinase of *Escherichia coli* autophosphorylates by an intramolecular reaction. *J. Bacteriol.* **2010**, *192*, 1735–1739. [CrossRef]
97. Sun, H.; Song, Y.; Chen, F.; Zhou, C.; Liu, P.; Fan, Y.; Zheng, Y.; Wan, X.; Feng, L. An ArcA-modulateds RNA in pathogenic *Escherichia coli* K1. *Front. Microbiol.* **2020**, *11*, 574833. [CrossRef]
98. Xi, D.; Yang, S.; Liu, Q.; Li, Y.; Li, Y.; Yan, J.; Wang, X.; Ning, K.; Cao, B. The response regulator ArcA enhances biofilm formation in the vpsT manner under the anaerobic condition in *Vibrio cholerae*. *Microb. Pathog.* **2020**, *144*, 104197. [CrossRef] [PubMed]
99. Yan, J.; Li, Y.; Guo, X.; Wang, X.; Liu, F.; Li, A.; Cao, B. The effect of ArcA on the growth, motility, biofilm formation, and virulence of *Plesiomonas shigelloides*. *BMC Microbiol.* **2021**, *21*, 266. [CrossRef] [PubMed]
100. Zheng, M.; Storz, G. Redox sensing by prokaryotic transcription factors. *Biochem. Pharmacol.* **2000**, *59*, 1–6. [CrossRef]
101. Zheng, M.; Aslund, F.; Storz, G. Activation of the OxyR transcription factor by reversible disulfide bond formation. *Science* **1998**, *279*, 1718–1721. [CrossRef]
102. Figurski, D.H.; Fine, D.H.; Perez-Cheeks, B.A.; Grosso, V.W.; Kram, K.E.; Hua, J.; Xu, K.; Hedhli, J. Targeted mutagenesis in the study of the tightadherence (tad) locus of *Aggregatibacter actinomycetemcomitans*. In *Genetic Manipulation of DNA and Protein*; David, F., Ed.; IntechOpen: Rijeka, Croatia, 2013; p. Ch. 3.
103. Ramsey, M.M.; Whiteley, M. Polymicrobial interactions stimulate resistance to host innate immunity through metabolite perception. *Proc. Natl. Acad. Sci. USA* **2009**, *106*, 1578–1583. [CrossRef]
104. Valentin-Hansen, P.; Hojrup, P.; Short, S. The primary structure of the DeoR repressor from *Escherichia coli* K-12. *Nucleic Acids Res.* **1985**, *13*, 5927–5936. [CrossRef]
105. Ishihama, A. Prokaryotic genome regulation: Multifactor promoters, multitarget regulators and hierarchic networks. *FEMS Microbiol. Rev.* **2010**, *34*, 628–645. [CrossRef]
106. Saglie, F.R.; Carranza, F.A., Jr.; Newman, M.G.; Cheng, L.; Lewin, K.J. Identification of tissue-invading bacteria in human periodontal disease. *J. Periodontal Res.* **1982**, *17*, 452–455. [CrossRef]
107. Chen, Y.C.; Chang, S.C.; Luh, K.T.; Hsieh, W.C. *Actinobacillus actinomycetemcomitans* endocarditis: A report of four cases and review of the literature. *QJM An. Int. J. Med.* **1991**, *81*, 871–878. [CrossRef]
108. Mintz, K.P.; Fives-Taylor, P.M. Adhesion of *Actinobacillus actinomycetemcomitans* to a human oral cell line. *Infect. Immun.* **1994**, *62*, 3672–3678. [CrossRef]
109. Schreiner, H.C.; Sinatra, K.; Kaplan, J.B.; Furgang, D.; Kachlany, S.C.; Planet, P.J.; Perez, B.A.; Figurski, D.H.; Fine, D.H. Tight-adherence genes of *Actinobacillus actinomycetemcomitans* are required for virulence in a rat model. *Proc. Natl. Acad. Sci. USA* **2003**, *100*, 7295–7300. [CrossRef]
110. Fine, D.H.; Goncharoff, P.; Schreiner, H.; Chang, K.M.; Furgang, D.; Figurski, D. Colonization and persistence of rough and smooth colony variants of *Actinobacillus actinomycetemcomitans* in the mouths of rats. *Arch. Oral. Biol.* **2001**, *46*, 1065–1078. [CrossRef] [PubMed]
111. Kram, K.E.; Hovel-Miner, G.A.; Tomich, M.; Figurski, D.H. Transcriptional regulation of the tad locus in *Aggregatibacter actinomycetemcomitans*: A termination cascade. *J. Bacteriol.* **2008**, *190*, 3859–3868. [CrossRef] [PubMed]

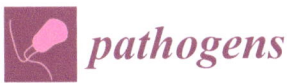

Article

Presence and Immunoreactivity of *Aggregatibacter actinomycetemcomitans* in Rheumatoid Arthritis

Anna Svärd [1,2], Riccardo LoMartire [1,3], Klara Martinsson [4], Carina Öhman [5], Alf Kastbom [2,4] and Anders Johansson [5,*]

1 Center for Clinical Research Dalarna, Uppsala University, 791 82 Falun, Sweden; anna.svard@regiondalarna.se (A.S.); riccardo.lomartire@regiondalarna.se (R.L.)
2 Department of Rheumatology, Linköping University Hospital, 581 85 Linköping, Sweden; alf.kastbom@liu.se
3 School of Health and Welfare, Dalarna University, 791 88 Falun, Sweden
4 Division of Inflammation and Infection, Department of Biomedical and Clinical Sciences, Linköping University, 581 83 Linköping, Sweden; klara.martinsson@liu.se
5 Department of Odontology, Umeå University, 901 87 Umeå, Sweden; carina.ohman@umu.se
* Correspondence: anders.p.johansson@umu.se; Tel.: +46-90-7856291

Abstract: The presence of periodontal pathogens is associated with an increased prevalence of rheumatoid arthritis (RA). The systemic antibody response to epitopes of these bacteria is often used as a proxy to study correlations between bacteria and RA. The primary aim of the present study is to examine the correlation between the presence of *Aggregatibacter actinomycetemcomitans* (Aa) in the oral cavity and serum antibodies against the leukotoxin (LtxA) produced by this bacterium. The salivary presence of Aa was analyzed with quantitative PCR and serum LtxA ab in a cell culture-based neutralization assay. The analyses were performed on samples from a well-characterized RA cohort ($n = 189$) and a reference population of blood donors ($n = 101$). Salivary Aa was present in 15% of the RA patients and 6% of the blood donors. LtxA ab were detected in 19% of RA-sera and in 16% of sera from blood donors. The correlation between salivary Aa and serum LtxA ab was surprisingly low (rho = 0.55 [95% CI: 0.40, 0.68]). The presence of salivary Aa showed no significant association with any of the RA-associated parameters documented in the cohort. A limitation of the present study is the relatively low number of individuals with detectable concentrations of Aa in saliva. Moreover, in the comparison of detectable Aa prevalence between RA patients and blood donors, we assumed that the two groups were equivalent in other Aa prognostic factors. These limitations must be taken into consideration when the result from the study is interpreted. We conclude that a systemic immune response to Aa LtxA does not fully reflect the prevalence of Aa in saliva. In addition, the association between RA-associated parameters and the presence of Aa was negligible in the present RA cohort.

Keywords: *Aggregatibacter actinomycetemcomitans*; salivary concentrations; rheumatoid arthritis; systemic biomarker

Citation: Svärd, A.; LoMartire, R.; Martinsson, K.; Öhman, C.; Kastbom, A.; Johansson, A. Presence and Immunoreactivity of *Aggregatibacter actinomycetemcomitans* in Rheumatoid Arthritis. *Pathogens* **2024**, *13*, 368. https://doi.org/10.3390/pathogens13050368

Academic Editor: Daniel H. Fine

Received: 29 March 2024
Revised: 24 April 2024
Accepted: 26 April 2024
Published: 29 April 2024

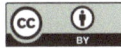

1. Introduction

Rheumatoid arthritis (RA) is an inflammatory disease that can display autoantibody production and systemic disease manifestations [1,2]. Autoantibodies to citrullinated proteins (ACPAs) are specific markers of RA and are usually assayed as antibodies to citrullinated peptides (anti-CCP) [3]. For many years, RA has been suggested to be clinically and pathologically associated with periodontitis [4]. Periodontitis is a bacteria-induced inflammatory disease that degrades the tooth-supporting structures, alveolar bone and connective tissue [5]. Interestingly, Konig and co-workers [6] showed that the citrullinome in periodontitis sometimes reflected patterns of hypercitrullination observed in the rheumatoid joint. Among the periodontal pathogens, *Aggregatibacter actinomyctemecomitans* (Aa), but not other bacterial species, induced hypercitrullination in host neutrophils [6]. It was shown that the molecular mechanism by which Aa triggers the dysregulated activation of citrullinating enzymes in neutrophils mimics autoantigen citrullination in the RA joint. Aa is a Gram-negative facultative anaerobic bacterial species that is associated with aggressive forms of periodontitis [7,8].

Due to the high genetic diversity of Aa, the bacterium exists as a harmless commensal and as an exogene pathogen [9]. A highly virulent genotype of the bacterium is the JP2, which has an enhanced production of a leukotoxin (LtxA) [10]. Detection of the JP2 genotype of Aa was initially restricted to some regions of Africa, while it today can be sporadically found in patients of many different geographic origins around the world [11]. Adolescents carrying the JP2 genotype of Aa are at significantly enhanced risk to develop periodontitis [12]. LtxA produced by this bacterium is closely linked to the initiation of degenerative processes involved in many diseases, like periodontitis and rheumatoid arthritis [13,14]. The toxin is a large pore-forming protein that specifically binds to the β_2 integrin LFA-1 (CD11a/CD18) expressed by human leukocytes [15]. The interaction of LtxA with human neutrophiles induces an extracellular release of trap-like structures that contain citrullinated proteins [6,16]. The NLRP3 inflammasome is activated by LtxA and is important in the pathogenesis of both RA and periodontitis [17,18]. These properties of the periodontal pathogen Aa and its LtxA indicate a potential relationship between RA and the prevalence of Aa [19]. It has been reported that an RA patient with periodontitis colonized with the highly leukotoxic JP2 genotype of Aa one year after the eradication of Aa remained free of arthritis and anti-CCP antibodies [20]. A commonly used strategy for the determination of Aa prevalence on an individual basis is an analysis of systemic antibodies against surface epitopes unique for this bacterium [21]. Systemic antibodies with reactivity against LtxA have shown to be significantly enhanced in RA patients compared with healthy controls when examined in a US population [6]. Contrary to this observation, systemic LtxA antibodies, when analyzed in a Swedish cohort, were not significantly associated to RA [22]. Moreover, one previous study on a Japanese population showed that systemic IgG responses to Aa in patients with RA were significantly lower than those in controls [23].

In addition to the immunodetection of Aa-LtxA antibodies, the systemic capacity to neutralize the activity of LtxA has been analyzed [24–26]. The presence of systemic LtxA-neutralizing capacity has been shown to correlate significantly with the occurrence of LtxA antibodies, while the association with periodontitis has not been established [27–29]. We have previously examined the prevalence of systemic LtxA neutralization in relation to RA and associated systemic risk markers without any conclusive result for the associations between LtxA neutralization and RA development [30]. Aa has been shown to produce virulence factors with the capacity to affect a proper host response against this bacterium [31,32]. However, it is not yet known how the presence of systemic LtxA antibodies correlates with the amount of Aa in the oral cavity. RA has been associated with an impaired host response in vaccine studies [33,34]. Taken together, these findings indicate the importance of investigating whether systemic antibodies against Aa and its LtxA reflect the prevalence of the bacterium in the oral cavity in RA patients.

The primary aim of the present study is to examine the correlation between the amount of Aa in the oral cavity and the level of systemic Aa-LtxA antibodies in serum. A secondary aim is to examine the salivary presence of Aa in relation to the occurrence of RA-associated serological and clinical parameters.

2. Materials and Methods

2.1. Study Populations and Samples

The study populations have previously been described in detail [35]. Briefly, 196 individuals with established RA from the County of Dalarna, Sweden, were included in the cross-sectional "Secretory antibodies in Rheumatoid Arthritis" (SARA) study with enrolment 2012–2013. RA patients were randomly selected among planned follow-up visits at the Rheumatology Clinic, Falun Hospital, Sweden. Healthy blood donors ($n = 101$) were recruited from the local blood donor center and referred to the Rheumatology Clinic for blood and saliva sampling. Demographic and clinical parameters of the two study cohorts are summarized in Table 1. Participants were required to provide at least 0.5 mL of saliva during a 10-min sampling time; otherwise, they were excluded from the study. Paired saliva and serum samples were collected at the same visit at the Rheumatology Clinic. Participants were asked to restrain from eating, drinking other liquids than water, brushing teeth, or smoking 1 h before saliva sampling. Passive secretion was used for saliva sampling, i.e., the study participant leaned forward and drooled for 10 min into a test tube placed on ice. After the disruption of mucus fibers by pipetting a few times, the saliva samples were centrifuged for 5 min at $5000\times g$. Serum samples were also centrifuged for 5 min at $5000\times g$. Subsequently, serum and saliva samples were stored at $-80\,°C$ until further analyses.

Table 1. Demographic and clinical parameters of the two study cohorts.

	RA Patients	Blood Donors
Number	196	101
Age $\pm$ SD	64(13)	49(14)
Men	40 (20%)	47 (47%)
Smoking	101 (52%)	36 (36%)
Oral health problems *	96 (50%)	23 (23%)
Oral treatment §	53 (33%)	18 (18%)

* Self-reported experienced gum problem. § Having been subject to treatment of periodontal gum problem.

RA patients' disease activity was registered on the day of sampling and measured by the Disease Activity Score of 28 joints (DAS28) using erythrocyte sedimentation rate (ESR).

Information on smoking and oral health was obtained using a self-report questionnaire provided by the Epidemiological Investigations in RA (EIRA) Study [36].

2.2. Analysis of Total IgA in Saliva

The total IgA in saliva was quantified using commercially available immune assays (IBL International, Hamburg, Germany).

2.3. Autoantibody Analyses

IgG ACPAs in serum were analyzed previously, using the second-generation anti-CCP immunoassay (Svar Life Science, Malmö, Sweden). IgA ACPAs in serum and saliva were also analyzed previously in a similar way but using an anti-human α-chain antibody as secondary antibody [37].

Serum secretory component-containing (SC) ACPAs were measured by modifying commercially available anti-CCP ELISA kits (Euro-Diagnostica, Malmö, Sweden) as described elsewhere [38]. Briefly, SC ACPA were analyzed by diluting serum samples 1:25, and the detection antibody was diluted 1:2000 (polyclonal goat antibody conjugated to horseradish peroxidase, GAHu/SC/PO, Nordic Biosite, Sweden). Incubation and washing were performed according to instructions by the manufacturer. A 7-step standard curve was calculated by diluting a serum sample high in SC ACPAs.

2.4. Leukotoxin (LtxA) Antibody Assay

Anti-LtxA antibodies in serum were analyzed for their LtxA neutralizing capacity, which was detected as a reduction in cell damage and subsequent inhibited leakage of neutral red upon exposure to purified LtxA [39]. THP-1 cells in RPMI-10% fetal bovine serum (FBS)-50 nM phorbol myristate acetate were seeded at 1×10^6 cells/mL in flat 96-well plates and incubated at $37\,°C$ 5% CO_2 overnight. The cells were washed with RPMI, patient serum and LtxA added in triplicates and incubated for 2 h at $37\,°C$ 5% CO_2. The medium was removed, and 0.04 mg/mL neutral red diluted in RPMI-10% FBS was added, incubated 90 min at 37 °C 5% CO_2 and washed with PBS pH 7.4. Then, 50% EtOH with 1% acetic acid was added to lyse the cells. After 10 min of incubation, the optical density (OD) was read at 650 nm (TECAN Sunrise, CA, USA). The anti-LtxA antibody neutralization capacity in percent was calculated by dividing the serum sample OD with the maximum cell viability OD (incubation with FBS only) × 100. Serum samples inhibiting LtxA cell lysis ≥30% were classified as positive and <30% were classified as negative regarding anti-LtxA presence [27].

2.5. qPCR-Based Quantification of Salivary A. actinomycetemcomitans

This method has been previously described in detail [40]. Briefly, stimulated saliva was collected and the Viral DNA extraction kit (DiaSorin AB, Dublin, Ireland) was used for the DNA isolation, and for the procedure, an automated extraction instrument was used (Liaison® IXT, Diasorin AB, Ireland). DNA was extracted from 550 μL of the sample mixture and eluted in a volume of 100 μL. Standard suspensions of the Aa (JP2 genotype HK1651) (10^8–10^1 cells/mL), prepared in PBS buffer, were treated as described above. The samples and the standard solutions were stored at +4 °C until use. Quantification of the total concentration of *A. actinomycetemcomitans* in the DNA samples was performed according to Claesson et al., 2019 (PMID: 30847232). Briefly, the PCR mixture (10 μL) contained 5 μL Kapa Syber Green (KK 4601; Kapa Biosystems, Boston USA), 4 μL template, and 1 μL of a primer mix specific for the LtxA (0.5 μM/primer, F: CTAGGTATTGCGAAACAATTT, R: CCTGAAATTAAGCTGGTAATC). The PCR program was as follows: hold/time 95°/10 m, cycling/time 95°/10 s, cycling/time 55°/5 s and 45 cycles.

2.6. Ethics

The ethics review board in Uppsala, Sweden, approved of the study, and all participants signed written informed consent (Uppsala: 2011/159).

2.7. Statistical Analyzes

The prevalence point estimate (Wilson's 95% confidence interval) of both detectable salivary Aa ≥ 100 bacteria/mL and detectable serum LtxA ab ≥ 30% was computed for the RA cohort and blood donors separately (DescTools v0.99.48 in R v4.2.3). To test the equality of the prevalence between the cohorts, we used a z-test of two independent proportions (R v4.2.3). Next, the monotonic correlation between salivary Aa and serum LtxA ab was quantified using Spearman's rho on left-censored data at the detection limit [41] with confidence intervals based on the bias-corrected and adjusted bootstrap method with 10,000 replications (boot v1.3-28.1 in R v4.2.3) [42]. In the final phase, we restricted the analyses to the RA patients. Within this subset, we first quantified the correlation between detectable salivary Aa and RA-associated risk markers using Spearman's rho; then, we estimated the association between detectable salivary Aa and detectable ACPA using Pearson's chi-square test and finally compared both DAS28 and total IgA in saliva between patients with and without detectable salivary Aa using the Mann–Whitney U test. All computations were based on complete cases.

3. Results

3.1. Salivary A. actinomycetemcomitans and Serum LtxA Antibodies in Both Cohorts

Salivary Aa ≥ 100 bacteria/mL was found in 14.8% (95% CI: 10.5%, 20.6%) of RA patients and in 5.9% (95% CI: 2.8%, 12.4%) of blood donors. Meanwhile, LtxA-neutralizing antibodies ≥ 30% inhibition in serum were found in 18.8% of RA patients (95% CI: 13.9%, 25.0%) and 16.0% (95% CI: 10.1%, 24.4%) of blood donors (Table 2).

Table 2. Prevalence of salivary Aa and LtxA-neutralizing antibodies positive individuals in the two analyzed study cohorts.

	Saliva Aa		Serum LtxA ab	
	Total Analyzed (Missing)	Number Pos (%)	Total Analyzed (Missing)	Number Pos (%)
All	290 (7)	34 (11.7)	286 (11)	51 (17.8)
Blood donors	101 (0)	6 (5.9)	100 (1)	16 (16.0)
RA-cohort	189 (7)	28 (14.8)	186 (10)	35 (18.8)

3.2. Association between Salivary Aa and Systemic LtxA ab in Both Cohorts

Based on data from 279 individuals, we observed a moderately strong positive correlation of 0.55 (95% CI: 0.40, 0.68) between salivary Aa and LtxA-neutralizing antibodies, which is illustrated in Figure 1. Correlation coefficients were similar when estimated separately for RA patients (rho = 0.54; 95% CI: 0.36, 0.69) and blood donors (rho = 0.60; 95% CI: 0.38, 0.80).

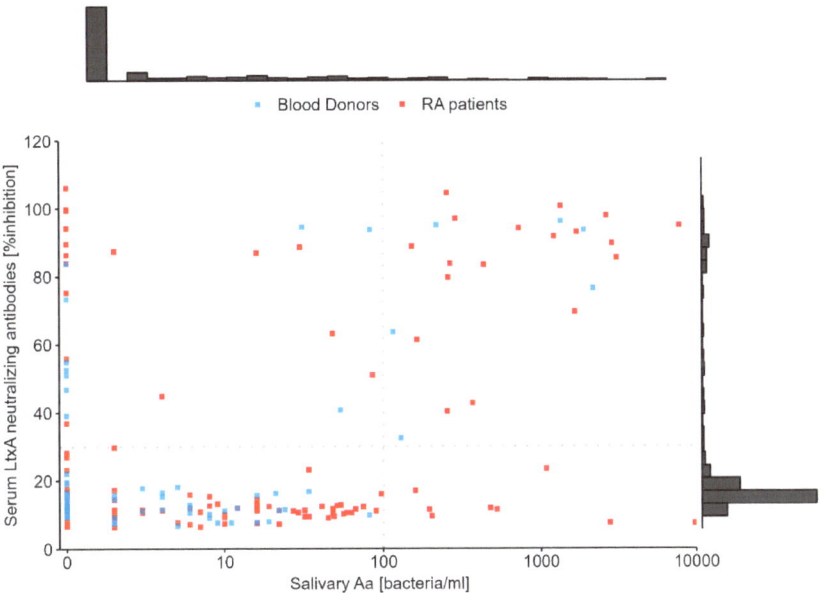

Figure 1. Relationship between salivary Aa and systemic LtxA ab in patients with RA (red points) and healthy blood donors (blue points). Salivary Aa is presented on the natural log scale with a constant of one added to zero values before transformation. The dotted lines mark the detection limit for each variable, and each variable´s distribution is illustrated by the marginal histograms.

Among the 34 individuals that tested positive for Aa in saliva, 24 also tested positive for LtxA-neutralizing antibodies in serum, while eight tested negative and two had no recorded data. Interestingly, the eight incongruent individuals, with Aa in saliva but no LtxA antibody in serum, were all RA patients. Moreover, they were females 49–66 years old and 6/8 were smokers. The median (interquartile range) of total IgA in saliva for these eight individuals was 90 µg/mL (106) compared to 55 µg/mL (50) for the 24 individuals that were positive for both saliva Aa and serum LtxA ab.

3.3. Association between Aa and ACPA, Disease Activity and Treatment in RA Patients

Among RA patients, 80% were positive for IgG ACPA in serum, 45% for IgA ACPA in serum and 12% for IgA ACPA in saliva. When comparing ACPA status between RA patients with and without Aa in saliva, no differences of importance were observed (Table 3). Also, DAS28 was similar among RA patients with Aa in saliva (median: 2.8; IQR: 1.9) and RA patients without Aa in saliva (median: 3.2; IQR: 1.3; P = 0.27).

Table 3. Levels of serum ACPA and saliva IgA stratified by detectable salivary Aa. No differences of importance in levels between the two groups were detected.

	RA Patients with Aa in Saliva	RA Patients without Aa in Saliva
Positive serum IgG ACPA	22 (79%)	128 (80%)
Positive serum IgA ACPA	12 (43%)	74 (46%)
Positive saliva IgA ACPA	2 (7%)	18 (11%)
Total IgA in saliva, median µg/mL (IQR)	61 (53)	62 (50)
SC ACPA in serum, median µg/mL (IQR)	52 (44)	68 (46)

Correlations between detectable salivary Aa and ESR, CRP, oral health and RA treatment were also investigated among the RA patients, as illustrated in Figure 2. No correlations of clinical importance were observed for salivary Aa or LtxA-neutralizing antibodies, besides the moderately strong positive correlation between the two as mentioned above.

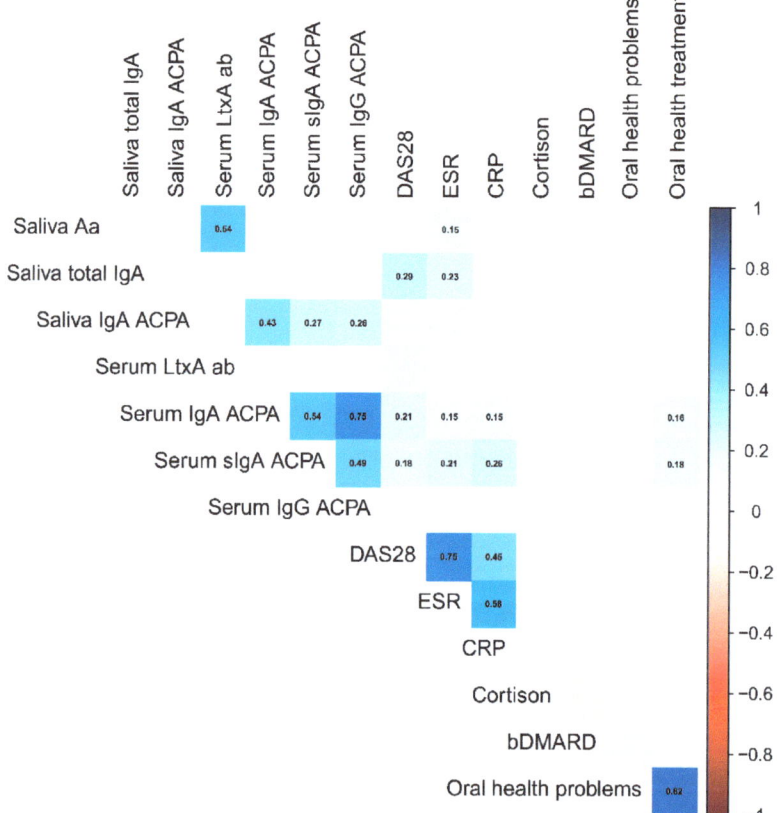

Figure 2. Plot of monotonic correlations between Aa markers and RA-associated parameters based on data left censored at the detection level. Blue color and red color indicate positive and negative correlations, respectively. Point estimates shown for correlations significant at 0.05 level only. The different parameters are described in material and methods (Sections 2.1–2.3).

4. Discussion

The association between RA and periodontitis is well established, while the role of the periodontal pathogens still is unclear [19,43]. In the present study, we examined the prevalence of Aa in saliva samples from two different cohorts: one consisted of patients diagnosed with RA and one consisted of healthy blood donors [35]. The prevalence of salivary Aa was 15% in the RA cohort and 6% among the blood donors. Aa LtxA-neutralizing ab in serum was detected in 19% of the RA patients and in 16% of the blood donors. The prevalence of salivary Aa and serum LtxA ab corresponds to levels previously found in periodontally healthy individuals rather than in periodontitis patients [44,45]. The correlation between saliva Aa and serum LtxA ab in the present study was surprisingly low, indicating that systemic immunoreactivity against Aa epitopes does not fully reflect the presence of this bacterium in the oral cavity. This indicates that collected biobank samples of plasma or serum do not fully reflect the oral presence of the periodontal pathogens. Systemic antibodies to Aa or LtxA reflect previous immunoreactivity against the bacterium, while detection of the bacterium in the oral cavity shows the presence at the time for sampling [21,29]. These circumstances have to be considered in the interpretation of data from diseases like RA that involve treatment strategies with immunosuppressive effects [46].

Findings from the present study did not support a correlation between the prevalence of Aa and the levels of different RA-associated parameters documented in the RA patients (ACPAs, DAS28, ESR, CRP, self-reported oral health, treatment with glucocorticoids or bDMARDs). A limitation in the present study is the lack of periodontal registrations. In addition, our results need to be interpreted in light of the low prevalence of detectable salivary Aa. However, the low prevalence of Aa and self-reported oral health problems in the present cohort indicates a generally good periodontal status among the study participants. A recent case-control study in a Chinese population showed that the presence of Aa was more devasting for RA patients with periodontitis compared to periodontally healthy RA patients [47]. This indicates that differences in the periodontal conditions between various studies might contribute to the diverging results on the correlation between RA-associated parameters and presence of periodontal pathogens [6,22]. Periodontitis-associated bacteria can be detected in the oral cavity of both periodontally healthy individuals and in periodontitis patients [5]. In periodontitis, the epithelial barrier function is impaired, which promotes the translocation of periodontal bacteria to the peripheral circulation [48]. The distribution of periodontal microbes into the peripheral circulation is associated with extra-oral inflammation and with several systemic diseases [49]. DNA of periodontal pathogens has been detected in synovial fluid, which indicated that these bacteria may play a role in the pathogenesis of RA [50,51].

There is a need for a suitable alternative to complete clinical periodontal examinations, which are both time consuming and expensive [52]. Radiographic periodontal bone loss shows a strong correlation to periodontitis and might be a suitable tool to simplify periodontal registrations in future population studies [44]. This technique has been successfully used to determine the correlation between periodontitis and RA; however, this study lacks data regarding the presence of periodontal microbes [53]. Aa produces molecules with virulence mechanisms that are closely linked to the pathogenesis of RA [6]. The association of Aa with RA is focused on the production of a leukotoxin (LtxA) with the capacity to induce dysbiosis in the host response [51]. The LtxA-induced virulence mechanisms involve the capacity to promote the citrullination of host proteins [54]. Aa can be found in the oral cavity of both periodontally healthy and periodontally diseased individuals [5,55].

Interestingly, in comparative analyses between the prevalence of Aa in saliva and serum LtxA, eight of the individuals from the two cohorts with Aa in saliva lacked serum LtxA ab. All these eight individuals were from the RA cohort, indicating a possible dysregulation of immune responses and subsequent impaired microbial host response in these RA patients. The association of RA with dysregulated immune response and autoimmunity may indicate impaired microbial host response [56]. In addition, Aa exhibit virulence

Pathogens **2024**, 13, 368

properties that might contribute to avoid host response [31]. Among these properties, the bacterium can invade periodontal tissues and the ability to produce LtxA with the capacity to specifically activate and kill leukocytes [13,57]. The immunosuppressive effect of Aa has been reported by an enhanced systemic immune response to LtxA in a patient treated with antibiotics that eradicated the bacteria [20]. However, the observation of an impaired systemic immune response of Aa-colonized RA patients is based on few individuals and needs to be further confirmed in larger studies.

In conclusion, systemic immunoreactivity to the Aa bacterium does not completely reflect Aa in saliva. This is important knowledge when designing studies on Aa and possibly other periodontal pathogens. Also, we conclude that salivary Aa was not significantly associated with the levels of RA-associated parameters in serum from the RA cohort. However, these results need to be interpreted with care due to the low number of Aa-positive individuals.

Author Contributions: Conceptualization, A.J., A.S., R.L. and A.K.; methodology, A.J., K.M. and C.Ö.; software, R.L.; validation, A,.J., A.S. and A.K.; formal analysis, C.Ö. and K.M.; investigation, A.S. and A.K.; resources, A.J., A.S. and A.K.; data curation, R.L., A.S. and A.K.; writing—original draft preparation, A.J.; writing—review and editing, A.J., A.S., R.L., A.K., K.M. and C.Ö.; funding acquisition, A.J., A.S. and A.K. All authors have read and agreed to the published version of the manuscript.

Funding: This research was funded by TUA grants from the County Council of Västerbotten, Sweden (A.J.; 7003193), the Thuréus Foundation for periodontal research, ALF grants from Region Östergötland, King Gustav V 80-year Foundation, the Swedish Rheumatism Association, and Center for Clinical Research, Dalarna, Uppsala University.

Institutional Review Board Statement: The ethics review board in Uppsala, Sweden, approved of the study, and all participants provided written informed consent (Uppsala: 2011/159).

Informed Consent Statement: Written informed consent has been obtained from the participants in the study.

Data Availability Statement: At Center for Clinical Research Dalarna, Uppsala University, Sweden.

Acknowledgments: We thank all the study participants in the two cohorts for their consent to participate in the study.

Conflicts of Interest: The authors declare no conflicts of interest.

References

1. Pisetsky, D.S. Annals of the Rheumatic Diseases collection on autoantibodies in the rheumatic diseases: New insights into pathogenesis and the development of novel biomarkers. *Ann. Rheum. Dis.* **2023**, *82*, 1243–1247. [CrossRef] [PubMed]
2. Lopez-Oliva, I.; Malcolm, J.; Culshaw, S. Periodontitis and rheumatoid arthritis-Global efforts to untangle two complex diseases. *Periodontology 2000* **2024**. [CrossRef]
3. Trier, N.H.; Houen, G. Anti-citrullinated protein antibodies as biomarkers in rheumatoid arthritis. *Expert Rev. Mol. Diagn.* **2023**, *23*, 895–911. [CrossRef] [PubMed]
4. Potempa, J.; Mydel, P.; Koziel, J. The case for periodontitis in the pathogenesis of rheumatoid arthritis. *Nat. Rev. Rheumatol.* **2017**, *13*, 606–620. [CrossRef]
5. Belibasakis, G.N.; Belstrøm, D.; Eick, S.; Gursoy, U.K.; Johansson, A.; Könönen, E. Periodontal microbiology and microbial etiology of periodontal diseases: Historical concepts and contemporary perspectives. *Periodontology 2000* **2023**. [CrossRef]
6. Konig, M.F.; Abusleme, L.; Reinholdt, J.; Palmer, R.J.; Teles, R.P.; Sampson, K.; Rosen, A.; Nigrovic, P.A.; Sokolove, J.; Giles, J.T.; et al. Aggregatibacter actinomycetemcomitans-induced hypercitrullination links periodontal infection to autoimmunity in rheumatoid arthritis. *Sci. Transl. Med.* **2016**, *8*, 369ra176. [CrossRef] [PubMed]
7. Fine, D.H.; Patil, A.G.; Velusamy, S.K. Aggregatibacter actinomycetemcomitans (Aa) Under the Radar: Myths and Misunderstandings of Aa and Its Role in Aggressive Periodontitis. *Front. Immunol.* **2019**, *10*, 728. [CrossRef] [PubMed]
8. Hbibi, A.; Bouziane, A.; Lyoussi, B.; Zouhdi, M.; Benazza, D. Aggregatibacter actinomycetemcomitans: From Basic to Advanced Research. *Adv. Exp. Med. Biol.* **2022**, *1373*, 45–67. [CrossRef]
9. Nedergaard, S.; Jensen, A.B.; Haubek, D.; Nørskov-Lauritsen, N. Multilocus Sequence Typing of Aggregatibacter actinomycetemcomitans Competently Depicts the Population Structure of the Species. *Microbiol. Spectr.* **2021**, *9*, e0108521. [CrossRef]

10. Jensen, A.B.; Lund, M.; Nørskov-Lauritsen, N.; Johansson, A.; Claesson, R.; Reinholdt, J.; Haubek, D. Differential Cell Lysis Among Periodontal Strains of JP2 and Non-JP2 Genotype of Aggregatibacter actinomycetemcomitans Serotype B Is Not Reflected in Dissimilar Expression and Production of Leukotoxin. *Pathogens* **2019**, *8*, 211. [CrossRef]
11. Khzam, N.; Miranda, L.A.; Kujan, O.; Shearston, K.; Haubek, D. Prevalence of the JP2 genotype of Aggregatibacter actinomycetemcomitans in the world population: A systematic review. *Clin. Oral Investig.* **2022**, *26*, 2317–2334. [CrossRef] [PubMed]
12. Haubek, D.; Ennibi, O.K.; Poulsen, K.; Vaeth, M.; Poulsen, S.; Kilian, M. Risk of aggressive periodontitis in adolescent carriers of the JP2 clone of Aggregatibacter (Actinobacillus) actinomycetemcomitans in Morocco: A prospective longitudinal cohort study. *Lancet* **2008**, *371*, 237–242. [CrossRef] [PubMed]
13. Johansson, A. Aggregatibacter actinomycetemcomitans leukotoxin: A powerful tool with capacity to cause imbalance in the host inflammatory response. *Toxins* **2011**, *3*, 242–259. [CrossRef]
14. Krutyhołowa, A.; Strzelec, K.; Dziedzic, A.; Bereta, G.P.; Łazarz-Bartyzel, K.; Potempa, J.; Gawron, K. Host and bacterial factors linking periodontitis and rheumatoid arthritis. *Front. Immunol.* **2022**, *13*, 980805. [CrossRef] [PubMed]
15. Lally, E.T.; Kieba, I.R.; Sato, A.; Green, C.L.; Rosenbloom, J.; Korostoff, J.; Wang, J.F.; Shenker, B.J.; Ortlepp, S.; Robinson, M.K.; et al. RTX toxins recognize a beta2 integrin on the surface of human target cells. *J. Biol. Chem.* **1997**, *272*, 30463–30469. [CrossRef] [PubMed]
16. Hirschfeld, J.; Roberts, H.M.; Chapple, I.L.; Parčina, M.; Jepsen, S.; Johansson, A.; Claesson, R. Effects of Aggregatibacter actinomycetemcomitans leukotoxin on neutrophil migration and extracellular trap formation. *J. Oral Microbiol.* **2016**, *8*, 33070. [CrossRef] [PubMed]
17. Kelk, P.; Moghbel, N.S.; Hirschfeld, J.; Johansson, A. Aggregatibacter actinomycetemcomitans Leukotoxin Activates the NLRP3 Inflammasome and Cell-to-Cell Communication. *Pathogens* **2022**, *11*, 159. [CrossRef] [PubMed]
18. Murakami, T.; Nakaminami, Y.; Takahata, Y.; Hata, K.; Nishimura, R. Activation and Function of NLRP3 Inflammasome in Bone and Joint-Related Diseases. *Int. J. Mol. Sci.* **2022**, *23*, 5365. [CrossRef] [PubMed]
19. Looh, S.C.; Soo, Z.M.P.; Wong, J.J.; Yam, H.C.; Chow, S.K.; Hwang, J.S. Aggregatibacter actinomycetemcomitans as the Aetiological Cause of Rheumatoid Arthritis: What Are the Unsolved Puzzles? *Toxins* **2022**, *14*, 50. [CrossRef]
20. Mukherjee, A.; Jantsch, V.; Khan, R.; Hartung, W.; Fischer, R.; Jantsch, J.; Ehrenstein, B.; Konig, M.F.; Andrade, F. Rheumatoid Arthritis-Associated Autoimmunity Due to Aggregatibacter actinomycetemcomitans and Its Resolution With Antibiotic Therapy. *Front. Immunol.* **2018**, *9*, 2352. [CrossRef]
21. Ebersole, J.L.; Hamzeh, R.; Nguyen, L.; Al-Sabbagh, M.; Dawson, D., 3rd. Variations in IgG antibody subclass responses to oral bacteria: Effects of periodontal disease and modifying factors. *J. Periodontal Res.* **2021**, *56*, 863–876. [CrossRef] [PubMed]
22. Gomez-Bañuelos, E.; Johansson, L.; Konig, M.F.; Lundquist, A.; Paz, M.; Buhlin, K.; Johansson, A.; Rantapää-Dahlqvist, S.; Andrade, F. Exposure to Aggregatibacter actinomycetemcomitans before Symptom Onset and the Risk of Evolving to Rheumatoid Arthritis. *J. Clin. Med.* **2020**, *9*, 1906. [CrossRef] [PubMed]
23. Okada, M.; Kobayashi, T.; Ito, S.; Yokoyama, T.; Komatsu, Y.; Abe, A.; Murasawa, A.; Yoshie, H. Antibody responses to periodontopathic bacteria in relation to rheumatoid arthritis in Japanese adults. *J. Periodontol.* **2011**, *82*, 1433–1441. [CrossRef] [PubMed]
24. Johansson, A.; Johansson, I.; Eriksson, M.; Ahrén, A.M.; Hallmans, G.; Stegmayr, B. Systemic antibodies to the leukotoxin of the oral pathogen Actinobacillus actinomycetemcomitans correlate negatively with stroke in women. *Cerebrovasc. Dis.* **2005**, *20*, 226–232. [CrossRef]
25. Johansson, A.; Eriksson, M.; Ahrén, A.M.; Boman, K.; Jansson, J.H.; Hallmans, G.; Johansson, I. Prevalence of systemic immunoreactivity to Aggregatibacter actinomycetemcomitans leukotoxin in relation to the incidence of myocardial infarction. *BMC Infect. Dis.* **2011**, *11*, 55. [CrossRef] [PubMed]
26. Johansson, A.; Buhlin, K.; Sorsa, T.; Pussinen, P.J. Systemic Aggregatibacter actinomycetemcomitans Leukotoxin-Neutralizing Antibodies in Periodontitis. *J. Periodontol.* **2017**, *88*, 122–129. [CrossRef]
27. Brage, M.; Holmlund, A.; Johansson, A. Humoral immune response to Aggregatibacter actinomycetemcomitans leukotoxin. *J. Periodontal Res.* **2011**, *46*, 170–175. [CrossRef] [PubMed]
28. Johansson, A.; Buhlin, K.; Koski, R.; Gustafsson, A. The immunoreactivity of systemic antibodies to Actinobacillus actinomycetemcomitans and Porphyromonas gingivalis in adult periodontitis. *Eur. J. Oral Sci.* **2005**, *113*, 197–202. [CrossRef] [PubMed]
29. Damgaard, C.; Reinholdt, J.; Enevold, C.; Fiehn, N.E.; Nielsen, C.H.; Holmstrup, P. Immunoglobulin G antibodies against Porphyromonas gingivalis or Aggregatibacter actinomycetemcomitans in cardiovascular disease and periodontitis. *J. Oral Microbiol.* **2017**, *9*, 1374154. [CrossRef]
30. Martinsson, K.; Di Matteo, A.; Öhman, C.; Johansson, A.; Svärd, A.; Mankia, K.; Emery, P.; Kastbom, A. Antibodies to leukotoxin A from the periodontal pathogen Aggregatibacter actinomycetemcomitans in patients at an increased risk of rheumatoid arthritis. *Front. Med.* **2023**, *10*, 1176165. [CrossRef]
31. Oscarsson, J.; Claesson, R.; Lindholm, M.; Höglund Åberg, C.; Johansson, A. Tools of Aggregatibacter actinomycetemcomitans to Evade the Host Response. *J. Clin. Med.* **2019**, *8*, 1079. [CrossRef] [PubMed]
32. Shahoumi, L.A.; Saleh, M.H.A.; Meghil, M.M. Virulence Factors of the Periodontal Pathogens: Tools to Evade the Host Immune Response and Promote Carcinogenesis. *Microorganisms* **2023**, *11*, 115. [CrossRef]

33. Christoph, R.; Giovanni, A.; Arne, S.; Sebastian, V.; Gerhard, D.; Angelika, M.; Marc, S.; Sonja, H.; Marie, S.; Lydia, J.; et al. Immunogenicity of tick-borne-encephalitis-virus-(TBEV)-vaccination and impact of age on humoral and cellular TBEV-specific immune responses in patients with rheumatoid arthritis. *Vaccine* **2024**, *42*, 745–752. [CrossRef]
34. Hertzell, K.B.; Pauksens, K.; Rombo, L.; Knight, A.; Vene, S.; Askling, H.H. Tick-borne encephalitis (TBE) vaccine to medically immunosuppressed patients with rheumatoid arthritis: A prospective, open-label, multi-centre study. *Vaccine* **2016**, *34*, 650–655. [CrossRef] [PubMed]
35. Roos Ljungberg, K.; Börjesson, E.; Martinsson, K.; Wetterö, J.; Kastbom, A.; Svärd, A. Presence of salivary IgA anti-citrullinated protein antibodies associate with higher disease activity in patients with rheumatoid arthritis. *Arthritis Res. Ther.* **2020**, *22*, 274. [CrossRef] [PubMed]
36. Stolt, P.; Bengtsson, C.; Nordmark, B.; Lindblad, S.; Lundberg, I.; Klareskog, L.; Alfredsson, L. Quantification of the influence of cigarette smoking on rheumatoid arthritis: Results from a population based case-control study, using incident cases. *Ann. Rheum. Dis.* **2003**, *62*, 835–841. [CrossRef] [PubMed]
37. Svärd, A.; Kastbom, A.; Sommarin, Y.; Skogh, T. Salivary IgA antibodies to cyclic citrullinated peptides (CCP) in rheumatoid arthritis. *Immunobiology* **2013**, *218*, 232–237. [CrossRef] [PubMed]
38. Kastbom, A.; Roos Ljungberg, K.; Ziegelasch, M.; Wetterö, J.; Skogh, T.; Martinsson, K. Changes in anti-citrullinated protein antibody isotype levels in relation to disease activity and response to treatment in early rheumatoid arthritis. *Clin. Exp. Immunol.* **2018**, *194*, 391–399. [CrossRef] [PubMed]
39. Repetto, G.; del Peso, A.; Zurita, J.L. Neutral red uptake assay for the estimation of cell viability/cytotoxicity. *Nat. Protoc.* **2008**, *3*, 1125–1131. [CrossRef]
40. Ennibi, O.K.; Claesson, R.; Akkaoui, S.; Reddahi, S.; Kwamin, F.; Haubek, D.; Johansson, A. High salivary levels of JP2 genotype of Aggregatibacter actinomycetemcomitans is associated with clinical attachment loss in Moroccan adolescents. *Clin. Exp. Dent. Res.* **2019**, *5*, 44–51. [CrossRef]
41. Helsel, D.R. *Statistics for Censored Environmental Data Using Minitab and R*, 2nd ed.; John Wiley & Sons: Hoboken, NJ, USA, 2012; ISBN 978-1-118-16276-7.
42. Tibshirani, R.J.; Efron, B. *An Introduction to the Bootstrap. Monographs on Statistics and Applied Probability*, 1st ed.; Chapman & Hall: London, UK; CRS Press: Boca Raton, FL, USA, 1994; Volume 57, ISBN 0412042312.
43. Kobayashi, T.; Bartold, P.M. Periodontitis and periodontopathic bacteria as risk factors for rheumatoid arthritis: A review of the last 10 years. *Jpn. Dent. Sci. Rev.* **2023**, *59*, 263–272. [CrossRef] [PubMed]
44. Lindholm, M.; Claesson, R.; Löf, H.; Chiang, H.M.; Oscarsson, J.; Johansson, A.; Åberg, C.H. Radiographic and clinical signs of periodontitis and associated bacterial species in a Swedish adolescent population. *J. Periodontol.* **2023**, *94*, 630–640. [CrossRef] [PubMed]
45. Volkov, M.; Dekkers, J.; Loos, B.G.; Bizzarro, S.; Huizinga, T.W.J.; Praetorius, H.A.; Toes, R.E.M.; van der Woude, D. Comment on "Aggregatibacter actinomycetemcomitans-induced hypercitrullination links periodontal infection to autoimmunity in rheumatoid arthritis". *Sci. Transl. Med.* **2018**, *10*, eaan8349. [CrossRef] [PubMed]
46. Koh, Y.R.; Cummings, K.C., 3rd. Newer Immunosuppressants for Rheumatologic Disease: Preoperative Considerations. *Anesthesiol. Clin.* **2024**, *42*, 131–143. [CrossRef] [PubMed]
47. Huang, Y.; Ni, S. Aggregatibacter Actinomycetemcomitans With Periodontitis and Rheumatoid Arthritis. *Int. Dent. J.* **2024**, *74*, 58–65. [CrossRef] [PubMed]
48. Li, Z.; Huang, Q.; Wang, Z.; Huang, L.; Gu, L. Effects of Porphyromonas gingivalis and Aggregatibacter actinomycetemcomitans on Modeling Subgingival Microbiome and Impairment of Oral Epithelial Barrier. *J. Infect. Dis.* **2024**, *229*, 262–272. [CrossRef]
49. Gualtero, D.F.; Lafaurie, G.I.; Buitrago, D.M.; Castillo, Y.; Vargas-Sanchez, P.K.; Castillo, D.M. Oral microbiome mediated inflammation, a potential inductor of vascular diseases: A comprehensive review. *Front. Cardiovasc. Med.* **2023**, *10*, 1250263. [CrossRef] [PubMed]
50. Reichert, S.; Haffner, M.; Keyßer, G.; Schäfer, C.; Stein, J.M.; Schaller, H.G.; Wienke, A.; Strauss, H.; Heide, S.; Schulz, S. Detection of oral bacterial DNA in synovial fluid. *J. Clin. Periodontol.* **2013**, *40*, 591–598. [CrossRef] [PubMed]
51. Kulkarni, A.; Beckler, M.D.; Amini, S.S.; Kesselman, M.M. Oral Microbiome in Pre-Rheumatoid Arthritis: The Role of Aggregatibacter Actinomycetemcomitans in Bacterial Composition. *Cureus* **2022**, *14*, e32201. [CrossRef]
52. Salvi, G.E.; Roccuzzo, A.; Imber, J.C.; Stähli, A.; Klinge, B.; Lang, N.P. Clinical periodontal diagnosis. *Periodontology 2000* **2023**, *93*, 236–253. [CrossRef]
53. Kindstedt, E.; Johansson, L.; Palmqvist, P.; Koskinen Holm, C.; Kokkonen, H.; Johansson, I.; Rantapää Dahlqvist, S.; Lundberg, P. Association Between Marginal Jawbone Loss and Onset of Rheumatoid Arthritis and Relationship to Plasma Levels of RANKL. *Arthritis Rheumatol.* **2018**, *70*, 508–515. [CrossRef] [PubMed]
54. González-Febles, J.; Sanz, M. Periodontitis and rheumatoid arthritis: What have we learned about their connection and their treatment? *Periodontology 2000* **2021**, *87*, 181–203. [CrossRef] [PubMed]
55. Fine, D.H.; Schreiner, H.; Velusamy, S.K. Aggregatibacter, A Low Abundance Pathobiont That Influences Biogeography, Microbial Dysbiosis, and Host Defense Capabilities in Periodontitis: The History of A Bug, And Localization of Disease. *Pathogens* **2020**, *9*, 179. [CrossRef] [PubMed]

56. Wu, Q.; Zhang, W.; Lu, Y.; Li, H.; Yang, Y.; Geng, F.; Liu, J.; Lin, L.; Pan, Y.; Li, C. Association between periodontitis and inflammatory comorbidities: The common role of innate immune cells, underlying mechanisms and therapeutic targets. *Int. Immunopharmacol.* **2024**, *128*, 111558. [CrossRef]

57. Saglie, F.R.; Marfany, A.; Camargo, P. Intragingival occurrence of Actinobacillus actinomycetemcomitans and Bacteroides gingivalis in active destructive periodontal lesions. *J. Periodontol.* **1988**, *59*, 259–265. [CrossRef]

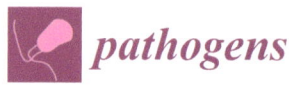

pathogens

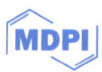

Article

Aggregatibacter actinomycetemcomitans Cytolethal Distending Toxin Induces Cellugyrin-(Synaptogyrin 2) Dependent Cellular Senescence in Oral Keratinocytes

Bruce J. Shenker [1,*], Jonathan Korostoff [2], Lisa P. Walker [1], Ali Zekavat [1], Anuradha Dhingra [1], Taewan J. Kim [2] and Kathleen Boesze-Battaglia [1]

[1] Department of Basic and Translational Sciences, School of Dental Medicine, University of Pennsylvania, Philadelphia, PA 19104, USA; lism@dental.upenn.edu (L.P.W.); seyed20@dental.upenn.edu (A.Z.); dhingra@upenn.edu (A.D.); battagli@dental.upenn.edu (K.B.-B.)

[2] Department of Periodontics, School of Dental Medicine, University of Pennsylvania, Philadelphia, PA 19104, USA; jkorosto@upenn.edu (J.K.); taewank@upenn.edu (T.J.K.)

* Correspondence: shenker@upenn.edu; Tel.: +1-215-898-5959

Abstract: Recently, we reported that oral-epithelial cells (OE) are unique in their response to *Aggregatibacter actinomycetemcomitans* cytolethal distending toxin (Cdt) in that cell cycle arrest (G2/M) occurs without leading to apoptosis. We now demonstrate that Cdt-induced cell cycle arrest in OE has a duration of at least 7 days with no change in viability. Moreover, toxin-treated OE develops a new phenotype consistent with cellular senescence; this includes increased senescence-associated β-galactosidase (SA-β-gal) activity and accumulation of the lipopigment, lipofuscin. Moreover, the cells exhibit a secretory profile associated with cellular senescence known as the senescence-associated secretory phenotype (SASP), which includes IL-6, IL-8 and RANKL. Another unique feature of Cdt-induced OE senescence is disruption of barrier function, as shown by loss of transepithelial electrical resistance and confocal microscopic assessment of primary gingival keratinocyte structure. Finally, we demonstrate that Cdt-induced senescence is dependent upon the host cell protein cellugyrin, a homologue of the synaptic vesicle protein synaptogyrin. Collectively, these observations point to a novel pathogenic outcome in oral epithelium that we propose contributes to both *A. actinomycetemcomitans* infection and periodontal disease progression.

Keywords: *Aggregatibacter actinomycetemcomitans*; cytolethal distending toxin; senescence; oral keratinocytes; cellugyrin; synaptogyrin-2; periodontal disease

Citation: Shenker, B.J.; Korostoff, J.; Walker, L.P.; Zekavat, A.; Dhingra, A.; Kim, T.J.; Boesze-Battaglia, K. *Aggregatibacter actinomycetemcomitans* Cytolethal Distending Toxin Induces Cellugyrin-(Synaptogyrin 2) Dependent Cellular Senescence in Oral Keratinocytes. *Pathogens* **2024**, *13*, 155. https://doi.org/10.3390/pathogens13020155

Academic Editor: Daniel H. Fine

Received: 20 December 2023
Revised: 25 January 2024
Accepted: 30 January 2024
Published: 8 February 2024

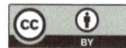

1. Introduction

Aggregatibacter actinomycetemcomitans has been linked to systemic disorders, including endocarditis and brain abscesses, among others [1]. In the oral cavity, the organism has long been associated with what prior to 2017 was referred to as localized aggressive periodontitis (LAP), a complex disorder involving risk factors of both host and microbial origin [2–8]. Although LAP no longer exists as a disease classification, the clinical manifestations remain part of the new classification corresponding to aggressive molar-incisor pattern periodontitis (MIPP). *A. actinomycetemcomitans* was previously thought to function as the causative agent of LAP. It is now believed that the initial colonization of supragingival biofilms by *A. actinomycetemcomitans* represents a risk factor for the onset of gingival inflammation. As an accessory pathogen, *A. actinomycetemcomitans* eventually translocates from the gingival margin through the gingival epithelium into the underlying connective tissue, a process associated with the conversion from health to disease [1,2,6]. In this regard, *A. actinomycetemcomitans* exhibits virulence properties that contribute to this new role as an accessory pathogen; these include tissue invasiveness, the ability to create an environment facilitating the accumulation of other organisms, evasion or subversion of host defenses and the capacity to promote inflammation. Collectively, these pathogenic attributes contribute to the accumulation of inflammophilic organisms that mediate downstream events in the pathogenesis of periodontitis (reviewed in [1,2,7]. Importantly, *A. actinomycetemcomitans* expresses two exotoxins, cytolethal distending toxin (Cdt) and leukotoxin [1,9–11], which are capable of subverting host cell function [1,2,8,12].

A. actinomycetemcomitans cyolethal distending toxin (*Aa*Cdt) is encoded by three genes, cdtA, cdtB, and cdtC, encoding three polypeptides designated as CdtA, CdtB and CdtC with molecular masses of 23–30, 28–32 and 19–20 kDa, respectively. The three proteins associate with one another to form a holotoxin [10,13–17] that functions as an AB2 toxin. Subunits CdtA and CdtC comprise the cell-binding (B) component, and CdtB is the active subunit. It is noteworthy that Cdts represent a highly distributed and conserved family of putative virulence factors produced by more than 30 γ- and ε-Proteobacteria, which are responsible for chronic infections and inflammatory diseases that typically affect mucocutaneous tissue (reviewed in [11]). Cdts, regardless of bacterial origin, cause similar effects on proliferating cells: cell cycle arrest (typically G2/M) and eventually apoptotic cell death [10,14,18–26]. Recent observations suggest that Cdt is also capable of inducing functional alterations in the absence of cell death in non-proliferating cells [27–30].

We propose that Cdt contributes to several virulence properties of *A. actinomycetem-comitans* as it functions as a tri-perditious toxin that affects lymphocyte, macrophage, mast cell and epithelial function, thereby altering acquired and innate immunity as well as epithelial barrier integrity [11,31]. Cdt is able to exhibit these diverse effects and intoxicate multiple cell types by virtue of three unique properties that we have identified: (1) exploitation of a ubiquitous cell receptor, cholesterol [32–34]; (2) utilization of a novel host protein, cellugyrin, for cell entry and trafficking [35,36], and (3) utilization of a molecular mode of action that disrupts phosphatidylinositol-3 kinase (PI-3K) signaling, a pathway utilized by virtually all cells to regulate an array of functions [27,29,37,38].

Recently, we demonstrated that oral-epithelial cells (OE) are unique in their response to *Aa*Cdt [39]. Assessment of the effect of *Aa*Cdt on two immortalized OE lines as well as primary gingival keratinocytes (PGKs) showed that all three cell types were sensitive to *Aa*Cdt-induced cell cycle arrest as toxin-treated cells accumulated in the G2/M phase within 24 h of exposure to low Cdt concentrations (pg/mL) [39]. Similar to other cell types, toxin-treated cells also exhibited PI-3K signaling blockade, leading to glycogen synthase kinase 3β (GSK3β) activation, a requirement for Cdt-induced cell cycle arrest. However, unlike other cells, which typically undergo apoptosis following Cdt-induced cell cycle arrest, epithelial cell G2/M arrest did not lead to cell death [39]. We have now extended these observations and demonstrated that Cdt-induced cell cycle arrest in OE is durable. Moreover, OEs develop a phenotype typical of senescent cells, increased senescence-associated β-galactosidase (SA-β-gal) activity, accumulation of the lipopigment, lipofuscin, a product of oxidative processes, and the senescence-associated secretory phenotype (SASP), typified by enhanced production of IL-6, IL-8, and RANKL. We also show that senescent OEs exhibit a breakdown in barrier function, a unique characteristic of senescent cells. Finally, we determined that Cdt-induced cellular senescence is dependent upon the host cell protein cellugyrin. Collectively, these observations point to a novel pathogenic outcome in the oral epithelium that likely contributes to altered epithelial integrity and thereby promotes both *A. actinomycetemcomitans* infection and disease progression.

2. Materials and Methods

2.1. Oral Keratinocyte Culture and Gene Editing

The TIGK cell line was established from human gingival epithelial cells and immortalized with bmi1-transduction followed by human telomerase reverse transcriptase (hTERT) (kindly provided by RJ Lamont) [40]. TIGK cells were incubated in DermaLife K Basal Medium (Lifeline Cell Technology, Frederick, MD, USA) supplemented with glutamine, extract P, epinephrine, rh TGF, hydrocortisone hemisuccinate, rh insulin, apo-transferrin and calcium chloride.

Primary human gingival keratinocytes (PGK) were derived from discarded healthy gingival tissue obtained from patients undergoing crown lengthening procedures as previously described [39,41]. Briefly, tissue was washed in a HAMS F12 nutrient mixture (ThermoFisher Scientific, Waltham, MA, USA) containing 1% penicillin/streptomycin and 1% ampthotericin and then cut into 0.3 cm^2 fragments. The pieces of gingiva were incubated in HAMS F12 medium described above and also containing 2% dispase (Sigma Aldrich Co.; Burlington, MA, USA) for 24 h at 37 °C. Tissue was then separated with vigorous pipetting in 0.05% trypsin/EDTA (Life Technologies; Carlsbad, CA, USA), and the cell suspension was centrifuged, resuspended and incubated in Keratinocyte serum free medium (K-SFM; Life Technologies) containing bovine pituitary extract (BPE) (5 ng/mL), epidermal growth factor (10 μg/mL), and 2% penicillin/streptomycin.

We employed pLentiCRISPR V2 to generate cellugyrin-deficient TIGK cells (TIGK^{Cg-}) [39]. Briefly, two separate CRISPR-Cas9 guide sequences for cellugyrin were inserted into plentiCRISPR V2 plasmids, in which the puromycin resistance cassette was replaced with a neomycin resistance cassette (GTACATCTGCTTAGACTCGT, CGCGTCGACCACCAA-GAAGA) (Genscript, Piscataway, NJ, USA). Plasmids were co-transfected into HEK-293T cells, and viral supernatants were collected for introduction into cells. Virus was added to cells at a MOI of 4 and incubated overnight; cells were washed, then incubated for an additional 24 h before being selected with 250 ng/mL neomycin. Cells were plated for single-cell cloning, and cellugyrin-negative lines were generated from selected clones.

2.2. Preparation of Cdt

The construction and expression of the plasmid containing the *cdt* genes for the holotoxin (pUCAacdtABChis) have previously been reported [42]. The histidine-tagged holotoxin was isolated by nickel affinity chromatography, as previously described [15].

2.3. Assessment of Cell Proliferation

To measure Cdt-induced cell cycle distribution, replicate cultures of TIGK cells (10^5) were incubated for the time indicated, harvested (TIGK cells required trypsin digestion), washed, and fixed for 60 min with cold 80% ethanol [43]. Cells were stained with 10 μg/mL propidium iodide containing 1 mg/mL RNase (Sigma Aldrich Co.) for 30 min. Samples were analyzed on a Becton-Dickinson LSRII flow cytometer (BD Biosciences; San Jose, CA, USA); a minimum of 15,000 events were collected for each sample. Cell cycle analysis was performed using Modfit 6.0 (Verity Software House; Topsham, ME, USA).

Bromodeoxyuridine (BrdU) incorporation was assessed in TIGK cultures set up as described above with and without Cdt for 72 h. BrdU (10 μM; BrdU Kit; Thermofisher) was added to TIGK cultures for the last 4 h of incubation. Cells were harvested, fixed in 80% EtOH for 30 min and then treated with 2N HCl containing 0.5%Triton X-100. Following centrifugation, cells were resuspended in 0.1 M $Na_2B_4O_7$ for 5 min, and then in PBS containing 2% BSA and 0.05% Tween 20 (BioRad; Hercules, CA, USA). Cells were stained with anti-BrdU-FITC (Invitrogen, Waltham, MA, USA) for 1 h at RT, washed and stained with propidium iodide. Cells were analyzed by multiparametric flow cytometry on a Becton-Dickinson LSRII flow cytometer (BD Biosciences; San Jose, CA, USA); fluorochromes were excited with a 488 nm laser, and fluorescence was detected using a 530/30 filter (FITC) and a 575/26 filter (propidium iodide). A minimum of 15,000 events were collected for each sample, and analysis was performed using WinList 9.0.1 (Verity Software House).

Analysis of cell proliferation was also assessed on TIGK cells using ViaFluor 488 (Biotium; Fremont, CA, USA). Cell cultures were established in 24-well plates, as described above; cells were pre-treated with medium alone or medium containing Cdt (20 pg/mL) for 16 h. ViaFluor was added to each well for 15 min, according to the manufacturer's directions after which cells were washed and incubated for 72 h. Cells were then harvested by trypsinization and analyzed for fluorescence as described above.

2.4. Assessment of SA-β-Gal Activity

TIGK cells (10^5) were added to 24 well plates in the media described above; cells received media or Cdt for the time indicated. SA-β-gal activity was measured using the Senescence β-galactosidase activity assay kit (Cell Signaling, Danvers, MA, USA) as described by the manufacturer. Briefly, media was removed from cells and bafilomycin (to prevent acidification) was added for 1 h; the cell permeable fluorogenic substrate was added and the cells incubated for an additional 4 h at 37 °C. Cells were trypsinized and washed. Fluorescence resulting from hydrolysis of the substrate was analyzed by flow cytometry using a 488 nm laser and fluorescence emission assessed through a 530/30 nm filter. At least 10,000 events were analyzed.

2.5. Assessment of Lipofuscin Content

TIGK cells were established in 24-well plates as described above; at the times indicated, cells were stained using the SenTraGor reagent according to the manufacturer's recommendation (Lab Supplies Scientific; Athens, Greece). Briefly, media was removed and cells harvested following trypsinization. Cells were fixed in 4% formaldehyde at RT for 20 min, washed, permeabilized in 0.01% Triton X-100 for 15 min, washed sequentially in 50% and 70% EtOH, and then incubated for 8 min with SenTraGor. Cells were washed with 50% EtOH and then stained with anti-biotin antibody conjugated to AF488 (Santa Cruz Biotechnology; Santa Cruz, CA, USA) or isotype (IgG1) control antibody (Santa Cruz Biotechnology) for 1 h at RT; after washing, cells were analyzed by flow cytometry using a 488 nm laser. Fluorescence emission was measured through a 530/30 filter; at least 10,000 cells were analyzed.

2.6. Analysis of Cytokine Release from TIGK Cells

TIGK cultures were set up as described above; cytokine production was measured in TIGK supernatants 72 h after exposure to medium with or without Cdt. In some experiments, cells were pre-exposed to necrosulfonamide [(NSA); Millipore Sigma, Burlington, MA, USA] for one h prior to the addition of Cdt. Culture supernatants were collected and analyzed by ELISA for IL-6, IL-8 and RANKL using commercially available kits according to the manufacturer's instructions (Peprotech; Cranberry, NJ, USA) [27]. In each instance, the amount of cytokine present in the supernatant was determined using a standard curve.

2.7. Analysis of Epithelial Barrier Integrity

Assessment of Trans-Epithelial Electrical Resistance (TEER) is a widely accepted quantitative technique to measure the integrity of the barrier function of OE culture models [44]. Polarized PGKs (1.5×10^5) were grown on 12-well transwell inserts (Corning; Corning, NY, USA) in the medium described above. Cells were grown to confluence and monitored for the establishment of TEER with the STX2 electrode (Epithelial Volt/Ohm Meter; World Precision Instruments, Sarasota, FL, USA). Cdt or media were then added to cultures, and TEER was measured at 24 h intervals.

PGKs were grown as above on transwell dishes and treated with Cdt (10 pg/mL, 48 h) or medium only, washed in PBS, and fixed in 4% PFA for 15 min at room temperature. The cells were permeabilized and blocked in 5% BSA and 0.2% Triton X-100 in PBS (PBST) at 37 °C for 1 h. Cells were then incubated with a 1:100 dilution of anti-ß-catenin antibody (Cell Signaling) diluted in blocking solution at 4 °C overnight, washed three times with PBST, incubated with donkey anti-rabbit Alexa Fluor 488 (1:1000; Invitrogen) and Hoechst 33258 (1:10,000; Invitrogen) at 37 °C for 1 h, washed and mounted in Prolong Gold Antifade reagent (P36930, Invitrogen). Confocal Z-stack images were acquired on a Nikon A1R laser scanning confocal microscope with a 60X (water) objective at 18 °C, and the data were analyzed using Nikon software (NIS Elements AR 5.30.03) [30].

3. Results

3.1. Cdt Induces a Senescent Cell Phenotype in Oral Epithelial Cells

We previously reported that the oral keratinocyte cell lines TIGK and OKF6 as well as PGKs exposed to Cdt exhibited cell cycle arrest (G2/M) that persisted for at least 72 h; notably, the arrest occurred in the absence of any evidence of DNA damage or apoptotic cell death [39]. In those studies, cell cycle arrest was determined by assessing DNA content with propidium iodide to measure cell distribution within the cell cycle. In our current study, we have expanded the assessment of Cdt-induced growth arrest by first utilizing dual parameter flow cytometric analysis to simultaneously measure G0/G1 and G2/M with propidium iodide and more accurately assess the S-phase with bromodeoxyuridine (BrdU), a synthetic nucleoside analogue with a chemical structure similar to thymidine. Representative results are shown in Figure 1; cells were exposed to Cdt or medium alone for 72 h. BrdU was added to the cultures for the last 4 h; 6.8% of untreated (no toxin) TIGK cells exhibited positive BrdU fluorescence (Figure 1A). During the same time period, cells treated with 20 pg/mL Cdt exhibited fewer S-phase cells, as only 1.3% were BrdU positive (Figure 1B); these results further support the conclusion that exposure of OEs to Cdt leads to growth arrest. Consistent with earlier studies, Cdt treatment resulted in an increase in the percentage of G2/M cells to 59.2% relative to untreated cells, which contained 5.8% G2/M cells. The percentage of cells in G0/G1 decreased from 77.1% in control cells to 32.6% in cells treated with Cdt.

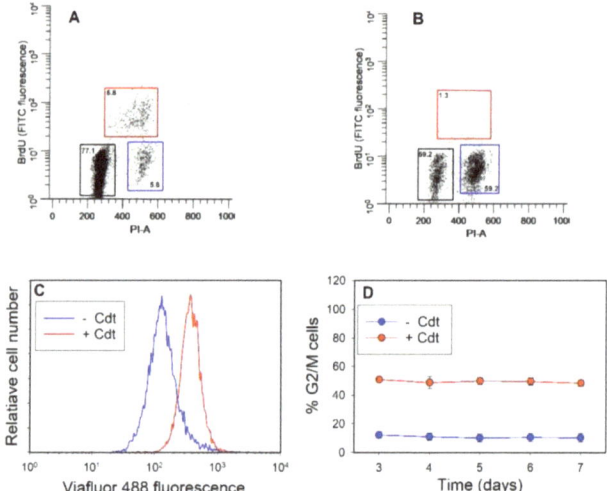

Figure 1. Cdt induces durable cell cycle arrest in OE. TIGK cells were treated with Cdt for varying periods of time as indicated and then monitored for cell cycle arrest. Panels (**A**) (control cells) and (**B**) (Cdt-treated cells) show the effect of Cdt (20 pg/mL) on TIGK proliferation after 72 h. Cell cycle progression was assessed using dual parameter flow cytometry; DNA content was assessed by monitoring propidium iodide fluorescence (PI-A) and incorporation of BrdU-FITC. Boxes indicate gates for cell cycle analysis: G1/G0 (black), G2/M (blue) and S (red); numbers indicate the percentage of cells within each gated box. Panel (**C**) shows the analysis of cell cycle progression in control (blue line) and toxin-treated (red line) cells stained with Viafluor 488 and incubated for 72 h. The results for panels (**A–C**) are each representative of three experiments. Panel (**D**) shows cell cycle analysis of TIGK cells treated with medium (blue) and Cdt [20 pg/mL; (red)] for 3–7 days using propidium iodide. Cells were analyzed for cell phase as described in Section 2; the percentage of G2/M cells is plotted versus time. Results are compiled from three experiments and represent the mean ± SEM; all data points for Cdt-treated cells are significantly different from those observed in control cells ($p < 0.01$). Individual cell cycle histograms are shown in Figure S1.

In a complementary approach, we utilized Viafluor 488 to assess the effect of Cdt on cell proliferation. Cells were treated with Cdt (or medium) and then labeled with Viafluor as described in Section 2. Fluorescence was assessed 72 h later; each round of cell division results in a reduction in fluorescence as the probe is distributed to daughter cells. Control and toxin-treated cells were compared based upon their level of fluorescence and designated as either high Viafluor fluorescence (Viafluor^{high}) or low Viafluor fluorescence (Viafluor^{low}). Control TIGK cells progressed through the cell cycle, resulting in a transition to a population characterized as Viafluor^{low} [mean channel fluorescence (MCF) 135] when compared to Cdt-treated TIGK cells (Figure 1C). The toxin-treated cells underwent cell cycle arrest, which was reflected in their retaining higher levels of Viafluor and hence exhibited brighter fluorescence given that the dye was not diluted out into daughter cells; the Viafluor^{high} exhibited a MCF of 430.

In a third assessment, the durability of Cdt-induced cell cycle arrest was analyzed using propidium iodide to determine cell cycle distribution at days 3–7-post toxin treatment (Figure 1D). We previously reported that Cdt-treated TIGK cells exhibited G2/M arrest as early as 24 h, and the percentage of G2/M cells remained elevated at 72 h. In our current analysis, the proliferating TIGK control cells routinely contained 10.3 ± 2.8 to $12.2 \pm 2.1\%$ G2/M cells; this is consistent with a distribution of normal proliferating cells (see Figure S1 for cell cycle profiles). In contrast, the percentage of G2/M Cdt-treated cells increased to $50.9 \pm 2.1\%$ at day 3, as previously reported [39]; the accumulation of G2/M cells remained at this level throughout days 4–7 of analysis. Collectively, these experiments indicate that OEs exposed to Cdt undergo a sustained, or durable, cell cycle arrest in the G2/M phase of the cell cycle.

Durable cell cycle arrest in an otherwise replication-competent cell is a critical feature of cellular senescence but not necessarily a defining feature alone. Cellular senescence is also associated with the acquisition of a new phenotype characterized by other common traits such as increased SA-β-gal activity and lipofuscin accumulation [45–47]. Therefore, we next utilized flow cytometry to assess Cdt-treated cells for changes in SA-β-gal activity by monitoring the hydrolysis of a cell-permeable fluorogenic substrate (see Section 2). As shown in Figure 2A, cells treated with Cdt for 72 h exhibited a significant dose-dependent increase in SA-β-gal activity, as the MCF increased to 156.7 ± 16.5 (2 pg/mL Cdt) and 191.1 ± 13.8 (10 pg/mL Cdt); this compares to a MCF of 99.5 ± 7.5 in control cells. Exposure to 25 pg/mL Cdt did not result in any further increase in SA-β-gal activity as the MCF was 190.4 ± 14.8. It should be noted that these levels remained elevated for 7 days (see Figure 2A inset). Experiments were also conducted with PGKs, which exhibited similar elevations in SA-β-gal activity (Figure 2B) when treated with 10 pg/mL (MCF 174 ± 33) and 25 pg/mL Cdt (MCF 187 ± 29) relative to untreated cells (MCF 122 ± 27).

Another feature of the senescent cell phenotype is the accumulation of lipofuscin, which we analyzed with SenTraGor™, a highly lipophilic and biotinylated analog of Sudan Black B that is detectable with an anti-biotin antibody conjugated with AF488 [48–50]. TIGK cells were incubated with medium or 20 pg/mL Cdt for 3–7 days and processed as described in Section 2. As shown in Figure 2C, the MCF for control cells was 19.9 ± 4.0 (3 days), 21.5 ± 1.8 (4 days), and 28.5 ± 5.6 (7 days). In the presence of Cdt, fluorescence increased in a time-dependent manner: 28.0 ± 8.0 (3 days), 34.5 ± 2.3 (4 days), and almost doubling at day 7 to 47.8 ± 7.1. PGK cells were also assessed for lipofuscin following exposure to Cdt (Figure 2D); cells treated with 10 and 25 pg/mL Cdt exhibited increased fluorescence with MCFs of 41.2 ± 5.4 and 40.2 ± 4.0 compared to 25.8 ± 5.2 in control cells. Results from earlier time points are shown in Figure S2.

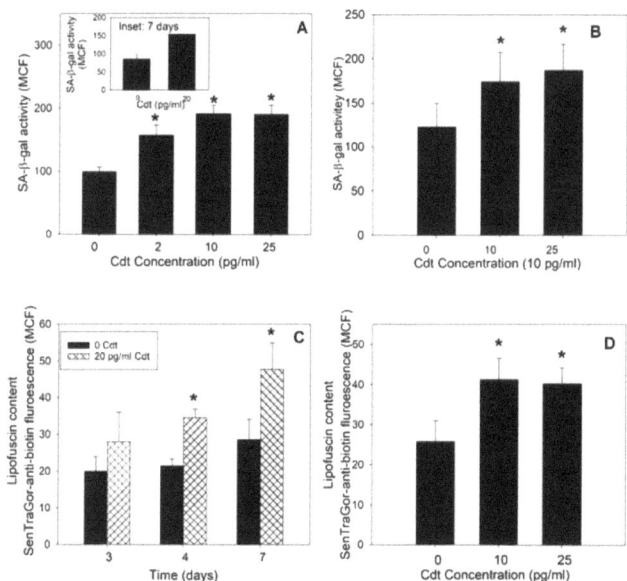

Figure 2. Cdt induces a cellular senescent phenotype in OEs characterized by increases in both SA-β-gal activity and lipofuscin content. TIGK cells were treated with 0–25 pg/mL Cdt for 72 h and then analyzed for SA-β-gal activity as described in Section 2. Data are plotted as fluorescence (MCF) vs. Cdt concentration. The inset (panel (**A**)) shows results for exposure to Cdt for 7 days. Panel (**B**) shows the effect of Cdt on SA-β-gal activity in toxin-treated PGK cells following 3 days of exposure to Cdt. Panel (**C**) shows the effect of Cdt (20 pg/mL) on lipofuscin levels in TIGK cells following 3–7 days of exposure to toxin. Lipofuscin was detected using biotinylated SenTraGor, followed by staining with an anti-biotin antibody conjugated to AF488. Results are plotted as fluorescence (MCF) versus time of exposure to Cdt (days). Panel (**D**) shows the effect of Cdt on lipofuscin levels in PGK cells after 4 days of treatment with toxin. Results are plotted as the MCF (mean ± SEM) of three experiments; * indicates statistical significance ($p < 0.05$).

3.2. Cdt Induces Oral Epithelial Cells to Exhibit the Senescent Associated Secretory Phenotype (SASP)

In addition to both enhanced SA-β-gal activity and lipofuscin, senescent cells typically acquire a phenotype characterized by robust secretory activity known as SASP [46,47,51]. This secretory phenotype has been identified in almost all senescent cells and may include pro-inflammatory cytokines, chemokines, proteases and other biologically active agents. It is in this context that we next assessed Cdt-treated TIGK cell supernatants for IL-8 (Figure 3A), IL-6 (Figure 3B) and RANKL secretion (Figure 3C). All three cytokines exhibited dose-dependent increases when cells were exposed to 0–100 pg/mL Cdt. IL-8 secretion increased from 123.1 ± 13.8 pg/mL in control cells to 184.8 ± 35.5, 273.1 ± 55.7, 453.3 ± 95.1 and 780 ± 73.0 pg/mL in the presence of 10, 25, 50 and 100 pg/mL Cdt, respectively. Similarly, IL-6 levels increased from 4.7 ± 4.5 pg/mL in control cells to 19.2 ± 8.9, 108.7 ± 17.2, 168.3 ± 13.6 and 206.2 ± 23.6 pg/mL in the presence of the same doses of toxin (10–100 pg/mL). Significant increases in RANKL secretion were also observed in a dose-dependent manner; in the presence of 10, 25, 50 and 100 pg/mL, Cdt RANKL levels were 15 ± 6, 23.9 ± 2.0, 63.9 ± 4.5 and 108. ± 4.0 pg/mL, respectively. No detectable RANKL was observed in the supernatants of control cells.

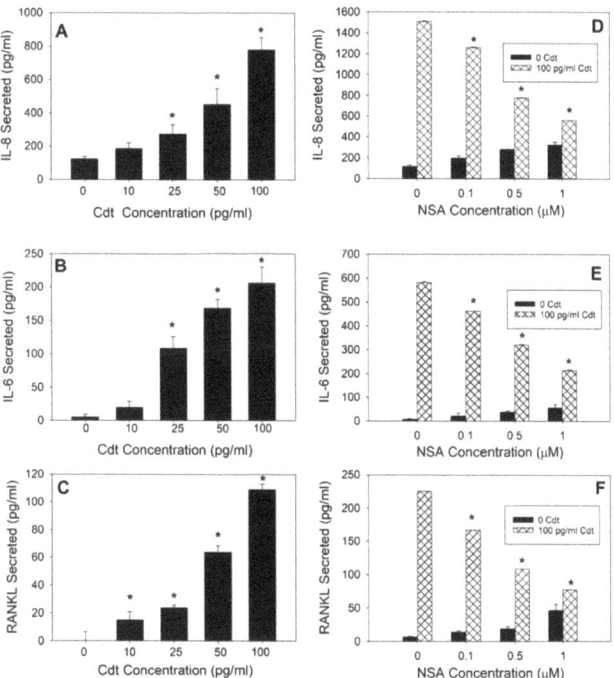

Figure 3. Cdt induces SASP in TIGK cells. TIGK cells were treated with Cdt (0–100 pg/mL) for 72 h; cell supernatants were harvested and analyzed by ELISA for release of IL-8 (panel (**A**)), IL-6 (panel (**B**)) and RANKL (panel (**C**)). In a second series of experiments, TIGK cells were pre-treated with the GSDMD inhibitor NSA (0–1 μM) for one h, followed by the addition of Cdt (100 pg/mL). Supernatants were harvested 72 h later and analyzed for release of IL-8 (panel (**D**)), IL-6 (panel (**E**)) and RANKL (panel (**F**)). Results are the mean ± SEM of three experiments; * indicates statistical significance ($p < 0.01$).

Recent studies have suggested that gasdermin D (GSDMD) activation is a key event leading to the release of senescence-associated proteins [52–57]. GSDMD is converted to an active fragment (GSDMD-NT), which causes nonlytic membrane pore formation. Small GSDMD-NT-dependent pores have recently been observed in a variety of senescent cells and are now considered a significant feature of cellular senescence [58]. To ascertain if GSDMD activation was involved in Cdt-induced cytokine release from TIGK cells, we employed the GSDMD inhibitor necrosulfonamide (NSA); results are shown in Figure 3D–F. Cells were pre-treated with 0.1–1.0 μM NSA for 60 min, followed by the addition of 100 pg/mL Cdt. Supernatants were analyzed by ELISA and demonstrated that IL-8, IL-6 and RANKL levels were reduced in a dose-dependent manner when cells were pretreated with 0.1, 0.5 and 1.0 μM NSA. Maximum inhibition occurred in the presence of the highest NSA dose employed in this study (1.0 μM), with all three cytokine levels reduced by >60%. Interestingly, we observed small increments of cytokine release in the presence of NSA alone; this was not due to NSA-induced changes in either cell viability or induction of senescence (Figure S3).

3.3. Cdt-Induced Senescent PGKs Exhibit Loss of Barrier Function

We next assessed Cdt-treated cells for alterations in epithelial barrier function. For this purpose, we measured transepithelial electrical resistance (TEER), which is a widely accepted quantitative technique to measure the integrity of cellular barriers in epithelial cell culture models [44]. This technique categorizes cell barriers as tight, intermediate, or leaky based upon TEER values. We have demonstrated that PGK monolayers reproducibly develop TEER with intermediate values ($429 \pm 30.9 \; \Omega \times cm^2$; Figure 4); moreover, after 48 h exposure to Cdt, the TEER values were significantly reduced to essentially the background levels observed with medium alone ($236 \pm 16.6 \; \Omega \times cm^2$).

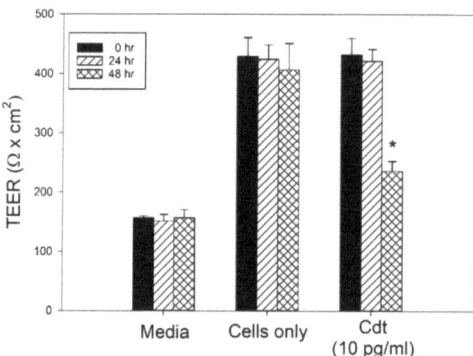

Figure 4. Cdt-induced OE senescent cells exhibit a breakdown in epithelial barrier function. PGKs were grown to confluence until a stable TEER was established. Medium or Cdt was then added and the cells assessed daily for changes in TEER as described in Section 2. Results of three experiments were plotted as mean resistance ($\Omega \times cm^2$) at 24 h (solid bars), 48 h (hatched bars) and 72 h (cross hatched bars); * indicates statistical significance ($p < 0.01$).

To further evaluate whether Cdt perturbs epithelial barrier function, cell–cell adhesion in PGKs was examined by immunostaining Cdt-treated (10 pg/mL) and untreated (control) cells for an adherans junction protein, ß-catenin [59]. There was distinct staining for ß-catenin adjoining the border between adjacent cells in the control cultures (Figure 5A–C left, Figure S4 top). Treatment of PGK cells with 10 pg/mL Cdt (48 h) resulted in an alteration of the staining pattern for ß-catenin; intense staining outlining the individual cells was detected while the junctions between the cells were largely devoid of ß-catenin (Figure 5A–C right, Figure S4 bottom). The linear intensity profile (Figure 5D) further highlights these ß-catenin negative gaps ($1.45 \; \forall \; 0.25 \; \mu m$; size ranging from 0.4–2.9 μm based upon analysis of 10 regions) between cells treated with Cdt. This result strongly points to Cdt-driven disruption of adherans junctions that can lead to compromised cell–cell communication and compromised barrier function.

3.4. Cdt-Induced Cellular Senescence Is Dependent on the Host Cell Protein Cellugyrin

In previous studies with lymphocytes and macrophages, we demonstrated that shortly after Cdt binds to cholesterol within lipid-enriched membrane microdomains, the host cell protein, cellugyrin, localizes to the same region. Following these events, Cdt subunits CdtB and CdtC are internalized and associate with cellugyrin, leading to their intracellular transport complexed to cellugyrin within the context of synaptic-like microvesicles (SLMVs) [35,36,38]. Importantly, reduced expression of cellugyrin in lymphocytes and macrophages protects cells from CdtB internalization and subsequent toxicity. Therefore, we assessed whether the susceptibility of TIGK cells to Cdt-induced senescence was also dependent on cellugyrin. CRISPR/Cas9 gene editing was employed using a pLentivirus V2 plasmid containing cellugyrin-specific sequences to establish a cellugyrin-deficient TIGK cell line (TIGK^{Cg-}). As shown in Figure 6A inset, TIGK^{Cg-} cells do not express detectable cellugyrin. Wildtype TIGK cells (TIGK^{WT}) and TIGK^{Cg-} cells were treated with Cdt for 48 h and assessed for cell cycle arrest (G2/M). Similar to our previous results [39], TIGK^{WT} cells exhibited a dose-dependent response to Cdt, as the accumulation of G2/M cells was $16.6 \pm 3.0\%$, $22.4 \pm 1.9\%$ and $35.8 \pm 2.9\%$ following exposure to 5, 10 and 20 pg/mL Cdt, compared to $9.3 \pm 2.8\%$ in untreated controls. In contrast, TIGK^{Cg-} cells were protected from Cdt-induced cell cycle arrest as the percentage of cells in the G2/M phase did not change from those values observed in control cells (8.6 ± 2.9%).

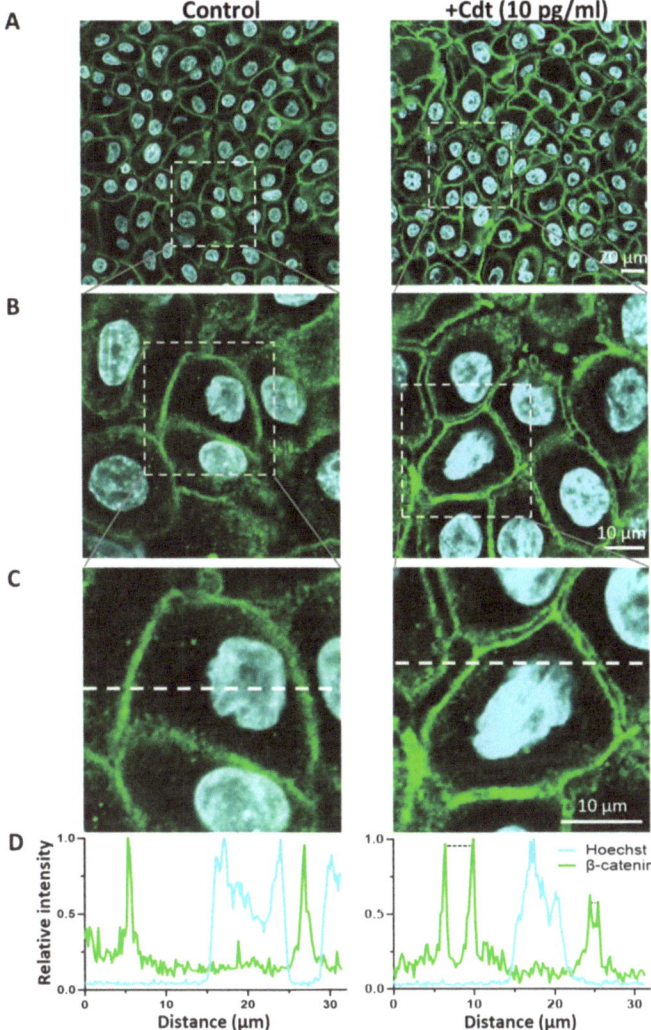

Figure 5. Cdt treatment alters cell–cell contacts in PGKs. (**A**) Confocal images showing control (untreated) and Cdt (10 pg/mL, 48 h)-treated PGKs immunostained with ß-catenin (green). Nuclei stained with Hoechst are pseudo-colored in cyan. (**B**) Boxed regions in the panel (**A**) were enlarged and shown. (**C**) The boxed regions in panel (**B**) were further enlarged, highlighting the appearance of distinct gaps between cells in the Cdt-treated set (right) relative to the control cells. (**D**) Line intensity profiles for ß-catenin (green) and Hoechst nuclear stain (cyan) across the white dotted line in panel (**C**). The gaps between the adjacent cells identified by the ß-catenin staining pattern are depicted by dotted black lines.

We then evaluated the susceptibility of TIGK^{Cg-} cells to Cdt-induced increases in SA-β-gal activity and lipofuscin accumulation. TIGK^{WT} and TIGK^{Cg-} cells were treated with 20 pg/mL Cdt, followed by analysis 72 h later for SA-β-gal activity as described earlier. TIGK^{WT} cells exhibited an increase in SA-β-gal activity (Figure 6B); MCF increased from 125 ± 27.5 in control cells to 261.4 ± 41.1 in Cdt-treated cells. In contrast, Cdt-treated

TIGK^{Cg-} cells did not exhibit any increase in fluorescence relative to control cells; the MCFs were 148.9 ± 31.8 (Cdt-treated) and 153.7 ± 34.1 (control). In a similar experiment, TIGK^{WT} and TIGK^{Cg-} cells were treated with Cdt and assessed 96 h later for changes in lipofuscin using the SenTraGor reagent and anti-biotin antibody conjugated to AF488 (Figure 6C). Toxin-treated TIGK^{WT} cells exhibited an increase in fluorescence, as MCFs were 20.3 ± 4.5 in control cells and 39.5 ± 9.7 in toxin-treated cells. Cdt-treated TIGK^{Cg-} cells failed to exhibit a change in fluorescence relative to control cells. These results confirm that, similar to other cell types examined to date, the susceptibility of OEs to Cdt is also dependent upon cellugyrin [35,36,38].

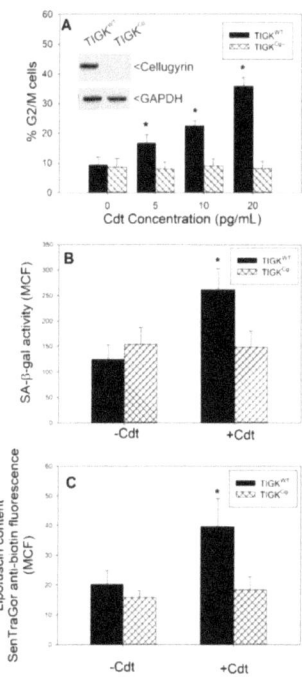

Figure 6. Cdt-induced cellular senescence is dependent on the host cell protein cellugyrin. Cellugyrin-deficient TIGK cells (TIGK^{Cg-}) were prepared using CRISPR/Cas9 gene editing (inset panel (**A**)). In panel A, TIGK^{Cg-} (cross-hatched bars) were compared with TIGK^{WT} cells (solid bars) for susceptibility to Cdt-induced cell cycle arrest. The percentage of G2/M cells was determined using propidium iodide fluorescence and flow cytometry; the results are plotted as the percentage of G2/M cells (mean ± SEM) versus Cdt concentration. Panel (**B**) compares the effect of Cdt (10 pg/mL) on TIGK^{WT} and TIGK^{Cg-} cell SA-β-gal activity after 72 h; the data are plotted as SA-β-gal fluorescence [MCF; (mean ± SEM)]. Panel (**C**) shows the effect of Cdt on lipofuscin content in TIGK^{WT} and TIGK^{Cg-} cells following 96 h exposure to the toxin; results are plotted as lipofuscin content [MCF; (mean ± SEM)]. * indicates statistical significance ($p < 0.05$) when compared to similarly treated TIGK^{WT} cells.

4. Discussion

Durable cell cycle arrest in the absence of cell death is a hallmark of cellular senescence; in this state, cells are no longer proliferating but remain metabolically active. Multiple types of cellular senescence have been described, including replicative, oncogenic, genotoxic and developmental, among others [60–62]. Moreover, the senescent phenotype has been implicated as a significant contributing factor to the pathogenesis of a wide range of disorders, including cancer, fibrosis, cardiovascular disease, diabetes, osteoarthritis and neurological disorders [46,63–65]. Recent studies have also demonstrated that pathogens, both bacterial and viral, are contributors to senescence [66,67]. Indeed, infection-induced senescence has been shown to involve toxins, viral capsids and flagella [67–71]. It should be noted that several studies have also demonstrated that bacterial factors such as *Porphyromonas gingivalis* lipopolysaccharide (LPS) can induce senescence in fibroblasts and dendritic cells, thereby contributing to periodontal disease-associated inflammation [72–75].

In this study, we demonstrated that, in addition to sustained G2/M arrest, *Aa*Cdt-treated OEs exhibit two of the most common hallmarks of senescent cells: elevated levels of SA-β-gal activity and the accumulation of oxidatively modified proteins and degraded lipid, commonly referred to as lipofuscin. Perhaps one of the most interesting, if not significant, features of senescent cells is that they also produce a secretome known as SASP, which contains pro-inflammatory mediators among other biologically active agents [46,47]. We have demonstrated that Cdt-treated OEs secrete IL-6, IL-8 and RANKL 72 h following exposure to toxin while remaining suspended in the G2/M phase of the cell cycle. Additionally, cytokine secretion exhibited dependence on GSDMD activation as the GSDMD inhibitor, NSA, blocked the toxin-induced release of all three cytokines. It should be noted that GSDMD activation as well as the formation of GSDMD-mediated nonlytic pores have recently been shown to be a feature shared by many senescent cells and are critical to senescence-associated secretory protein release [52–54].

The SASP is, perhaps, the most significant aspect of cellular senescence from a pathogenic perspective. The upregulated secretion of generally pro-inflammatory mediators allows senescent cells to: (1) induce senescence in neighboring cells (paracrine senescence), thereby further enhancing SASP secretome production and reducing the population of normal functioning (healthy) cells in involved tissue; (2) alter the local environment within the tissue, perhaps contributing to increased susceptibility to infection; and (3) promote recruitment and activation of inflammatory cells (reviewed in [46,47,67]. Thus, induction of cellular senescence represents a cell function vulnerable to hijacking and exploitation by pathogens; in this scenario, cellular senescence and SASP contribute to sustained infection and chronic inflammation [67]. Moreover, we demonstrate that senescent OEs exhibit another unique feature: breakdown of barrier function. Clearly, Cdt-induced cellular senescence can have a profound effect on oral epithelial tissue and contribute to disease initiation and/or progression. This axis of cellular toxicity may account for the significant role that *A. actinomycetemcomitans* has been reported to play in the conversion from periodontal health to disease, as has been observed for MIPP (previously reported as LAP) (reviewed in [1,2,6]). While direct evidence of a role for senescence in periodontal disease is currently limited, there is increasing acknowledgment of its potential participation in age-associated alterations within the periodontal environment as it relates to disease susceptibility [51,76,77]. Investigators have also demonstrated the presence of senescent osteocytes obtained from the alveoli of old mice, suggesting that these cells contribute to alveolar bone resorption [75]. As noted earlier, *P. gingivalis* LPS has also been reported to induce cellular senescence, further supporting the fact that the associated phenotypic changes are involved in the pathogenesis of periodontitis.

Senescence of various cells shares many attributes; however, it should be noted that they are not identical, as many of their novel features are dependent upon cell type and the pathway leading to senescence [45,62,78]. In this context, it is important to note that *Aa*Cdt-induced senescence in OEs is unique as it occurs in the absence of DNA damage [39]. Moreover, *Aa*Cdt-induced senescence is associated with a novel mechanism involving PI-3K signaling blockade and concomitant GSK3β activation, which mediates downstream phosphorylation of CDK1 (inactivation) [39]. *Haemophilus ducreyi* Cdt has been shown to also induce senescence in several cell lines [60,79–81]. In these studies, cells were exposed to relatively higher doses of toxin relative to those used in our current study, and senescence was associated with the activation of the DNA damage response.

Another unique feature of Cdt-induced toxicity, in general, and Cdt-induced senescence, in particular, is the dependence on the host cell protein cellugyrin (synaptogyrin-2). This protein belongs to the synaptogyrin family, a group of proteins that contain four transmembrane regions with a tyrosine-phosphorylated tail. Within cells, cellugyrin is embedded in SLMV^{Cg+} [35,36], which likely serve as sorting vesicles. These structures contain proteins essential for endocytic processing and are likely components of the trans-Golgi network (TGN) [82,83]. We have previously shown that both the CdtB and CdtC subunits are associated with cellugyrin and that intracellular transport of the Cdt subunits in macrophages and lymphocytes is dependent upon this association [35,36]. Moreover, we now demonstrate that, in addition to lymphocytes and macrophages, this dependence on cellugyrin extends to OEs. Specifically, epithelial cells rendered unable to express cellugyrin, TIGK^{Cg-} cells, were protected from Cdt-induced cell cycle arrest and senescence.

It is generally accepted that cellular senescence evolved as a protective mechanism to eliminate cells containing damaged DNA that escaped both repair and elimination by apoptosis [61,63]. However, it is now clear that this protective response represents another cell function vulnerable to exploitation by pathogens. As noted earlier, the colonization of supragingival biofilms by *A. actinomyetemcomitans* is not sufficient to cause periodontitis but represents a risk factor for the onset of gingival inflammation. Now considered an accessory pathogen, *A. actinomycetemcomitans* eventually translocates from the gingival margin through the gingival epithelium into the underlying connective tissue; this transition is associated with the conversion from periodontal health to disease [1,2,6]. There is extensive literature demonstrating a role for Cdt in the pathogenesis of disease, attributed to the wide range of Cdt-producing pathogens that are associated with sustained infection and promotion of inflammation in mucocutaneous tissues (reviewed in [11]). Moreover, evidence is accumulating to link *A. actinomyetemcomitans*-associated periodontitis with Cdt; for example, several studies demonstrate that a high percentage of *A. actinomyetemcomitans* isolates from LAP-diseased sites contain the *cdt* genotype and/or express active toxin [84–87]. There is growing evidence from studies employing human gingival explant models as well as in vivo animal models that demonstrate the ability of Cdt to induce cell cycle arrest, disrupt the epithelial barrier and penetrate the epithelium [88–90]. Ohara et al. [90] observed that Cdt-mediated cell cycle arrest occurs in vivo within basal cells of junctional and gingival epithelium; they propose that cell cycle blockade contributes to subsequent desquamation and detachment of junctional epithelial cells. Our current study is consistent with these observations, as it demonstrates that an important feature of the Cdt-induced epithelial senescent phenotype is associated with disruption of epithelial barrier function. Our TEER data and fluorescence microscopic analysis of epithelial cells indicate that this likely involves disruption of adherens junctions containing β-catenin.

To date, we have demonstrated that Cdt is a tri-perditious toxin that can profoundly affect acquired and innate immune cells as well as epithelial barrier function [27,28,30,39,43,91,92]. We propose that *Aa*Cdt-induced OE senescence is a significant contributing factor to *A. actinomycetemcomitans* infection and the subsequent development of chronic inflammation. As outlined in Figure 7, the initial effect of epithelial exposure to Cdt likely occurs while *A. actinomycetemcomitans* is present at the gingival margin. We propose that local secretion (or release within outer membrane vesicles) of the toxin leads to cell cycle arrest within the epithelium. Further acquisition of the senescent phenotype leads to breakdown of the epithelial barrier, which we propose enables *A. actinomycetemcomitans* to transit the epithelium and colonize the underlying connective tissue. Additionally, we suggest that sustained release of both the Cdt and SASP secretomes in this new location modifies the tissue such that it becomes supportive of not only *A. actinomycetemcomitans* infection but also of other inflammophilic organisms. Over time, the collective effects of sustained SASP, microbial infection and Cdt release contribute to a pro-inflammatory state. It is noteworthy that Belibasakis et al [93,94] previously reported that Cdt induces cell cycle arrest and IL-6 release from gingival fibroblasts; they did not relate these observations to senescence. As noted above, one of the unique properties of SASP is its ability to promote senescence in otherwise healthy adjacent cells. This property allows for both the amplification of senescence and the continued induction of senescence in the face of continual epithelial cell turnover. These events ensure that senescent cells remain continually present in the diseased tissue and that the altered environment contributes to the chronicity of *A. actinomycetemcomitans* infection and inflammatory disease.

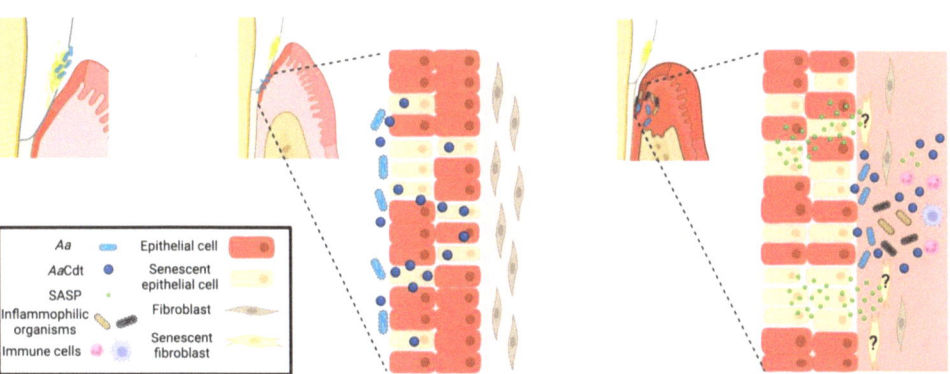

Figure 7. Model depicting the role of *Aa*Cdt-induced senescence in the pathogenesis of MIPP. The left panel shows healthy tissue at risk for MIPP due to the presence of supragingival *A. actinomycetem-comitans* (*Aa*). Initial exposure to *Aa*Cdt occurs while the bacteria are at the gingival margin, leading to cell cycle arrest and senescence within the epithelium and concomitant loss of barrier function indicated as distinct gaps between epithelial cells (middle panel). Continued exposure to Cdt along with OE-derived SASP-associated proinflammatory mediators further contribute to increased OE senescence and translocation of *A. actinomycetemcomitans* into the subgingival tissue (right panel); collectively, the mediators contribute to an altered gingival microenvironment conducive to supporting infection by inflammophilic organisms. Noteworthy, continued exposure to *Aa*Cdt and/or SASP perpetuates the induction of OE senescence (and possibly fibroblasts) in the face of constant epithelial turnover. Ultimately, these events lead to the recruitment of both innate and acquired immune cells, chronic inflammation and bone destruction.

In conclusion, the involvement of cellular senescence, in general, and pathogen-induced cellular senescence, in particular, in periodontal disease pathogenesis has several clinical implications. For example, these Cdt-mediated pathologic events account for many of the virulence characteristics ascribed to *A. actinomycetemcomitans*, including tissue invasiveness, the ability to create an environment that facilitates the accumulation of other organisms, the evasion of host defenses and the ability to promote inflammation. Moreover, senescent cell involvement in disease pathogenesis offers new opportunities for disease classification, diagnosis and therapy.

Supplementary Materials: The following supporting information can be downloaded at: https://www.mdpi.com/article/10.3390/pathogens13020155/s1, Figure S1: Representative cell cycle histogram profiles; Figure S2: Lipofuscin content in TIGK cells at 24 and 48 h; Figure S3: Viability and SA-β-gal activity assessed in TIGK cells exposed to Cdt and NSA; Figure S4: Tiled view of the confocal z-scan.

Author Contributions: Conceptualization, B.J.S. and K.B.-B.; Methodology, B.J.S., K.B.-B., L.P.W., A.Z. and A.D.; Validation, B.J.S., K.B.-B., L.P.W. and A.D.; Formal analysis, B.J.S., K.B.-B., L.P.W., A.Z. and A.D.; Investigation, L.P.W., A.Z. and A.D.; Resources, B.J.S., K.B.-B. and J.K.; Writing—Original Draft Preparation, B.J.S. and K.B.-B.; Writing—Review and Editing, J.K., A.D. and T.J.K.; Visualization, B.J.S., K.B.-B. and J.K.; Project Administration, B.J.S. and K.B.-B.; Data Curation, B.J.S., K.B.-B., L.P.W., A.Z., T.J.K. and A.D.; Funding acquisition, B.J.S. and K.B.-B. All authors have read and agreed to the published version of the manuscript.

Funding: This research was funded by grants DE006014 and DE023071 from the National Institute of Dental and Craniofacial Research at the National Institutes of Health.

Institutional Review Board Statement: This study was approved by the University of Pennsylvania Institutional Review Board protocol 162500.

Informed Consent Statement: Informed consent was obtained from all subjects involved in the study.

Data Availability Statement: Data are provided within the context of this article.

Acknowledgments: The authors wish to acknowledge the support and expertise of the PDM Flow Cytometry Facility and the Live-cell Confocal Imaging Core Facility.

Conflicts of Interest: The authors declare no conflicts of interests.

References

1. Herbert, B.A.; Novince, C.M.; Kirkwood, K.L. *Aggregatibacter actinomycetemcomitans*, a potent immunoregulator of the periodontal host defense system and alveolar bone homeostasis. *Mol. Oral. Microbiol.* **2016**, *31*, 207–227. [CrossRef] [PubMed]
2. Fine, D.H.; Patil, A.G.; Velusamy, S.K. *Aggregatibacter actinomycetemcomitans* (Aa) Under the Radar: Myths and Misunderstandings of Aa and Its Role in Aggressive Periodontitis. *Front. Immunol.* **2019**, *10*, 728. [CrossRef] [PubMed]
3. Teles, F.; Wang, Y.; Hajishengallis, G.; Hasturk, H.; Marchesan, J.T. Impact of systemic factors in shaping the periodontal microbiome. *Periodontol. 2000* **2021**, *85*, 126–160. [CrossRef] [PubMed]
4. Lamont, R.J.; Koo, H.; Hajishengallis, G. The oral microbiota: Dynamic communities and host interactions. *Nat. Rev. Microbiol.* **2018**, *16*, 745–759. [CrossRef] [PubMed]
5. Lamont, R.J.; Hajishengallis, G. Polymicrobial synergy and dysbiosis in inflammatory disease. *Trends Mol. Med.* **2015**, *21*, 172–183. [CrossRef] [PubMed]
6. Hajishengallis, G.; Lamont, R.J. Polymicrobial communities in periodontal disease: Their quasi-organismal nature and dialogue with the host. *Periodontol. 2000* **2021**, *86*, 210–230. [CrossRef] [PubMed]
7. Oscarsson, J.; Claesson, R.; Lindholm, M.; Hoglund Aberg, C.; Johansson, A. Tools of *Aggregatibacter actinomycetemcomitans* to Evade the Host Response. *J. Clin. Med.* **2019**, *8*, 1079. [CrossRef]
8. Belibasakis, G.N.; Maula, T.; Bao, K.; Lindholm, M.; Bostanci, N.; Oscarsson, J.; Ihalin, R.; Johansson, A. Virulence and Pathogenicity Properties of *Aggregatibacter actinomycetemcomitans*. *Pathogens* **2019**, *8*, 222. [CrossRef]
9. Lally, E.T.; Kieba, I.R.; Demuth, D.R.; Rosenbloom, J.; Golub, E.E.; Taichman, N.S.; Gibson, C.W. Identification and expression of the *Actinobacillus actinomycetemcomitans* leukotoxin gene. *Biochem. Biophys. Res. Commun.* **1989**, *159*, 256–262. [CrossRef]
10. Shenker, B.J.; McKay, T.; Datar, S.; Miller, M.; Chowhan, R.; Demuth, D. *Actinobacillus actinomycetemcomitans* immunosuppressive protein is a member of the family of cytolethal distending toxins capable of causing a G2 arrest in human T cells. *J. Immunol.* **1999**, *162*, 4773–4780. [CrossRef]
11. Scuron, M.D.; Boesze-Battaglia, K.; Dlakic, M.; Shenker, B.J. The Cytolethal Distending Toxin Contributes to Microbial Virulence and Disease Pathogenesis by Acting As a Tri-Perditious Toxin. *Front. Cell Infect. Microbiol.* **2016**, *6*, 168. [CrossRef] [PubMed]
12. DiFranco, K.M.; Gupta, A.; Galusha, L.E.; Perez, J.; Nguyen, T.K.; Fineza, C.D.; Kachlany, S.C. Leukotoxin (Leukothera(R)) targets active leukocyte function antigen-1 (LFA-1) protein and triggers a lysosomal mediated cell death pathway. *J. Biol. Chem.* **2012**, *287*, 17618–17627. [CrossRef] [PubMed]
13. Thelestam, M.; Frisan, T.A. Actinomycetemcomitans cytolethal distending toxin. *J. Immunol.* **2004**, *172*, 5813–5814. [CrossRef] [PubMed]
14. Shenker, B.J.; Hoffmaster, R.H.; Zekavat, A.; Yamaguchi, N.; Lally, E.T.; Demuth, D.R. Induction of apoptosis in human T cells by *Actinobacillus actinomycetemcomitans* cytolethal distending toxin is a consequence of G2 arrest of the cell cycle. *J. Immunol.* **2001**, *167*, 435–441. [CrossRef] [PubMed]
15. Shenker, B.J.; Hoffmaster, R.H.; McKay, T.L.; Demuth, D.R. Expression of the cytolethal distending toxin (Cdt) operon in *Actinobacillus actinomycetemcomitans*: Evidence that the CdtB protein is responsible for G2 arrest of the cell cycle in human T cells. *J. Immunol.* **2000**, *165*, 2612–2618. [CrossRef] [PubMed]
16. Pickett, C.L.; Whitehouse, C.A. The cytolethal distending toxin family. *Trends Microbiol.* **1999**, *7*, 292–297. [CrossRef] [PubMed]
17. De Rycke, J.; Oswald, E. Cytolethal distending toxin (CDT): A bacterial weapon to control host cell proliferation? *FEMS Microbiol. Lett.* **2001**, *203*, 141–148. [CrossRef] [PubMed]
18. Whitehouse, C.A.; Balbo, P.B.; Pesci, E.C.; Cottle, D.L.; Mirabito, P.M.; Pickett, C.L. Campylobacter jejuni cytolethal distending toxin causes a G2-phase cell cycle block. *Infect. Immun.* **1998**, *66*, 1934–1940. [CrossRef]
19. Sert, V.; Cans, C.; Tasca, C.; Bret-Bennis, L.; Oswald, E.; Ducommun, B.; De Rycke, J. The bacterial cytolethal distending toxin (CDT) triggers a G2 cell cycle checkpoint in mammalian cells without preliminary induction of DNA strand breaks. *Oncogene* **1999**, *18*, 6296–6304. [CrossRef]
20. Peres, S.Y.; Marches, O.; Daigle, F.; Nougayrede, J.P.; Herault, F.; Tasca, C.; De Rycke, J.; Oswald, E. A new cytolethal distending toxin (CDT) from Escherichia coli producing CNF2 blocks HeLa cell division in G2/M phase. *Mol. Microbiol.* **1997**, *24*, 1095–1107. [CrossRef]
21. Matangkasombut, O.; Wattanawaraporn, R.; Tsuruda, K.; Ohara, M.; Sugai, M.; Mongkolsuk, S. Cytolethal distending toxin from *Aggregatibacter actinomycetemcomitans* induces DNA damage, S/G2 cell cycle arrest, and caspase-independent death in a *Saccharomyces cerevisiae* model. *Infect. Immun.* **2010**, *78*, 783–792. [CrossRef] [PubMed]

22. De Rycke, J.; Sert, V.; Comayras, C.; Tasca, C. Sequence of lethal events in HeLa cells exposed to the G2 blocking cytolethal distending toxin. *Eur. J. Cell Biol.* **2000**, *79*, 192–201. [CrossRef] [PubMed]

23. Cortes-Bratti, X.; Chaves-Olarte, E.; Lagergard, T.; Thelestam, M. The cytolethal distending toxin from the chancroid bacterium Haemophilus ducreyi induces cell-cycle arrest in the G2 phase. *J. Clin. Investig.* **1999**, *103*, 107–115. [CrossRef] [PubMed]

24. Comayras, C.; Tasca, C.; Peres, S.Y.; Ducommun, B.; Oswald, E.; De Rycke, J. Escherichia coli cytolethal distending toxin blocks the HeLa cell cycle at the G2/M transition by preventing cdc2 protein kinase dephosphorylation and activation. *Infect. Immun.* **1997**, *65*, 5088–5095. [CrossRef] [PubMed]

25. Bielaszewska, M.; Sinha, B.; Kuczius, T.; Karch, H. Cytolethal distending toxin from Shiga toxin-producing Escherichia coli O157 causes irreversible G2/M arrest, inhibition of proliferation, and death of human endothelial cells. *Infect. Immun.* **2005**, *73*, 552–562. [CrossRef] [PubMed]

26. Jinadasa, R.N.; Bloom, S.E.; Weiss, R.S.; Duhamel, G.E. Cytolethal distending toxin: A conserved bacterial genotoxin that blocks cell cycle progression, leading to apoptosis of a broad range of mammalian cell lineages. *Microbiology* **2011**, *157*, 1851–1875. [CrossRef] [PubMed]

27. Shenker, B.J.; Walker, L.P.; Zekavat, A.; Dlakic, M.; Boesze-Battaglia, K. Blockade of the PI-3K signalling pathway by the *Aggregatibacter actinomycetemcomitans* cytolethal distending toxin induces macrophages to synthesize and secrete pro-inflammatory cytokines. *Cell Microbiol.* **2014**, *16*, 1391–1404. [CrossRef]

28. Shenker, B.J.; Walker, L.M.; Zekavat, Z.; Ojcius, D.M.; Huang, P.R.; Boesze-Battaglia, K. Cytolethal distending toxin-induced release of interleukin-1beta by human macrophages is dependent upon activation of glycogen synthase kinase 3beta, spleen tyrosine kinase (Syk) and the noncanonical inflammasome. *Cell Microbiol.* **2020**, *22*, e13194. [CrossRef]

29. Shenker, B.J.; Boesze-Battaglia, K.; Zekavat, A.; Walker, L.; Besack, D.; Ali, H. Inhibition of mast cell degranulation by a chimeric toxin containing a novel phosphatidylinositol-3,4,5-triphosphate phosphatase. *Mol. Immunol.* **2010**, *48*, 203–210. [CrossRef]

30. Kim, T.J.; Shenker, B.J.; MacElory, A.S.; Spradlin, S.; Walker, L.P.; Boesze-Battaglia, K. *Aggregatibacter actinomycetemcomitans* cytolethal distending toxin modulates host phagocytic function. *Front. Cell Infect. Microbiol.* **2023**, *13*, 1220089. [CrossRef]

31. Boesze-Battaglia, K.; Alexander, D.; Dlakic, M.; Shenker, B.J. A Journey of Cytolethal Distending Toxins through Cell Membranes. *Front. Cell Infect. Microbiol.* **2016**, *6*, 81. [CrossRef]

32. Boesze-Battaglia, K.; Walker, L.P.; Zekavat, A.; Dlakic, M.; Scuron, M.D.; Nygren, P.; Shenker, B.J. The *Aggregatibacter actinomycetemcomitans* Cytolethal Distending Toxin Active Subunit CdtB Contains a Cholesterol Recognition Sequence Required for Toxin Binding and Subunit Internalization. *Infect. Immun.* **2015**, *83*, 4042–4055. [CrossRef]

33. Boesze-Battaglia, K.; Brown, A.; Walker, L.; Besack, D.; Zekavat, A.; Wrenn, S.; Krummenacher, C.; Shenker, B.J. Cytolethal distending toxin-induced cell cycle arrest of lymphocytes is dependent upon recognition and binding to cholesterol. *J. Biol. Chem.* **2009**, *284*, 10650–10658. [CrossRef] [PubMed]

34. Boesze-Battaglia, K.; Besack, D.; McKay, T.; Zekavat, A.; Otis, L.; Jordan-Sciutto, K.; Shenker, B.J. Cholesterol-rich membrane microdomains mediate cell cycle arrest induced by *Actinobacillus actinomycetemcomitans* cytolethal-distending toxin. *Cell Microbiol.* **2006**, *8*, 823–836. [CrossRef] [PubMed]

35. Boesze-Battaglia, K.; Walker, L.P.; Dhingra, A.; Kandror, K.; Tang, H.Y.; Shenker, B.J. Internalization of the Active Subunit of the *Aggregatibacter actinomycetemcomitans* Cytolethal Distending Toxin Is Dependent upon Cellugyrin (Synaptogyrin 2), a Host Cell Non-Neuronal Paralog of the Synaptic Vesicle Protein, Synaptogyrin 1. *Front. Cell Infect. Microbiol.* **2017**, *7*, 469. [CrossRef] [PubMed]

36. Boesze-Battaglia, K.; Dhingra, A.; Walker, L.M.; Zekavat, A.; Shenker, B.J. Internalization and Intoxication of Human Macrophages by the Active Subunit of the *Aggregatibacter actinomycetemcomitans* Cytolethal Distending Toxin Is Dependent Upon Cellugyrin (Synaptogyrin-2). *Front. Immunol.* **2020**, *11*, 1262. [CrossRef] [PubMed]

37. Shenker, B.J.; Dlakic, M.; Walker, L.P.; Besack, D.; Jaffe, E.; LaBelle, E.; Boesze-Battaglia, K. A novel mode of action for a microbial-derived immunotoxin: The cytolethal distending toxin subunit B exhibits phosphatidylinositol 3,4,5-triphosphate phosphatase activity. *J. Immunol.* **2007**, *178*, 5099–5108. [CrossRef] [PubMed]

38. Huang, G.; Boesze-Battaglia, K.; Walker, L.P.; Zekavat, A.; Schaefer, Z.P.; Blanke, S.R.; Shenker, B.J. The Active Subunit of the Cytolethal Distending Toxin, CdtB, Derived from Both Haemophilus ducreyi and Campylobacter jejuni Exhibits Potent Phosphatidylinositol-3,4,5-Triphosphate Phosphatase Activity. *Front. Cell Infect. Microbiol.* **2021**, *11*, 664221. [CrossRef]

39. Shenker, B.J.; Walker, L.P.; Zekavat, A.; Korostoff, J.; Boesze-Battaglia, K. *Aggregatibacter actinomycetemcomitans* Cytolethal Distending Toxin-Induces Cell Cycle Arrest in a Glycogen Synthase Kinase (GSK)-3-Dependent Manner in Oral Keratinocytes. *Int. J. Mol. Sci.* **2022**, *23*, 11831. [CrossRef]

40. Moffatt-Jauregui, C.E.; Robinson, B.; de Moya, A.V.; Brockman, R.D.; Roman, A.V.; Cash, M.N.; Culp, D.J.; Lamont, R.J. Establishment and characterization of a telomerase immortalized human gingival epithelial cell line. *J. Periodontal Res.* **2013**, *48*, 713–721. [CrossRef]

41. Blasi, I.; Korostoff, J.; Dhingra, A.; Reyes-Reveles, J.; Shenker, B.J.; Shahabuddin, N.; Alexander, D.; Lally, E.T.; Bragin, A.; Boesze-Battaglia, K. Variants of Porphyromonas gingivalis lipopolysaccharide alter lipidation of autophagic protein, microtubule-associated protein 1 light chain 3, LC3. *Mol. Oral. Microbiol.* **2016**, *31*, 486–500. [CrossRef]

42. Shenker, B.J.; Besack, D.; McKay, T.; Pankoski, L.; Zekavat, A.; Demuth, D.R. *Actinobacillus actinomycetemcomitans* cytolethal distending toxin (Cdt): Evidence that the holotoxin is composed of three subunits: CdtA, CdtB, and CdtC. *J. Immunol.* **2004**, *172*, 410–417. [CrossRef] [PubMed]

43. Shenker, B.J.; Besack, D.; McKay, T.; Pankoski, L.; Zekavat, A.; Demuth, D.R. Induction of cell cycle arrest in lymphocytes by *Actinobacillus actinomycetemcomitans* cytolethal distending toxin requires three subunits for maximum activity. *J. Immunol.* **2005**, *174*, 2228–2234. [CrossRef] [PubMed]

44. Srinivasan, B.; Kolli, A.R.; Esch, M.B.; Abaci, H.E.; Shuler, M.L.; Hickman, J.J. TEER measurement techniques for in vitro barrier model systems. *J. Lab. Autom.* **2015**, *20*, 107–126. [CrossRef] [PubMed]

45. Zhou, D.; Borsa, M.; Simon, A.K. Hallmarks and detection techniques of cellular senescence and cellular ageing in immune cells. *Aging Cell* **2021**, *20*, e13316. [CrossRef] [PubMed]

46. Lopes-Paciencia, S.; Saint-Germain, E.; Rowell, M.C.; Ruiz, A.F.; Kalegari, P.; Ferbeyre, G. The senescence-associated secretory phenotype and its regulation. *Cytokine* **2019**, *117*, 15–22. [CrossRef] [PubMed]

47. Birch, J.; Gil, J. Senescence and the SASP: Many therapeutic avenues. *Genes. Dev.* **2020**, *34*, 1565–1576. [CrossRef] [PubMed]

48. Salmonowicz, H.; Passos, J.F. Detecting senescence: A new method for an old pigment. *Aging Cell* **2017**, *16*, 432–434. [CrossRef]

49. Myrianthopoulos, V.; Evangelou, K.; Vasileiou, P.V.S.; Cooks, T.; Vassilakopoulos, T.P.; Pangalis, G.A.; Kouloukoussa, M.; Kittas, C.; Georgakilas, A.G.; Gorgoulis, V.G. Senescence and senotherapeutics: A new field in cancer therapy. *Pharmacol. Ther.* **2019**, *193*, 31–49. [CrossRef]

50. Giatromanolaki, A.; Kouroupi, M.; Balaska, K.; Koukourakis, M.I. A Novel Lipofuscin-detecting Marker of Senescence Relates with Hypoxia, Dysregulated Autophagy and With Poor Prognosis in Non-small-cell-lung Cancer. *Vivo* **2020**, *34*, 3187–3193. [CrossRef]

51. Yue, Z.; Nie, L.; Zhao, P.; Ji, N.; Liao, G.; Wang, Q. Senescence-associated secretory phenotype and its impact on oral immune homeostasis. *Front. Immunol.* **2022**, *13*, 1019313. [CrossRef]

52. Zhao, P.; Yue, Z.; Nie, L.; Zhao, Z.; Wang, Q.; Chen, J.; Wang, Q. Hyperglycaemia-associated macrophage pyroptosis accelerates periodontal inflamm-aging. *J. Clin. Periodontol.* **2021**, *48*, 1379–1392. [CrossRef]

53. Yamagishi, R.; Kamachi, F.; Nakamura, M.; Yamazaki, S.; Kamiya, T.; Takasugi, M.; Cheng, Y.; Nonaka, Y.; Yukawa-Muto, Y.; Thuy, L.T.T.; et al. Gasdermin D-mediated release of IL-33 from senescent hepatic stellate cells promotes obesity-associated hepatocellular carcinoma. *Sci. Immunol.* **2022**, *7*, eabl7209. [CrossRef]

54. Fernandez-Duran, I.; Quintanilla, A.; Tarrats, N.; Birch, J.; Hari, P.; Millar, F.R.; Lagnado, A.B.; Smer-Barreto, V.; Muir, M.; Brunton, V.G.; et al. Cytoplasmic innate immune sensing by the caspase-4 non-canonical inflammasome promotes cellular senescence. *Cell Death Differ.* **2022**, *29*, 1267–1282. [CrossRef] [PubMed]

55. Kovacs, S.B.; Miao, E.A. Gasdermins: Effectors of Pyroptosis. *Trends Cell Biol.* **2017**, *27*, 673–684. [CrossRef] [PubMed]

56. He, W.T.; Wan, H.; Hu, L.; Chen, P.; Wang, X.; Huang, Z.; Yang, Z.H.; Zhong, C.Q.; Han, J. Gasdermin D is an executor of pyroptosis and required for interleukin-1beta secretion. *Cell Res.* **2015**, *25*, 1285–1298. [CrossRef] [PubMed]

57. Ding, J.; Wang, K.; Liu, W.; She, Y.; Sun, Q.; Shi, J.; Sun, H.; Wang, D.C.; Shao, F. Pore-forming activity and structural autoinhibition of the gasdermin family. *Nature* **2016**, *535*, 111–116. [CrossRef] [PubMed]

58. Evavold, C.L.; Kagan, J.C. Defying Death: The (W)hole Truth about the Fate of GSDMD Pores. *Immunity* **2019**, *50*, 15–17. [CrossRef] [PubMed]

59. Damek-Poprawa, M.; Korostoff, J.; Gill, R.; DiRienzo, J.M. Cell junction remodeling in gingival tissue exposed to a microbial toxin. *J. Dent. Res.* **2013**, *92*, 518–523. [CrossRef]

60. Mathiasen, S.L.; Gall-Mas, L.; Pateras, I.S.; Theodorou, S.D.P.; Namini, M.R.J.; Hansen, M.B.; Martin, O.C.B.; Vadivel, C.K.; Ntostoglou, K.; Butter, D.; et al. Bacterial genotoxins induce T cell senescence. *Cell Rep.* **2021**, *35*, 109220. [CrossRef]

61. Hernandez-Segura, A.; Nehme, J.; Demaria, M. Hallmarks of Cellular Senescence. *Trends Cell Biol.* **2018**, *28*, 436–453. [CrossRef]

62. Gorgoulis, V.; Adams, P.D.; Alimonti, A.; Bennett, D.C.; Bischof, O.; Bishop, C.; Campisi, J.; Collado, M.; Evangelou, K.; Ferbeyre, G.; et al. Cellular Senescence: Defining a Path Forward. *Cell* **2019**, *179*, 813–827. [CrossRef]

63. Munoz-Espin, D.; Serrano, M. Cellular senescence: From physiology to pathology. *Nat. Rev. Mol. Cell Biol.* **2014**, *15*, 482–496. [CrossRef] [PubMed]

64. He, S.; Sharpless, N.E. Senescence in Health and Disease. *Cell* **2017**, *169*, 1000–1011. [CrossRef] [PubMed]

65. Paez-Ribes, M.; Gonzalez-Gualda, E.; Doherty, G.J.; Munoz-Espin, D. Targeting senescent cells in translational medicine. *EMBO Mol. Med.* **2019**, *11*, e10234. [CrossRef] [PubMed]

66. Wei, W.; Ji, S. Cellular senescence: Molecular mechanisms and pathogenicity. *J. Cell Physiol.* **2018**, *233*, 9121–9135. [CrossRef] [PubMed]

67. Humphreys, D.; ElGhazaly, M.; Frisan, T. Senescence and Host-Pathogen Interactions. *Cells* **2020**, *9*, 1747. [CrossRef] [PubMed]

68. Blazkova, H.; Krejcikova, K.; Moudry, P.; Frisan, T.; Hodny, Z.; Bartek, J. Bacterial intoxication evokes cellular senescence with persistent DNA damage and cytokine signalling. *J. Cell Mol. Med.* **2010**, *14*, 357–367. [CrossRef] [PubMed]

69. Secher, T.; Samba-Louaka, A.; Oswald, E.; Nougayrede, J.P. Escherichia coli producing colibactin triggers premature and transmissible senescence in mammalian cells. *PLoS ONE* **2013**, *8*, e77157. [CrossRef]

70. Ibler, A.E.M.; ElGhazaly, M.; Naylor, K.L.; Bulgakova, N.A.; El-Khamisy, S.F.; Humphreys, D. Typhoid toxin exhausts the RPA response to DNA replication stress driving senescence and Salmonella infection. *Nat. Commun.* **2019**, *10*, 4040. [CrossRef]

71. Cougnoux, A.; Dalmasso, G.; Martinez, R.; Buc, E.; Delmas, J.; Gibold, L.; Sauvanet, P.; Darcha, C.; Dechelotte, P.; Bonnet, M.; et al. Bacterial genotoxin colibactin promotes colon tumour growth by inducing a senescence-associated secretory phenotype. *Gut* **2014**, *63*, 1932–1942. [CrossRef] [PubMed]

72. Karnam, S.; Girish, H.C.; Nayak, V.N. Senescent Fibroblast in Oral Submucous Fibrosis Aids in Disease Progression and Malignant Transformation. *J. Oral. Maxillofac. Pathol.* **2022**, *26*, 199–207. [CrossRef] [PubMed]
73. Elsayed, R.; Elashiry, M.; Liu, Y.; El-Awady, A.; Hamrick, M.; Cutler, C.W. Porphyromonas gingivalis Provokes Exosome Secretion and Paracrine Immune Senescence in Bystander Dendritic Cells. *Front. Cell Infect. Microbiol.* **2021**, *11*, 669989. [CrossRef] [PubMed]
74. Elashiry, M.; Elsayed, R.; Cutler, C.W. Exogenous and Endogenous Dendritic Cell-Derived Exosomes: Lessons Learned for Immunotherapy and Disease Pathogenesis. *Cells* **2021**, *11*, 115. [CrossRef] [PubMed]
75. Aquino-Martinez, R.; Eckhardt, B.A.; Rowsey, J.L.; Fraser, D.G.; Khosla, S.; Farr, J.N.; Monroe, D.G. Senescent cells exacerbate chronic inflammation and contribute to periodontal disease progression in old mice. *J. Periodontol.* **2021**, *92*, 1483–1495. [CrossRef]
76. Aquino-Martinez, R.; Rowsey, J.L.; Fraser, D.G.; Eckhardt, B.A.; Khosla, S.; Farr, J.N.; Monroe, D.G. LPS-induced premature osteocyte senescence: Implications in inflammatory alveolar bone loss and periodontal disease pathogenesis. *Bone* **2020**, *132*, 115220. [CrossRef] [PubMed]
77. Aquino-Martinez, R.; Khosla, S.; Farr, J.N.; Monroe, D.G. Periodontal Disease and Senescent Cells: New Players for an Old Oral Health Problem? *Int. J. Mol. Sci.* **2020**, *21*, 7441. [CrossRef]
78. Gonzalez-Gualda, E.; Baker, A.G.; Fruk, L.; Munoz-Espin, D. A guide to assessing cellular senescence in vitro and in vivo. *FEBS J.* **2021**, *288*, 56–80. [CrossRef]
79. Guidi, R.; Guerra, L.; Levi, L.; Stenerlow, B.; Fox, J.G.; Josenhans, C.; Masucci, M.G.; Frisan, T. Chronic exposure to the cytolethal distending toxins of Gram-negative bacteria promotes genomic instability and altered DNA damage response. *Cell Microbiol.* **2013**, *15*, 98–113. [CrossRef]
80. Guerra, L.; Guidi, R.; Frisan, T. Do bacterial genotoxins contribute to chronic inflammation, genomic instability and tumor progression? *FEBS J.* **2011**, *278*, 4577–4588. [CrossRef]
81. Frisan, T. Bacterial genotoxins: The long journey to the nucleus of mammalian cells. *Biochim. Biophys. Acta* **2016**, *1858*, 567–575. [CrossRef]
82. Janz, R.; Sudhof, T.C. Cellugyrin, a novel ubiquitous form of synaptogyrin that is phosphorylated by pp60c-src. *J. Biol. Chem.* **1998**, *273*, 2851–2857. [CrossRef]
83. Belfort, G.M.; Kandror, K.V. Cellugyrin and synaptogyrin facilitate targeting of synaptophysin to a ubiquitous synaptic vesicle-sized compartment in PC12 cells. *J. Biol. Chem.* **2003**, *278*, 47971–47978. [CrossRef] [PubMed]
84. Aberg, C.H.; Sjodin, B.; Lakio, L.; Pussinen, P.J.; Johansson, A.; Claesson, R. Presence of *Aggregatibacter actinomycetemcomitans* in young individuals: A 16-year clinical and microbiological follow-up study. *J. Clin. Periodontol.* **2009**, *36*, 815–822. [CrossRef] [PubMed]
85. Tan, K.S.; Song, K.P.; Ong, G. Cytolethal distending toxin of *Actinobacillus actinomycetemcomitans*. Occurrence and association with periodontal disease. *J. Periodontal Res.* **2002**, *37*, 268–272. [CrossRef]
86. Bandhaya, P.; Saraithong, P.; Likittanasombat, K.; Hengprasith, B.; Torrungruang, K. *Aggregatibacter actinomycetemcomitans* serotypes, the JP2 clone and cytolethal distending toxin genes in a Thai population. *J. Clin. Periodontol.* **2012**, *39*, 519–525. [CrossRef] [PubMed]
87. Åberg, C.H.; Antonoglou, G.; Haubek, D.; Kwamin, F.; Claesson, R.; Johansson, A. Cytolethal Distending Toxin in Isolates of *Aggregatibacter actinomycetemcomitans* from Ghanaian Adolescents and Association with Serotype and Disease Progression. *PLoS ONE* **2013**, *8*, e65781. [CrossRef]
88. Damek-Poprawa, M.; Haris, M.; Volgina, A.; Korostoff, J.; DiRienzo, J.M. Cytolethal distending toxin damages the oral epithelium of gingival explants. *J. Dent. Res.* **2011**, *90*, 874–879. [CrossRef] [PubMed]
89. DiRienzo, J.M. Breaking the Gingival Epithelial Barrier: Role of the *Aggregatibacter actinomycetemcomitans* Cytolethal Distending Toxin in Oral Infectious Disease. *Cells* **2014**, *3*, 476–499. [CrossRef] [PubMed]
90. Ohara, M.; Miyauchi, M.; Tsuruda, K.; Takata, T.; Sugai, M. Topical application of *Aggregatibacter actinomycetemcomitans* cytolethal distending toxin induces cell cycle arrest in the rat gingival epithelium in vivo. *J. Periodontal Res.* **2011**, *46*, 389–395. [CrossRef]
91. Shenker, B.J.; Demuth, D.R.; Zekavat, A. Exposure of lymphocytes to high doses of *Actinobacillus actinomycetemcomitans* cytolethal distending toxin induces rapid onset of apoptosis-mediated DNA fragmentation. *Infect. Immun.* **2006**, *74*, 2080–2092. [CrossRef]
92. Shenker, B.J.; Ojcius, D.M.; Walker, L.P.; Zekavat, A.; Scuron, M.D.; Boesze-Battaglia, K. *Aggregatibacter actinomycetemcomitans* cytolethal distending toxin activates the NLRP3 inflammasome in human macrophages, leading to the release of proinflammatory cytokines. *Infect. Immun.* **2015**, *83*, 1487–1496. [CrossRef]
93. Belibasakis, G.N.; Mattsson, A.; Wang, Y.; Chen, C.; Johansson, A. Cell cycle arrest of human gingival fibroblasts and periodontal ligament cells by *Actinobacillus actinomycetemcomitans*: Involvement of the cytolethal distending toxin. *APMIS* **2004**, *112*, 674–685. [CrossRef]
94. Belibasakis, G.N.; Johansson, A.; Wang, Y.; Chen, C.; Lagergård, T.; Kalfas, S.; Lerner, U.H. Cytokine responses of human gingival fibroblasts to *Actinobacillus actinomycetemcomitans* cytolethal distending toxin. *Cytokine* **2005**, *30*, 56–63. [CrossRef]

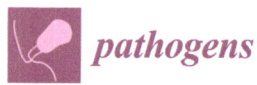

Article

Molecular Analysis of *Aggregatibacter actinomycetemcomitans* ApiA, a Multi-Functional Protein

Sera Jacob, Luciana Gusmao, Dipti Godboley, Senthil Kumar Velusamy, Nisha George, Helen Schreiner, Carla Cugini * and Daniel H. Fine *

Department of Oral Biology, Rutgers School of Dental Medicine, 110 Bergen, Newark, NJ 07103, USA; serageo14@gmail.com (S.J.); lgusmao@amnh.org (L.G.); godboldv@sdm.rutgers.edu (D.G.); senthil.velusamy@fujifilm.com (S.K.V.); nishageorge.george@gmail.com (N.G.); hschrein@sdm.rutgers.edu (H.S.)
* Correspondence: cc1337@sdm.rutgers.edu (C.C.); finedh@sdm.rutgers.edu (D.H.F.);
   Tel.: +1-973-972-7053 (D.H.F.)

Abstract: *Aggregatibacter actinomycetemcomitans* ApiA is a trimeric autotransporter outer membrane protein (Omp) that participates in multiple functions, enabling *A. actinomycetemcomitans* to adapt to a variety of environments. The goal of this study is to identify regions in the *apiA* gene responsible for three of these functions: auto-aggregation, buccal epithelial cell binding, and complement resistance. Initially, *apiA* was expressed in *Escherichia coli*. Finally, wild-type *A. actinomycetemcomitans* and an *apiA*-deleted version were tested for their expression in the presence and absence of serum and genes related to stress adaptation, such as oxygen regulation, catalase activity, and Omp proteins. Sequential deletions in specific regions in the *apiA* gene as expressed in *E. coli* were examined for membrane proteins, which were confirmed by microscopy. The functional activity of epithelial cell binding, auto-aggregation, and complement resistance were then assessed, and regions in the *apiA* gene responsible for these functions were identified. A region spanning amino acids 186–217, when deleted, abrogated complement resistance and Factor H (FH) binding, while a region spanning amino acids 28–33 was related to epithelial cell binding. A 13-amino-acid peptide responsible for FH binding was shown to promote serum resistance. An *apiA* deletion in a clinical isolate (IDH781) was created and tested in the presence and/or absence of active and inactive serum and genes deemed responsible for prominent functional activity related to *A. actinomycetemcomitans* survival using qRT-PCR. These experiments suggested that *apiA* expression in IDH781 is involved in global regulatory mechanisms that are serum-dependent and show complement resistance. This is the first study to identify specific *apiA* regions in *A. actinomycetemcomitans* responsible for FH binding, complement resistance, and other stress-related functions. Moreover, the role of *apiA* in overall gene regulation was observed.

Keywords: complement resistance; *Aggregatibacter actinomycetemcomitans*; factor H; epithelial cell binding; auto-aggregation; global regulation

Citation: Jacob, S.; Gusmao, L.; Godboley, D.; Velusamy, S.K.; George, N.; Schreiner, H.; Cugini, C.; Fine, D.H. Molecular Analysis of *Aggregatibacter actinomycetemcomitans* ApiA, a Multi-Functional Protein. *Pathogens* **2024**, *13*, 1011. https://doi.org/10.3390/pathogens13111011

Academic Editor: Longzhu Cui

Received: 11 September 2024
Revised: 1 November 2024
Accepted: 10 November 2024
Published: 18 November 2024

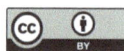

1. Introduction

In a complex biofilm, the interaction of individual microorganisms with other members of the diverse biofilm microbiome is multifaceted [1]. This is especially true when these complex associations are compounded by the effects of host factors [2]. In a microbiome at homeostasis, there are delicate interspecies interactions driven by the maintenance of intricate physical and metabolic associations that control host innate immune defenses, aimed at detoxifying the assaulting microbiome [3]. Periodontal disease is characterized by the formation of a dysbiotic biofilm and an outgrowth of key pathobionts, which can lead to host tissue destruction and, ultimately, periodontal pockets and bone loss [4]. *Aggregatibacter actinomycetemcomitans*, a well-studied member of the microbiome involved in Stage III Grade C periodontitis (previously called localized aggressive periodontitis; LAgP) which occurs predominantly in adolescents of African descent is of particular interest in dysbiotic associations [5]. *A. actinomycetemcomitans* is a Gram-negative, capnophilic, faculta-tive anaerobic member of the oral microbiota and a critical agent associated with the initial mucosal infection in periodontitis [6]. *A. actinomycetemcomitans* is unique because it has the ability to adapt to diverse environments for its own survival and for the protection of other less adaptable cohorts, especially in the subgingival environment [7]. Our group has studied several of A. *actinomycetemcomitans*'s virulence factors, including the widespread colonization island (WCI), which includes Flp [8], leukotoxin [9], cytolethal distending toxin [10], DispB [11,12], PNAG [13], Aae [14], and ApiA [15]. Of these A. *actinomycetem-comitans* virulence factors, ApiA and its relationship to complement resistance is perhaps the least understood, although recently more information has become available [16,17].

It is proposed that *A. actinomycetemcomitans* initially colonizes the oral mucosa by means of Aae, a monomeric autotransporter adhesin that binds at low concentrations to epithelial receptors in the supragingival domain [15]. Subsequently, when *A. actinomycetem-comitans* reaches higher levels numerically in the supragingival domain, ApiA, a trimeric autotransporter outer membrane protein (Omp), plays a major role in oral colonization, but this accumulation occurs in a linear fashion independent of receptor/adhesin interactions, suggesting auto-aggregation [15]. The successful migration and colonization of *A. acti-nomycetemcomitans* into the subgingival space occur as a result of *dspB*, an enzyme that disrupts the biofilm's protective shield and ejects cells from the inner core of the biofilm mass huge distances away from the original biofilm deposition [18]. *A. actinomycetemcomi-tans*'s subgingival migration is instrumental in the development of a consortia of bacteria that can lead to the destruction of periodontal tissue and the development of periodon-titis in susceptible individuals [19–22]. *A. actinomycetemcomitans*'s subgingival presence provokes an outpouring of gingival crevicular fluid, a serum exudate, which increases the inflammatory burden, resulting in additional colonization and proliferation at the site (5). The initial host response relies on serum-derived complements and host-derived cell-related toxins such as leukotoxin [23].

Many commensals and pathobionts have developed elegant strategies to subvert the cytotoxic effects of host defense systems, allowing for their persistence within this specific subgingival niche [24–27]. Several oral microbes display serum resistance and blunt the effects of the complement cascade, which can span the classical, lectin, and alternative pathways [24,28,29]. As compared to complement resistance in other pathobionts such as *Porphyromonas gingivalis*, studies of *A. actinomycetemcomitans* have fallen short, perhaps because ApiA, as a trimeric protein in nature, presents major structural challenges [16]. The alternative complement system, which is proposed to be triggered by *A. actinomycetemcomi-tans* ApiA, involves an enzymatic cascade that ultimately can activate a set of pore-forming proteins, leading to bacterial cell lysis [30]. The alternative pathway is governed by abun-dant levels of C3 protein, which undergoes a constant low level of spontaneous hydrolysis to C3a (anaphylatoxin) and C3b. In the absence of an antibody-guided response, C3b binds to cell wall components and lipopolysaccharides of "invading" cells [31]. A major regulator of the alternative complement pathway known to bind to and stabilize C3b is Factor H (FH). Factor H prevents convertase from activating the rest of the complement pathway [32,33].

A hallmark of *A. actinomycetemcomitans* biology is its early resistance to the effects of serum by the disruption of the complement cascade [24,34]. ApiA, a 295-amino-acid outer membrane protein, is conserved in *A. actinomycetemcomitans* species, with 99–100% of its nucleotide sequence identity and 100% of its amino acid identity shared among sequenced strains (accession number AB064943). Further *A. actinomycetemcomitans* is characterized by the interaction of ApiA (Omp100) with human Factor H [15,16,35], and since ApiA is randomly localized on the cell surface, it can facilitate binding to FH, which confers serum resistance [29,36,37]. In the absence of ApiA, *A. actinomycetemcomitans* has a reduced ability to survive the effects of serum, indicating a major role for *A. actinomycetemcomitans* ApiA in serum resistance [29,38,39]. There is precedent among other oral microbes, such as *Porphyromonas gingivalis* and *Treponema denticola*, to interact with proteins of the complement pathway [25,40–44].

The overriding goal of the first portion of this study was to determine regions in ApiA responsible for auto-aggregation, epithelial cell binding, and complement resistance. The premise of this study was that a deletion in an *apiA* gene region that failed to show a specific function, such as epithelial cell binding, was proposed to be responsible for that function. All findings were measured in a quantitative manner and were compared to the complete *apiA* gene expressed in *Esherichia coli* (the positive control) or to *E. coli* with an empty plasmid (the negative control). Following this logic, the deleted gene region that failed to show any complement resistance was proposed to be responsible for complement resistance via the alternative pathway. It has been suggested that *A. actinomycetemcomitans* also activates the classical pathway of complement resistance by means of *ompA-1* [38,45].

Outer membrane protein 100, a 100 kDa protein, later termed ApiA, was first identified by Komatsuzawa et al. in 2002 as one of six outer membrane proteins [36,46]. Since that time, it has been shown that ApiA is a multifunctional outer membrane protein that is involved in epithelial cell binding, auto-aggregation, and complement resistance [15]. This study was intentionally limited to surface-related proteins, and as such, our first aim was to visualize surface expression by means of fluorescence and immunogold labeled transmission electron microscopy. This was followed by studies of auto-aggregation and buccal epithelial cell binding to confirm the surface expression. Gene deletions in *apiA* were used to identify supplemental gene regions related to these supplemental functions. Finally, peptides, designed based on gene sequences deemed responsible for functionality, were used to confirm a region thought to be responsible for Factor H binding and complement resistance. This is the first research study to identify specific regions within ApiA potentially responsible for serum resistance in *A. actinomycetemcomitans,* which could be important in the modulation of immune responsiveness and early disease abatement. Further, the exploration of the *apiA* region in *A. actinomycetemcomitans,* IDH781, allowed us to examine the possibility that *apiA* could be involved in the global regulation of other genes critical for *A. actinomycetemcomitans* survival. These findings point to the potential influence of ApiA in *A. actinomycetemcomitans* adaptability in the face of environmental stressors.

2. Materials and Methods

2.1. Bacterial Strains and Growth Conditions

Bacterial strains used in this study are listed in Table 1. *A. actinomycetemcomitans* IDH781 and IDH781 *apiA* were routinely grown on brain heart infusion (BHI; Becton, Dickinson and company, Franklin Lakes, NJ, USA) agar and/or trypticase soy agar (TSA) supplemented with 0.6% yeast extract (Beckton Dickinson, Franklin Lakes, NJ, USA), 0.8% dextrose, and 0.4% sodium bicarbonate. For liquid cultures, *A. actinomycetemcomitans* was inoculated in BHI broth (Becton, Dickinson and company, Franklin Lakes, NJ, USA) or trypticase soy broth with 0.6% yeast extract (Becton, Dickinson and company, Franklin Lakes, NJ, USA), 0.8% dextrose, and 0.4% sodium bicarbonate. The strains were incubated at 37 °C in a 10% CO_2 incubator for 16–48 h or in an anaerobic chamber (10% CO_2, 10% H_2, and 80% N_2).

E. coli strains were revived from frozen stocks on Luria–Bertani (LB) plates supplemented with kanamycin (30 μg/mL) and incubated overnight at 37 °C. For expression of ApiA and variants in *E. coli*, each strain was inoculated into LB broth containing dextrose (0.5%) and kanamycin (30 μg/mL) and incubated overnight at 37 °C with shaking (220 rpm). After 16 h, the optical density at 600 nm (OD_{600}) of the overnight culture was measured. The strains were subcultured in LB broth supplemented with kanamycin (30 μg/mL) to an OD_{600} of 0.05. Once the culture reached an OD_{600} of 0.5, all strains were induced by adding isopropyl β-D-1-thiogalactopyranoside (IPTG; 0.1 mM). The culture was incubated for 45 min to allow for induction. Bacterial cells were pelleted by centrifugation (4000 rpm; 10 min) and washed three times with PBS (4000 rpm; 5 min). Bacterial cell pellets were then resuspended in 3 mL of PBS.

Table 1. Bacterial strains and plasmids.

E. coli Strains	Relevant Characteristics	Reference or Source
NEB5α	*fhuA2 Δ(argF-lacZ)U169 phoA glnV44 Φ80Δ (lacZ)M15 gyrA96 recA1 relA1 endA1 thi-1 hsdR17*	New England Biolabs
Mach1-T1^R	F- *φ80(lacZ)ΔM15 ΔlacX74 hsd*R(r$_K$-m$_K$+) *ΔrecA1398 endA1 tonA*	Invitrogen
Stellar	F–, *endA1, supE44, thi-1, recA1, relA1, gyrA96, phoA, Φ80d lacZΔ M15, Δ(lacZYA-argF) U169, Δ(mrr-hsdRMS-mcrBC), ΔmcrA, λ–*	Clontech
BL21(DE3)	*fhuA2 [lon] ompT gal (λ DE3) [dcm] ΔhsdS λ DE3 = λ sBamHIo ΔEcoRI-B int::(lacI::PlacUV5::T7 gene1) i21 Δnin5*	New England Biolabs
SJ100	BL21(DE3) containing plasmid pET29b (+)	This study
A. actinomycetemcomitans strains	Relevant characteristics	Reference or source
IDH781	Wild-type human *A. actinomycetemcomitans*, serotype d, spectinomycin-resistant	[47]
IDH781ΔapiA	Gene deletion of *apiA* in strain IDH781; SJ13	This study
Plasmid	Relevant characteristics	Reference or source
pJT1	Suicide vector, Spectinomycin-resistant	[48]
pET29b (+)	Expression vector, T7 promoter, Kanamycin-resistant	Novagen
pSJ101	pET29b+ containing full-length *apiA*; designated ApiA in text	[35]
pSJ102	pET29b+ containing truncated *apiA*; amino acids 28–33 deleted; designated Δ28–33 in text	This study
pSJ103	pET29b+ containing truncated *apiA*; amino acids 34–80 deleted; designated Δ34–80 in text	This study
pSJ104	pET29b+ containing truncated *apiA*; amino acids 81–100 deleted; designated Δ81–100 in text	This study
pSJ105	pET29b+ containing truncated *apiA*; amino acids 101–185 deleted; designated Δ101–185 in text	This study
pSJ106	pET29b+ containing truncated *apiA*; amino acids 186–217 deleted; designated Δ186–217 in text	[35]
pSJ107	pET29b+ containing truncated *apiA*; amino acids 81–185 deleted; designated Δ81–185 in text	This study
pSJ108	pET29b+ containing truncated *apiA*; amino acids 28–185 deleted; designated Δ28–185 in text	This study

2.2. Cloning of Full-Length apiA and Variants into pET-29(b)+

The pET-29(b)+ plasmid was purified from *E. coli* using the Qiagen Mini-Prep Kit (Germantown, MD, USA) as per the manufacturer's recommendation. The plasmid was subjected to double restriction digestion using NdeI and EcoRI high-fidelity restriction enzymes (New England Biolabs (NEB), Ipswich, MA, USA). Primers were designed to PCR amplify the *apiA* gene from IDH781 chromosomal DNA as the template and to include NdeI and EcoRI cleavage sites (Table 2). The desired fragment was amplified using PCR, after which the insert was digested by double digestion using NdeI and EcoRI. The digested inserts were ligated into the digested plasmid using the Instant Sticky-End Ligase Master Mix (New England Biolabs, Ipswich, MA, USA) to create the final ApiA clone. The ligation mixture was used to transform into commercially available chemically competent NEB 5a competent *E. coli* (non-expression host) (Table 1; New England Biolabs, Ipswich, MA, USA) following the manufacturer's recommendations. The inserted sequence was verified with commercially available T7 promoter and T7 terminator primers (Psomagen, Brooklyn, NY, USA, formerly Macrogen). The recombinant plasmid was transformed into commercially available chemically competent *E. coli* BL21 (DE3, expression host) (Table 1). The plasmid containing the full-length ApiA was designated SJ101 (Figure 1 and Table 1 [35]).

Table 2. Primers used in this study.

Oligonucleotides	Sequence (5′→3′)	Source
	Primers to amplify full-length *apiA*	
ApiA-NdeI-F	GGAATTCCATATGACATATCAATTATTTAA	[35]
ApiA-EcoRI-R	CGGAATTCTTACCACTCAAAGTTTAAACCG	[35]
	Amino acid 28–33 deletion in ApiA to construct pSJ102	
DNF 2	GTCGATGCATTGGCTAAAGACTCTGCTAATCTTCCACAACAA	This study
DNR 2	TTGTTGTGGAAGATTAGCAGAGTCTTTAGCCAATGCATCGAC	This study
	Amino acid 34–80 deletion in ApiA to construct pSJ103	
103F 2	GCTGAAAATCCTGGGGGGATCGATAGATTAGCTAAG	This study
103R 2	CTTTGCATTTCTATCGATCCCCCCAGGATTTTCAGC	This study
	Amino acid 81–185 deletion in ApiA to construct pSJ107	
DNF 3	GTATAGAAAAAGATGTTATGCGTAACACTTTTAGATCTTCAAGC	This study
DNR 3	GCTTGAAGATCTAAAAGTGTTACGCATAACATCTTTTTCTATAC	This study
	Amino acid 81–100 deletion in ApiA to construct pSJ104	
DNF 4	GTATAGAAAAAGATGTTATGCGTAACACTGAGTTAGATATTCAG	This study
DNR 4	CTGAATATCTAACTCAGTGTTACGCATAACATCTTTTTCTATAC	This study
	Amino acid 101–185 deletion in ApiA to construct pSJ105	
DNF 5	GATTACTAAAAATTTTAGATCTTCAAGCCAAAACATCGCG	This study
DNR 5	CGCGATGTTTTGGCTTGAAGATCTAAAATTTTTAGTAATC	This study
	pSJ13 sequence confirmation primers	
pJT1 F	CCT TGC CTA GGG CTA GCA TC	This study
pJT1 R	GGC TGC AGT AAC GAA TAC TAG	This study
	apiA gene deletion primers	
UF *Not*I	GGGCCCAATTAATGGCCGGTTTGAAATGCACGGTGG	This study
DR *Xho*I	TACTAGTTCGAATAACAGGCGCAG GAATCCGCC	This study
DF	TTAAGGATGAATTTTCACTTAAAGTGCGGTC	This study
UR	GACCGCACTTTAAGTGAAAATTCATCCTTAA	This study
	apiA gene deletion screening primers	
*apiA*ˆ F	GATATAGCCAGGTGTCTTCGGTGTCG	This study
*apiA*ˆ R	GAATCTTGACCGCGGTGAAGGCATTC	This study
	qPCR primers	
*pga*CF	GACGGTGATGCGGTATTGG	This study
*pga*CR	GACCGATGATGGAGCTGAA	This study
*api*AqF	GCCGAGTCAATGAATTAGACAAAG	This study
*api*AqR	CAACAGCTGCACTCAAGTTAAGG	This study
*rcp*AF	TGGGCATTAACTGGAGCCAC	This study
*rcp*AR	ATCCACCTCCGAAACCGAAG	This study
*omp*A1F	GAGATGGCTTGTTGAGAAAC	This study
*omp*A1R	AGGTTATACAGACCGTATCG	This study
*omp*A2 F	CAATATCCGGAGAATAGCGA	This study
*omp*A2 R	GGCATTACGTTTGGAGTATC	This study
*oxy*R F	CTGTAAGGTCGGTACGATATG	This study
*oxy*R R	GCAACCAAGGCAAAGATATG	This study
*kat*A F	GTTCAGCGATCGTGGTATTC	This study
*kat*A R	CGTTGTCGGCATTGATAAAG	This study
5SrRNAF	GCGGGGATCCTGGCGGTGACCTACT	This study
5SrRNAR	GCGATCTAGACCACCTGAAACCATACC	This study

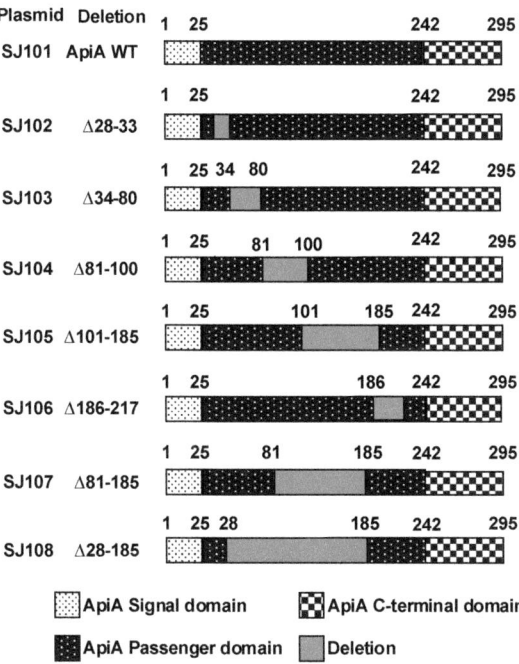

Inhibitor Peptide Sequences
Amino acids 101-185
P1 101 ELDIQKNTKSIAENTASIARIDGNLEGVNR
P2 131 VLQNVDVRSTENAARSRANEQKIAENKKAI
P3 161 ENKADKADVEKNRADIAANSRAIAT
Amino acids 186-217
P4 186 FRSSSQNIAA
P5 196 LTTKVDRNT
P6 205 ARIDRLDSRVNEL

Figure 1. Schematic of the various ApiA sequential deletions used in the functional assays.

To clone ApiA passenger domain variants, primers were designed to create the desired fragments using overlap extension PCR (Table 2; [48]). The mutants were created by an overlap extension PCR and cut by double restriction digestion using NdeI and EcoRI (Ipswich, MA, USA). The digested inserts were ligated into the digested plasmid using the Instant Sticky-End Ligase Master Mix (NEB, Ipswich, MA, USA) to create the recombinant plasmid. Further, these recombinant plasmids were transformed into commercially available chemically competent NEB 5-alpha-competent *E. coli* and *E. coli* BL21(DE3) (New England Biolabs) following the manufacturer's recommendations. PCR was performed on single colonies to confirm the insert contained the correct deletion. Plasmids were isolated for sequencing using the same growth conditions and plasmid preparation as previously described to verify the correct constructs. The verified constructs were transformed into commercially available chemically competent *E. coli* BL21(DE3) (New England Biolabs) following the manufacturer's recommendations for protein expression.

2.3. Construction of ApiA Deletion Strain in A. actinomycetemcomitans IDH781

A scarless, markerless deletion approach was used to construct an *apiA* isogenic mutant in strain IDH781 using plasmid pJT1 as previously described [48]. Primers were designed for the PCR amplification of the 1000 bp upstream (apiA NotI UF and apiA UR) and downstream (apiA DF and apiA XhoIR) fragments of *apiA*, which had 15 bp tails complementary to one another to enable fusion between the fragments (Accession: AB064943/IDH781) [47,48]. IDH781 genomic DNA served as the template (~5 ng). NotI and XhoI restriction sites were included in 5' and 3' ends of the flanking fragments, respectively, by PCR to enable infusion cloning (Takara Inc., Kusatsu, Japan) into pJT1. An overlap extension PCR (OEPCR) was performed as described previously with equimolar concentrations of the upstream and downstream flanking fragments without end primers [48,49]. The end primers were added, and the second step of PCR using 5 µL template from the first step of PCR was carried out to amplify the fusion product. The PCR fragment was ligated into NotI-XhoI double-digested pJT1 plasmid using an in-fusion cloning strategy (Takara Bio USA, Inc., San Jose, CA, USA). Colonies were screened by PCR for the insert and confirmed by sequencing. The resultant *apiA* deletion plasmid was designated as pSJ13 (Table 1).

Electroporation of pSJ13 into IDH781 was carried out as previously described [15,35,49]. IDH781 was grown for 24 h on BHI plates at 37 °C with supplements in a 10% CO_2 incubator. Cells were collected with a sterile cotton applicator and suspended in 20 mL ice-cold electroporation buffer (EB; 300 mM sucrose in 2.43 mM phosphate buffer; pH 7.2). These cells were washed three times with EB and centrifuged (8000 rpm) for 10 min at 4 °C. Cells were resuspended using 1/10 volume of EB. To make a homogenous suspension, a hand-held motorized pestle was used to disrupt the clumps. The OD_{600} was adjusted to 0.5–0.6. Forty microliters of washed IDH781 cells were incubated with ~500 ng of pSJ13 plasmid DNA on ice for 5 min and transferred to a 0.2 cm cuvette. The mixture was electroporated with 2.2 kV, 200 Ω, and 25 µF (Gene Pulsar; Bio-Rad, Hercules, CA, USA) and recovered in 1 mL of warm BHI media at 37 °C in a 10% CO_2 atmosphere for 5 h. Cells were centrifuged at 8000 rpm for 10 min and re- suspended in 300 µL of BHI broth. An aliquot of 100 µL of cells was plated on BHI plates supplemented with 50 µg/mL of spectinomycin. The plates were incubated in a 10% CO_2 incubator for 48 h [49]. Transformed cells containing plasmids integrated into the chromosome by a single homologous recombination event were selected on BHI plates supplemented with 50 µg/mL spectinomycin. Spectinomycin-resistant colonies were sub-cultured on BHI agar plates with no antibiotics. After sub-culturing for 3 days, the colonies were replicated on BHI agar with 1 mM IPTG. Spectinomycin-resistant clones were then grown in media without spectinomycin with the addition of 10% sucrose and IPTG to counter-select for double crossovers (the expression of *sacB* gene in pSJ13 makes the cells lethal in the presence of sucrose by forming fructo-polysaccharide). Colonies were streaked in BHI plates without antibiotics and BHI plates with 30 µg/mL of spectinomycin, and those that grew only on the former were selected [48,49]. The isolated recombinant plasmids with confirmed genomic deletion by PCR using the primers designed to amplify outside the 5' and 3' flanking regions were selected. This PCR product was also confirmed by sequencing. The resultant *apiA* isogenic mutant was designated as SJ13.

2.4. Immunofluorescence Microscopy

Growth and induction of *E. coli* harboring the plasmids were carried out as above. To immobilize cells for immunofluorescence assessment, 10 mL of each strain subculture was added into wells of the slide (Multitest Slide 8-Well, M.P Biomedicals LLC, Santa Ana, CA, USA) and air-dried. Ten microliters of primary antibody, anti-ApiA (0.7 mg/mL of rabbit polyclonal, Pocono Rabbit Farm and Lab, Canadensis, PA, USA), was added to each well at a 1:10 dilution in PBS and incubated for 2 h. After incubation, the slides were washed three times with PBS for 2–5 min each, and 10 µL of secondary antibody (1 mg/mL, goat anti-rabbit IgG FITC, Sigma-Aldrich, St. Louis, MI, USA) at a dilution of 1:80 in PBS was added and incubated for 1 h in the dark. After incubation, the slides were washed again three times with PBS for 2–5 min each and air-dried. The slides were then fixed using VECTASHIELD Antifade Mounting Medium (Vector Laboratories, Burlingame, CA, USA), covered with a coverslip, sealed, and examined and photographed using immunofluorescence microscopy (Confocal Imaging Facility, New Jersey Medical School, Newark, NJ, USA). Imaging was performed using Nikon A1R-A1 confocal microscope and Plan Apo VC 60× OIL NA-1.4 objective lens with 2.5× scanner zoom.

2.5. Electron Microscopy

Growth and induction of *E. coli* harboring the plasmids were carried out as above. Strains tested were pET-29b+ (negative control) and ApiA WT (full-length ApiA). Ten microliters of primary antibody, anti-ApiA (0.7 mg/mL of rabbit polyclonal antibody; Pocono Rabbit Farm), at a 1:10 dilution in PBS were added to bacterial cells and incubated for 2 h. Cells were washed three times with PBS and incubated with an immunogold-labeled secondary antibody (25 mg/mL, anti-rabbit IgG produced in goat and bound to gold particles (5 nm), Sigma-Aldrich) at 1:5 dilution for 1 h. Cells were washed with PBS and pelleted. The washed and pelleted cells were fixed with 2.5% glutaraldehyde (TED PELLA, Inc. Redding, CA, USA) for 2 h at RT and were washed again 3 times in PBS. Secondary fixation was carried out for 1 h with 1% osmium tetroxide (Sigma-Aldrich). The cells were again washed with PBS. A dehydration series was carried out with graded ethanol using 25%, 50%, 75%, and 100% ethanol each for 30 min. After the dehydration series, the samples were then transferred onto ultra-thin lacey carbon supported grid with 300 mesh (Sigma Aldrich) and imaged using a JEM-F200 transmission electron microscope (TEM) with a JEOL EDS detector and Gatan Oneview camera/DigiScan (Pleasanton, CA, USA). The images were taken under TEM (in transmission mode) at 200 kV and EDS under STEM mode (in scanning mode) at the Otto H. York Center for Environmental Engineering and Science (YCEES), New Jersey Institute of Technology (NJIT).

2.6. Auto-Aggregation Assay

Growth and induction of bacterial strains that included the empty plasmid and the full-length *apiA* gene with all deletions were carried out as previously described (see Figure 1). Quantitative assessment of the degree of auto-aggregation was determined by measuring the optical density of the supernatants at various time points. All strains were incubated in a shaker held at 37 °C for various time intervals after induction. Time 0 represents the OD 600 nm at time t = 45 min after induction. The OD 600 nm of the supernatant was measured using a NanoDrop One spectrophotometer (Thermo Fisher Scientific, Waltham, MA, USA) for 0, 35, 45, and 60 min following the induction period.

2.7. Buccal Epithelial Cell Culture

The TR146 human immortalized buccal epithelial cell line (10032305, Sigma-Aldrich) was grown in cell culture flasks (25 cm^2 Corning, NY, USA) using complete growth media (HAM's-F12 media supplemented with 10% of heat-inactivated fetal bovine serum (FBS; Gibco by Life Technologies, Grand Island, NY, USA) and 1X of Pen Strep Glutamine (Gibco by Life Technologies) at 37 °C with 5% CO_2. When cells reached approximately 85–90% confluency, the growth media were discarded, cells were washed with PBS, and they were detached by the addition of pre-warmed 0.05% trypsin-EDTA-1X (Gibco by Life Technologies). Equivalent volumes of pre-warmed complete growth medium were added, and cells were transferred to a 15 mL conical tube and pelleted by centrifugation at 200× *g* for 10 min. The pelleted cells were resuspended in 1 mL of pre-warmed complete growth medium. Cells were enumerated using the automated cell counter (Countess; Thermo Fisher Scientific).

2.8. Epithelial Cell Binding by Thymidine-Radiolabeled Bacteria

ApiA constructs, including the positive full-length *apiA* control and the negative empty plasmid control (pET29b+) and all the *apiA* deletions (Figure 1), were grown and induced as described above, with the addition of 10 µL 2′DeoxyThymidine 5′triphosphate and tetra Na salt [Methyl-3H] (1 mCi/mL, PerkinElmer, Waltham, MA, USA) to the overnight culture of buccal epithelial cells (BECs), which were prepared as described above. Radiolabeled bacterial cells (250 µL of the 3 mL subculture and induced cells) and BECs (250 µL) were combined and incubated for 5 min at 37 °C on a rotor shaker. The mix was pelleted for 2 min at $150 \times g$, and the pellet was washed twice using PBS and centrifuged for 2 min at $150 \times g$ to remove all unbound bacteria. The centrifugal speed allowed unbound bacteria to stay in suspension while pelleting the BECs. The pellet was resuspended in 200 µL of 0.1% Triton X and transferred to scintillation vials (Fisher Scientific), which were filled with Ecosiant A Scintillation solution (National Diagnostics, Charlotte, NC, USA). The amount of radioactivity was measured using an LS 6500 multi-purpose scintillation counter (Beckman Coulter, Brea, CA, USA) in the Office of Radiation Safety at Rutgers University. For all strains (Figure 1), the assay was carried out in technical quintuplicates. The entire experiment was repeated independently three times.

2.9. Complement Resistance Assays

Complement resistance assays were performed for both the *E. coli* strains expressing all *apiA* variants as well as an *A. actinomycetemcomitans* IDH781 wild-type and *apiA*-deleted strain of IDH781. For all the *E. coli* variants (Figure 1), cells were grown and induced as described above. The bacterial strains were incubated with normal human serum (NHS; Sigma Aldrich) and heat-inactivated human serum (HIS; Sigma Aldrich). For *E. coli* cells, a bacterial suspension of 10 µL was added to either 200 µL of 5% NHS or 5% HIS and incubated for 2 h at 37 °C. After incubation, 100 µL of each sample was serially diluted and plated on LB agar supplemented with 30 µg/mL kanamycin. Colony-forming units (CFU/mL) were calculated.

For *A. actinomycetemcomitans* experiments, wild-type IDH781 strain and the *apiA*-deleted IDH781 strain (SJ13) were initially grown on BHI agar supplemented with 0.6% yeast extract (Beckton Dickinson (BD), Franklin Lakes, NJ, USA), 0.8% dextrose, and 0.4% sodium bicarbonate. Colonies were picked from plates and checked for purity. Plates were scraped to obtain sufficient starting cultures and then inoculated into BHI broth (Beckton Dickinson) supplemented with 6% yeast extract (BD). Cells were subjected to centrifugation for 10 min at 4000 rpm, washed with PBS, and re-suspended to achieve an OD_{600nm} of 1.00. An aliquot of 10 µL from each strain (IDH781 and SJ13) was subjected to tests in the presence of a control where no human serum was used and grown for 2 h under anaerobic conditions. In a second set of experiments, both IDH781 and SJ13 were tested either in the presence of 50% normal human serum (NHS) or in the presence of heat-inactivated serum (HIS) and grown for two hours in an anaerobic chamber [29]. All samples were serially diluted and plated onto BHI agar plates for colony enumeration. IDH781, IDH781HIS, SJ13, and SJ13HIS results were normalized to cells in HIS as compared to NHS.

2.10. ELISA to Identify the ApiA Passenger Domain That Binds to Recombinant Factor H

Growth and induction of all the various *apiA* deletions and controls were performed as previously described in this study. One ml of bacterial cell suspension was incubated with 2 µg/mL of human FH (Complement Technology Inc., Tyler, TX, USA) for 30 min at 37 °C with vigorous shaking (850 rpm). The bacterial suspension was pelleted and washed three times using PBS then re-suspended in PBS, and the final concentration was adjusted to 10^8 bacteria/mL. From this bacterial suspension, 60 µL were transferred to 96-well enzyme-linked immunosorbent assay (ELISA) plate wells (Nunc PolySorp, Thermo Fisher Scientific), which were allowed to dry overnight at 37 °C. The ELISA plate wells were washed three times with PBS, blocked with 100 µL of 5% skim milk in PBS for 1 h at 37 °C. The wells were washed again three times with PBS and incubated with 50 µL of anti-FH monoclonal antibody (1 mg/mL, EPR6225, Abcam, Cambridge, MA, USA) diluted at a ratio of 1:500 in 5% skim milk for 1 h at RT. Wells were washed three times with PBS and incubated with HRP-conjugated goat anti-rabbit super clonal antibodies (0.0625 µg/mL, Thermo Fisher Scientific) for 1 h at RT. The wells were washed again 3 times with PBS, and 50 µL of TMB (3,3′,5,5′-tetramethylbenzidine) substrate (Thermo Scientific Pierce 1-Step Ultra TMB ELISA Substrate) solution was added. After 10 min of incubation, the reaction was stopped using 2 M H_2SO_4, and the absorbance at 450 nm was determined using a Tecan plate reader. Experiments were repeated three times in duplicate.

2.11. Peptide Effects on Complement Sensitivity Due to Factor H Binding

Peptides were designed to target the D101-217 amino acids of ApiA (Figure 1; EZBiolab, Carmel, IN, USA). This peptide was 85 amino acids in length, and it was divided into 3 peptides 25–30 amino acids in length. A second peptide set (Biomatik, Wilmington, DE, USA) consisting of 32 amino acids was designed to replicate the deleted sequence in variant D186-217, because it did not bind to FH in the ELISA assay, suggesting that this region was critical for FH binding. To test the ability of these peptides to affect complement activity, *E. coli* BL21 with pET21b+ was grown and induced as previously described. The peptides 1–6 (1 mg/mL) were incubated with 5% NHS for 1 h at 37 °C with rotation. Bacterial cells were then washed, added to this mixture, and incubated for 2 h at 37 °C to determine if the peptides added to serum were binding to C3b and FH, which would reduce their availability to attack the plasmid-containing bacteria. This would reduce the sensitivity of the strain to complement. The cells were serially diluted and plated as previously described. As a control, bacterial cells with no peptides or serum were also included. Experiments were performed in triplicate and repeated three times.

2.12. Growth Conditions for RNA Extractions

Cells were grown using two growth conditions: (1) IDH781 and IDH781Δ*apiA* (SJ13) in the absence of serum were grown on BHI agar plates and grown under anaerobic conditions (10% CO_2, 10% H_2, and 80% N_2) for 48 h, and (2) IDH781 and IDH781Δ*apiA* were exposed to 50% NHS or 50% HIS for 2 h under anaerobic conditions. Cells were collected from plates, re-suspended, grown in BHI broth, and then used for RNA extractions, as outlined below. Cells were uniformly distributed by vigorous vortexing, and OD_{600} was measured. The strains were subjected to 50% NHS or were grown in the absence of serum for 2 h (under anaerobic conditions). Cells were collected for RNA extraction as outlined below.

2.13. RNA Extractions and qRT-PCR

RNA was harvested from two growth conditions described above: (1) IDH781 and IDH781Δ*apiA* grown on BHI agar plates with no serum added for 48 h; and (2) IDH781 and IDH781Δ*apiA* exposed to 50% NHS or no serum for 2 h. Cells were collected from wild-type IDH781 and SJ13 in BHI broth. RNA isolation was carried out as previously described [13,50]. To stabilize the bacterial RNA, ice-cold 0.9% saline supplemented with 1/10th volume of 95% ethanol and 5% citric acid saturated phenol (Sigma Aldrich, Burlington, MA, USA) was added. The cells were centrifuged at 10,000 rpm for 5 min at 4 °C, and the cell pellets were flash-frozen in liquid nitrogen and stored at −80 °C until further use. RNA was isolated from the *A. actinomycetemcomitans* strains by the hot phenol method with the following modifications [50]. Glass beads were added to frozen pelleted cells followed by the addition of 700 μL ice-cold suspension buffer (30 mM sodium acetate at pH of 4.3, containing 1% β-mercaptoethanol, 2 mM aluminum ammonium sulfate, and 2 mM EDTA (Sigma Aldrich)). The cell suspension was bead-beaten (Biospec Products, Bartlesville, OK, USA) for 10 s to make sure the cells were dispersed evenly. A volume of 102 μL of preheated (65 °C) lysis buffer (300 mM sodium acetate at pH of 4.3, 10% β-mercaptoethanol, 8% SDS, and 16 mM EDTA at pH of 8.0) was added, bead-beaten for 20 s, and incubated at 65 °C for 3 min. An equal volume of preheated acidic phenol saturated with citrate buffer at pH of 4.0 (65 °C) was added and bead-beaten for 20 s (5Xs) with 1 min intervals maintaining the temperature at 65 °C. The phenol mixture was centrifuged at 14,000 rpm for 20 min at 4 °C. After repeating acidic phenol extraction, the aqueous phase was extracted with ice-cold chloroform (Sigma Aldrich) (2 times). The RNA was precipitated with the addition of 10% sodium acetate and 100% ethanol (2.5 volumes). The ethanol precipitated RNA was pelleted down by centrifugation at 14,000 rpm for 20 min and washed twice with 70% ethanol. The RNA pellet was air-dried and re-suspended in RNAse-free water. Total RNA was quantitated using a NanoDrop One Lite spectrophotometer (Thermo Fisher Scientific). The quality of the RNA was determined by the ratio of absorbance at 260/280 nm. To improve the quality of the total RNA, samples were passed through Micro Bio-Spin P-30 Gel Columns (Bio-RAD, Cat No. 732-6250).

After the gel filtration step, RNA samples were quantitated, and 500 ng of total RNA was mixed with RNA sample loading buffer (Sigma Aldrich), denatured at 65 °C for 10 min, ice-cooled, and analyzed on 1% TAE agarose gel. The RNA integrity was confirmed by visualizing the staining intensity difference between 23S and 16S rRNA and using the Agilent TapeStation system (Molecular Resource Facility, Rutgers, Newark). The purified total RNA samples were stored at −80 °C until further use. The total RNA (5 μg) was subjected to DNase I treatment to remove the contaminant genomic DNA using an RNA purification kit (Zymo Research, Irvine, CA, USA). As a negative control, complete DNA removal was confirmed in all the samples by PCR using *apiA* primers (Table 2) before subjecting the samples to qPCR.

2.14. Quantitative RT-PCR

cDNA was obtained from the isolated DNA-free RNA using a high-capacity reverse transcription kit (Applied biosystems, CA, USA) according to the manufacturer's instructions. One μg of RNA was converted into cDNA. qPCR reactions were performed in the CFX Opus 96 Real-Time PCR System (BIO-RAD) using PowerUp SYBR green master mix (Applied Biosystems, Carlsbad, CA, USA). Twenty-five microliter reactions were performed each time. cDNA was used in a dilution of 1:250 for reference gene 5SrRNA. Initial denaturation was performed at 94 °C for 10 min followed by 40 cycles of amplification (94 °C, 20 s; 56 °C, 20 s; and 72 °C, 20 s). Specificity of the products was assessed by melting curve analysis [13,49,50]. Negative control reaction with no reverse transcriptase was included in each run. Data were analyzed using Bio-Rad CFX Maestro software version 2.0 (Cambridge, MA, USA). The differential gene expression between IDH781 and SJ13 strains was calculated based on $2^{-\Delta\Delta C_T}$ value compared to 5S rRNA using three biological replicates, each of which had three technical replicates. The results were subjected to Student's *t*-test for statistical significance ($p < 0.05$).

2.15. Statistical Analysis

All experiments were performed on at least three separate occasions, with two or three technical replicates in each experiment. Statistical analysis comparing data was performed using one-way ANOVA for statistical significance with a confidence interval of 5% ($p < 0.05$) and Tukey–Kramer HSD for pairwise comparisons (JMP software package, version 12.0.1). Student's *t*-test was performed to compare the qRT-PCR results, and Bonferroni corrections were applied.

3. Results

3.1. Immunofluorescence and Transmission Electron Microscopy

To confirm the surface expression of ApiA and variants of *E. coli*, antibody staining was performed using a polyclonal anti-full-length ApiA antibody. The control strains, BL21 with pET21b+, failed to be recognized by the antibody. In contrast, full-length *apiA*, Δ34–80, and D186-217 showed immunofluorescence. The remaining gene regions expressed in *E. coli* failed to show immunofluorescence. To further assess the surface expression of ApiA in *E. coli*, TEM was used to examine the BL21 strains with pET21b+ (the negative control) and the ApiA full-length gene. The TEM results showed electron-dense immunogold areas in the full-length ApiA on the outer membrane as compared to the E. coli strain containing the empty plasmid, which failed to show immunogold labeling (Figure 2B).

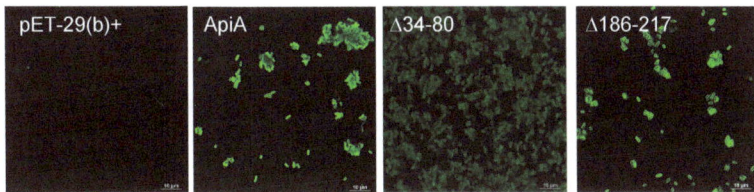

A

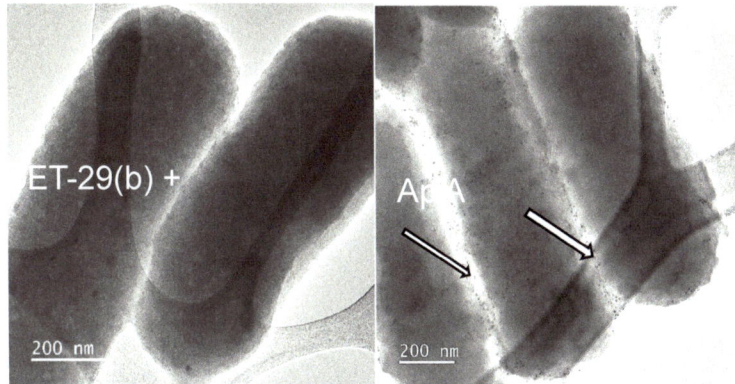

B

Figure 2. Immunofluorescence and TEM showing membrane labeling. Upper panels (left to right): pET29b+ empty plasmid, full-length ApiA (apple green), D34-80, and D186-217 (apple green) (**A**). Transmission electron microscopic images of immunogold particles are shown in right panel (**B**) (see arrows).

3.2. Auto-Aggregation Assay

A quantitative assessment of the auto-aggregation of the *E. coli* strains was performed based on the optical density measurements over 45 min post-induction (Table 3). The higher the optical density in the supernatants indicates the inability of the bacteria to auto-aggregate since the supernatants remain in a homogenous solution. The control strain, BL21 with pET21b+, failed to aggregate. Full-length ApiA and ApiA WT showed a significant change in the optical density and precipitated to form a pellet at the bottom of the test tube. Δ81–100 and Δ186–217 displayed similar results to those of full-length ApiA, indicating the missing region had no effect on their ability to auto-aggregate. ApiA variants Δ28–33, Δ34–80, Δ101–185, Δ81–185, and Δ28–185 showed reduced auto-aggregation. These results suggest the aggregation domain is contained in regions 28–80 and 101–185 of the passenger domain, which is feasible given the repeat regions located at 26–73, 74–122, and 148–184 (Figure 1).

Table 3. Auto-aggregation quantified as a measurement of optical density at different time intervals for different strains of *E. coli* expressing variants of *apiA*.

ApiA Construct	0 Min	35 Min	45 Min	60 Min
pET29b+	0.82 ± 04	0.91 ± 03	0.82 ± 04	0.83 ± 05
ApiA WT	0.39 ± 05	0.32 ± 03	0.32 ± 0.1	0.11 ± 12
Δ28–33	0.62 ± 08	0.67 ± 14	0.62 ± 0.1	0.52 ± 28
Δ34–80	0.62 ± 06	0.60 ± 04	0.52 ± 06	0.51 ± 03
Δ81–100	0.45 ± 06	0.14 ± 07	0.16 ± 11	0.19 ± 0.1
Δ101–185	0.56 ± 02	0.55 ± 06	0.61 ± 09	0.59 ± 26
Δ186–217	0.30+0.23	0.13 ± 08	0.15 ± 07	0.17 ± 05
Δ81–185	0.58 ± 08	0.43 ± 36	0.53 ± 24	0.47 ± 18
Δ28–185	0.49 ± 07	0.50 ± 09	0.58 ± 04	0.50 ± 09

3.3. Buccal Epithelial Cell Binding by Thymidine-Radiolabeled Bacteria

Epithelial cell binding was assessed by analyzing radioactively labeled bacteria and their ability bind to BECs. The percentage of binding was calculated by measuring the ratio of the radioactive counts per minute of bound bacterial cells to the total bacterial input counts per minute. As expected, the negative control, BL21 with pET21b+, failed to bind (Figure 3A). Variant Δ34–80 displayed the lowest level of binding, indicating the BEC binding site is likely within that region. pET29b+ (the empty plasmid vector) showed the lowest level of binding, while the full-length ApiA showed high levels of binding. The lowest binders were the empty plasmid, Δ34–80, Δ101–185, and Δ28–185. The most relevant amino acid deletions that contribute to binding therefore were Δ34–80 and Δ101–185.

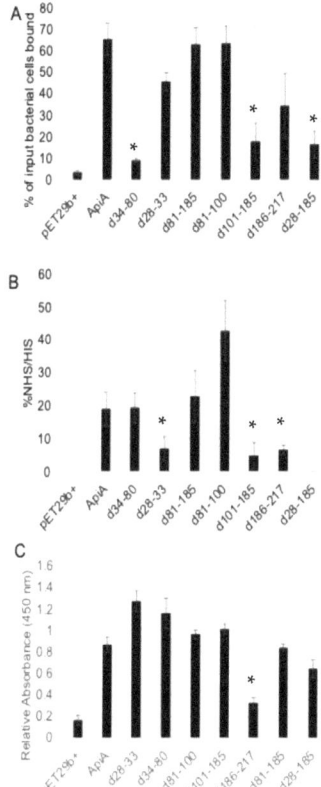

Figure 3. Buccal epithelial cell binding (**A**). Serum survival = % survival of the various strains when treated with 5% NHS and 5% HIS. (**B**). Factor H binding (**C**). ELISA was used to determine if *E. coli* strains treated with Factor H had the ability to interact or bind with Factor H. * represents $p \leq 0.01$.

3.4. Complement Resistance Assays

A quantitative assessment by CFU/mL plating for the complement resistance of the *E. coli* strains was performed by evaluating their survival in 5% normal human serum (NHS) relative to heat-inactivated serum (HIS). The negative control, BL21 with pET21b+, and Δ28–185 did not survive in the presence of NHS; however, *apiA*, D34-80, D81-185, and D81-100 were not sensitive to the serum. The results are shown in Figure 3B.

As per Figure 3B, IDH781 and the *apiA* deletion strain (SJ13) were also evaluated for their complement resistance, and IDH781 showed 45% resistance while SJ13 showed 17.2% resistance in comparison to the IDH781 control as determined by the CFU/mL plating of cells exposed to 50% NHS and HIS under anaerobic conditions ($p \leq 0.05$) (Figure 4). IDH781 is a well-maintained serotype d rough strain, and its growth was under anaerobic conditions, which might result in differences between our study and other studies [15,29,35].

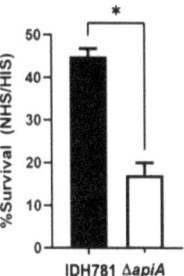

Figure 4. *A. actinomycetemcomitans*'s sutvival in serum showing ratio of surivival in normal serum as compared to heat-inactivated serum. * indicating significant difference ($p \leq 0.05$).

3.5. ELISA to Identify the ApiA Passenger Domain That Binds to Recombinant Factor H

The proposed mechanism of serum resistance is through the binding of the regulatory protein Factor H. Here, using an ELISA, recombinant variants were immobilized and assessed for their ability to bind purified Factor H (Figure 3C). Full-length ApiA and the variants Δ28–33, Δ34–80, Δ81–100, Δ101–185, Δ81–185, and Δ28–185 showed binding to Factor H. Variant Δ186–217 displayed a reduced binding ability in comparison to the other strains and the positive full-length ApiA, indicating the binding region is likely within amino acids 186–217. The control strain, BL21 with pET21b+, failed to bind.

3.6. Peptides' Effects on Complement Sensitivity

The addition of peptide P1 to the pETb+ empty plasmid control strain showed a nearly 900-fold increase in survival over that of the serum with the no-peptide-added control (Figure 5). In contrast, the addition of peptides P2, P3, P4, and P5 showed no significant difference in colony-forming units as compared to the control. The addition of peptide 6 provided the cells with about a 450-fold increase in survival in the presence of serum as compared to when no peptides were added (Figure 5).

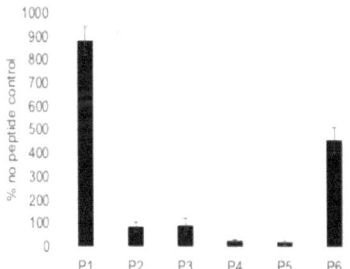

Figure 5. Indirect measurement of peptide binding to Factor H. Higher bacterial survival in the presence of peptides (1–6), the higher the level of interference with FH availability.

3.7. Quantitative RT-PCR of Cells Grown with and Without Serum

The relative expression of selected genes like *omp*A1 and *omp*A2, which are responsible for conferring complement resistance, were analyzed to gain a better understanding of how the deletion of *apiA* would affect the expression of these genes. qRT-PCR was used to assess the expression levels of genes involved in attachment and biofilm formation, like *rcp*B and *pga*C, as well as genes like *oxy*R and *kat*A, which are critical for stress resistance. In the first experiment WT-IDH 781 was compared to SJ13 (IDH with the *apiA* deletion. Here IDH 781 showed elevation for all genes tested in the absence of serum (Figure 6A). In the second set of experiment both WT-IDH 781 strain and SJ13 (IDH with the *apiA* deletion were tested in the presence or absence of serum (Figure 6B,C). Here IDH781 consistently showed elevation in expression of the genes assessed (Figure 6B) while SJ13 consistently showed a depression in gene expression in the presence of serum (Figure 6C). The significance levels were calculated by means of a Student's t-test and showed that the level of difference reached ($p < 0.001$) when the wild-type strain was compared to the apiA-deleted strain SJ13.

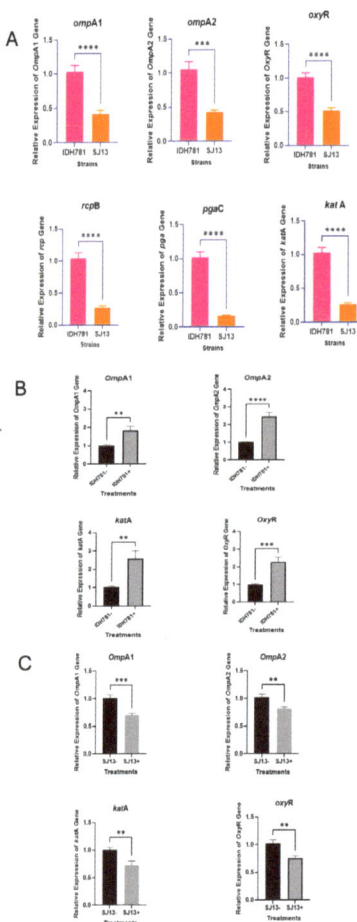

Figure 6. qRT-PCR assessment comparing expression of specific genes in the absence or presence of serum. These assessment were made in the absence of any serum treatment (**A**). The next group compared serum treatment to no treatment in, IDH 781 (**B**). And the final comparison was in SJ13 (IDH with an *apiA* deletion comparing serum treatment to no serum treatment (**C**). Note that stars indicate significant differences at a minimum of ($p \leq 0.05$).

The relative expression levels of the selected genes, *ompA1*, *ompA2*, *kat*A, and *oxyR*, were assessed in response to serum treatment in wild-type IDH781 (IDH781+ = serum added; IDH781 = no serum added) using qRT-PCR for the expression levels of genes. A similar assessment was conducted with the $\Delta apiA$ strain (SJ13), and the qRT-PCR showed that all the assessed genes were upregulated in IDH781 in the presence of serum and downregulated in the SJ13 *apiA*-deleted strain (Figure 6B). All reading showed significant differences in their expression profiles of *oxyR* ($p = 0.01$), *kat*A ($p = 0.01$), *omp*A1 ($p = 0.01$), and *omp*A2 ($p = 0.01$)

4. Discussion

A. actinomycetemcomitans contributes to periodontitis in both the early and later stages of the disease process [51]. The colonization of teeth and soft tissue occurs early in life, and *A. actinomycetemcomitans* utilizes many strategies to colonize soft tissues prior to tooth eruption [52,53]. Key among the adhesins known to influence these binding characteristics is the widespread colonization island of genes responsible for fimbrial structures and extracellular polysaccharides that lead to non-specific binding to abiotic surfaces such as enamel [8]. In addition, Aae and ApiA are two autotransporter proteins that enable *A. actinomycetemcomitans* to bind to soft tissue such as the gingival epithelium [14,15,54]. These two omps have very different structures, with Aae being monomeric and non-aggregating, and ApiA being trimeric with auto-aggregation or clumping [16]. Efforts to gain a better understanding of ApiA's diverse functional activity have been difficult largely because auto-aggregation complicates accurate quantitative assessments. Clumping has been shown to be associated with the C-terminus of ApiA, and as a result, a hybrid protein was created that merged the C-terminus of the monomeric form of Aae to the passenger domain of trimeric ApiA. Using this strategy, cellular clumping was minimal, which allowed for the exploration of soft tissue binding, auto-aggregation, and biofilm formation in the fused protein expressed in an *E. coli* host [16]. Sequential deletions were created in the passenger domain, and each deletion was examined for its effect on auto-aggregation, tissue binding, and biofilm formation. These experiments led to the conclusion that the C-terminus of ApiA was required for trimerization, auto-aggregation, and biofilm formation, although it was possible that the gene-deleted regions as expressed in the *E. coli* host in the monomeric protein were not truly representative of the functional activities exhibited in the trimeric autotransporter protein. Nevertheless, the results of the hybrid fusion experiments were helpful in efforts to re-examine deleted areas in the N-terminal passenger domain of the trimeric autotransporter, especially in the case of highly relevant complement resistance and Factor H binding [16]. The impact that *A. actinomycetemcomitans* has on the damage/response process can be likened to AIDS, in that its effect on the host dampens the immunological response, permitting other microbes to persist and thrive in an immunologically compromised host domain [55,56]. In the early stages of disease, *A. actinomycetemcomitans* has an impact on the innate immune system by virtue of its effect on (1) the epithelial barrier (cytolethal distending toxin [57]), (2) serum-derived complement resistance (Omp and ApiA) [38], and (3) leukocytes and monocytes (leukotoxins) [58,59]. The least understood of these virulence traits is complement resistance, a trait that occurs in the earliest stages of disease [17]. This study has been developed to better understand the role of ApiA as a trimeric autotransporter protein in complement resistance as well as auto-aggregation and epithelial cell binding [15,16].

ApiA, a trimeric multifunctional protein, has been proposed to be a critical virulence factor in periodontitis, occurring in children and young adolescents [15]. Most importantly, *A. actinomycetemcomitans* ApiA is thought to affect the early stages of disease in patients who suffer from Stage III Grade C (LAgP) periodontitis [16]. As a multifunctional omp, ApiA is uniquely positioned for auto-aggregation and biofilm formation as well as epithelial cell binding [18]. When *A. actinomycetemcomitans* migrates subgingivally, it is confronted by crevice fluid, a serum exudate containing complement protein [45]. ApiA was first characterized by Asakawa in 2003 [29]. While these studies have provided some insight into the importance of ApiA (e.g., Omp100), the specific identification of regions of interest in the gene locus and the functionality of the gene remained unresolved [15,17,29]. Defining these regions could help develop potent vaccine candidates and/or peptides related to active sites that could be used to interfere with local complement activity.

This study has helped identify regions within the passenger domain of *apiA* that are critical for the multi-functional capability of ApiA. Disease progression is not caused by microorganisms alone but is due to the way in which the host immune response modulates the challenge, which could either amplify or reduce disease progression [27,33,60,61]. Microbes are known to protect themselves from complement-related cell surface destruction by hijacking host complement regulators from plasma or other body fluids [25]. Pathogens use a range of strategies that allow them to survive and disseminate in the host. A strategy of immune evasion through molecular mimicry can provide bacteria with the ability to imitate host surface proteins, permitting them to persist within the host so as to avoid destruction by complement proteins [62,63]. *A. actinomycetemcomitans* displays serum resistance and immune evasion by binding to the complement protein FH by means of its outer membrane protein, ApiA [46]. Essentially, sequestering Factor H allows the bacterium to masquerade as a mammalian cell so as to avoid clearance via complement activity [27]. It is generally hypothesized that upon binding Factor H, the alternative complement pathway is downregulated, promoting host innate immune evasion [61]. Tricking the complement system, particularly the alternative complement pathway, enhances microbial virulence and is spontaneously activated on non-protected surfaces that would be vulnerable. Many bacterial pathobionts like *Neisseria meningitidis, Yersinia pestis,* and *Treponema denticola* have a variety of strategies to mimic host cell surface molecules, like heparin or glycosaminoglycan, which cause the complement regulator protein FH to bind to their outer membrane protein, thereby downregulating the complement system in order to allow for survival in the host [64–66].

Over years of evolution, FH binding as developed in human cells has been replicated in bacterial cells such that there is now competition for the sequestration of FH between specific bacterial cells and host cells [65]. Identifying the domain required for the interaction with FH could help develop substances (such as small peptides) to help to strengthen the resistance to complement sensitivity. This study identified ApiA domains responsible for binding to buccal epithelial cells, auto-aggregation, and the domain that is responsible for serum resistance. The examination of *A. actinomycetemcomitans*-related ApiA expression and functionality in an *E. coli* host has enabled the identification of regions responsible for surface expressed proteins that can be induced, isolated, analyzed, and functionally characterized. The focus of this study was on the surface expression of ApiA. Auto-aggregation and buccal epithelial cell binding can only take place if surface interactions occur. To ensure that these functional activities were due to the surface expression of ApiA, fluorescent antibody detection, followed by a TEM examination of gold-labeled antibody directed to the passenger domain of ApiA, was carried out. These tools provided visual evidence that ApiA was surface-expressed. After assurance that the surface expression was reproducible, the functional activities of surface expressed proteins were examined using the quantitation of auto-aggregation and epithelial cell binding. In all cases, ApiA expression proteins induced in *E. coli* showed distinctive and quantitatively reproducible functionality. ApiA binding to FH was used to select the most likely region of the *apiA* gene responsible for complement resistance and FH binding. It was revealing to discover that polyclonal antibody and a particular monoclonal antibody proposed to detect FH had little to no specificity and, as such, bound to all cell surfaces (including a host containing an empty plasmid that failed to express surface proteins). In contrast, one monoclonal antibody bound to the full-length ApiA as expressed in *E. coli* as well as to a very specific region containing 32 amino acids. To confirm the specificity of binding to the complement region of interest, peptides associated with the critical 32 amino acid region were made and then three peptide sequences within this 32-amino-acid region were designed. These peptides were added to untreated serum containing complement protein and revealed that a particular sequence containing a set of 13 amino acids blocked serum-related complement activity. This completed our efforts to identify the *apiA* region of interest in *E. coli*. Our attention was then focused on deleting the *apiA* gene in *A. actinomycetemcomitans* IDH 781 to determine its effect on complement resistance as well as how this deletion affected the expression of several auxiliary genes that regulated the expression of genes of functional prominence.

Reacting IDH781, the *A. actinomycetemcomitans* WT strain, with serum resulted in 45% serum resistance when compared to HIS and 38% when compared to the *apiA*-deleted strain (SJ13). Other recent studies suggested that OmpA-1 could provide added protection against complement proteins [17]. Studies have also shown that membrane vesicles secreted by strains of *A. actinomycetemcomitans* can also contribute to complement resistance [38,51]. These forays into complement resistance in *A. actinomycetemcomitans* indicate that this form of immune avoidance is potentially greater than currently imagined. In addition, experiments have not been extended to serotype b JP2 strains, most likely because of cloning difficulties in serotype b strains [67,68]. In spite of these shortcomings, the results of *A. actinomycetemcomitans* serotype a and d strains, strains which are not related to disease and which were grown in a manner in the laboratory that may have limited their translatability to their real-world activity, our data provide a good starting point. Also, the fact that the isolation of membrane vesicles from *A. actinomycetemcomitans* shows complement activity supports the concept that this activity can be more widespread in vivo [17,38]. Further, our focus on these restricted experimental conditions was due to the fact that previous studies have failed to make headway in ApiA-related complement resistance. Within the confines of the limitations of this study design, we feel that the data as presented provide a good starting point for future investigations.

The second aim of this study was to determine whether there were genes that were co-regulated with *A. actinomycetemcomitans apiA* in its interaction with serum. Using qRT-PCR, a series of candidate genes were examined, which included *ompA1*, *ompA2*, *oxyR*, and several other genes responsible for homeostatic equilibrium. For example, when *ompA1* and *ompA2* gene expression was assessed in wild-type IDH781 as compared to the *apiA*-deleted strain (SJ13) in the absence of serum, there was an approximate increase in gene expression by 50% in the wild-type strain. In comparison, *katA* and *OxyR* and *ompA1* and *ompA2* were all upregulated in the presence of serum, while these genes were all downregulated in the presence of serum in SJ13, suggesting that the *apiA* gene is not just responsible for serum sensitivity but could also be responsible for other more globally regulatory gene responses.

Overall, these data suggest that not only does the increased expression of *apiA* in the presence of serum result in a reduction in serum sensitivity for itself and its community partners, but this response to serum also provides *A. actinomycetemcomitans* with added ways of avoiding environmental hazards by upregulating genes for biofilm formation, attachment, and oxygen resistance. While much more work is required, these interactions imply that a multifaceted/coordinated response is a pre-requisite for life in a complex ecological environment. *A. actinomycetemcomitans* appears to possess many ways of addressing its need for adaptability, including leukotoxin, cytolethal distending toxin production, and complement resistance, but extrapolation from the data presented above suggests that many other interactions are required for survival in a complex ecosystem and that these unanswered questions warrant continued and expanded research.

Several limitations of this study are clear and include but are not limited to the following: (1) the need to assess varying growth media, (2) the need to assess different stages of growth, and (3) the need to assess various strains and species of *A. actinomycetemcomitans*. In the future, the JP2 serotype b strain of *A. actinomycetemcomitans* could be examined. Since the goal in this study was to provide initial data, future studies could use site-directed mutagenesis once the critical amino acids required for various functions related to *A. actinomycetemcomitans* survival have been identified. In addition, a more precise definition of FH binding could determined by using alanine substitutions in the regions of the 13-mer amino acid that has been found to be responsible for Factor H binding in this study. Furthermore, data related to peptide 1 provide clues that ApiA may be involved in additional ways, interfering with complement pathways such as the lectin or classical pathways [24,69]. For example, elevated levels of ompA1 and ompA2 in the presence of serum support the work by Lindblom and associates and can potentially represent added ways in which *A. actinomycetemcomitans* shows adaptive capabilities [17,69].

5. Conclusions

(1) Studies designed to examine the specific region in the *A. actinomycetemcomitans apiA* gene responsible for complement resistance were assessed using an *E. coli* vector to examine its complement resistance. Sequential gene deletions in *apiA* were examined by

immunofluorescence and immunogold transmission electron microscopy for surface expression and were confirmed by measuring auto-aggregation and buccal epithelial binding to assess the functional surface expression of *apiA*;

(2) *E. coli*-deleted regions (Δ34–80 and Δ186–217) failed to show epithelial cell binding (Δ34–80) and complement resistance (Δ186–217);

(3) Factor H binding, critical for complement resistance via the alternative pathway, was used to probe the region(s) most likely responsible for complement resistance, and a 32-amino-acid protein within the Δ186–217 deletion was identified;

(4) Peptides were designed for further testing within this 32-amino-acid region, and a 13-amino-acid segment provided preliminary evidence that this area was responsible for complement resistance;

(5) *apiA* was deleted in *A. actinomycetemcomitans* IDH781, and qRT-PCR was used to identify several other relevant genes in *A. actinomycetemcomitans* that were either up- or downregulated in the presence or absence of serum in wild-type *A. actinomycetemcomitans* or in Δ*apiA. actinomycetemcomitans*. It was proposed that *apiA* could be associated with global regulation or some other regulatory manner that could affect the expression of prominent stress-related genes that could play a role in overall *A. actinomycetemcomitans* adaptability and stress survival;

(6) This is the first study to identify a specific region within *apiA* responsible for complement resistance via the alternative pathway and, as such, provides a good starting point for future studies that can achieve a more in-depth model of complement resistance and the role of *apiA* in the global regulation of *A. actinomycetemcomitans*.

Author Contributions: Conceptualization, C.C., D.H.F. and H.S.; Data curation, C.C., D.H.F. and H.S.; Formal analysis, C.C., S.K.V., S.J. and H.S.; Funding acquisition, C.C. and D.H.F.; Investigation, S.K.V., S.J., D.G., L.G. and H.S.; Methodology, C.C., D.H.F. and H.S.; Project administration, H.S.; Resources, C.C., D.H.F. and N.G.; Supervision, D.H.F. and H.S.; Validation, C.C., D.H.F., S.K.V., S.J. and H.S.; Visualization, C.C. and S.J.; Writing—original draft, C.C., D.H.F. and H.S.; Writing—review and editing, C.C., D.H.F. and H.S. All authors have read and agreed to the published version of the manuscript.

Funding: This research was funded in part by the New Jersey Health Foundation, grant number PC31-15, and the National Institutes of Dental and Craniofacial Research, grant number DE-016306.

Institutional Review Board Statement: The study was conducted in accordance with the Declaration of Helsinki, and approved by the Institutional Review Board of Rutgers University protocol code Pro 0120050257 on 21 December 2023.

Informed Consent Statement: Written informed consent has been obtained from the patient(s) to publish this paper.

Data Availability Statement: Data will be made available upon request.

Acknowledgments: This study was conducted as part of the PhD awarded to S. Jacob.

Conflicts of Interest: The authors declare no conflicts of interest.

References

1. Marsh, P.D.; Zaura, E. Dental biofilm: Ecological interactions in health and disease. *J. Clin. Periodontol.* **2017**, *44* (Suppl. S18), S12–S22. [CrossRef] [PubMed]
2. Hajishengallis, G.; Lamont, R.J.; Koo, H. Oral polymicrobial communities: Assembly, function, and impact on diseases. *Cell Host Microbe* **2023**, *31*, 528–538. [CrossRef] [PubMed]
3. Bamashmous, S.; Kotsakis, G.A.; Kerns, K.A.; Leroux, B.G.; Zenobia, C.; Chen, D.; Trivedi, H.M.; McLean, J.S.; Darveau, R.P. Human variation in gingival inflammation. *Proc. Natl. Acad. Sci. USA* **2021**, *118*, e2012578118. [CrossRef] [PubMed]
4. Socransky, S.S.; Haffajee, A.D.; Cugini, M.A.; Smith, C.; Kent, R.L., Jr. Microbial complexes in subgingival plaque. *J. Clin. Periodontol.* **1998**, *25*, 134–144. [CrossRef]
5. Shaddox, L.M.; Spencer, W.P.; Velsko, I.M.; Al-Kassab, H.; Huang, H.; Calderon, N.; Aukhil, I.; Wallet, S.M. Localized aggressive periodontitis immune response to healthy and diseased subgingival plaque. *J. Clin. Periodontol.* **2016**, *43*, 746–753. [CrossRef]
6. Zambon, J.J. *Actinobacillus actinomycetemcomitans* in human periodontal disease. *J. Clin. Periodontol.* **1985**, *12*, 707–711. [CrossRef]

7. Fine, D.H.; Schreiner, H.; Velusamy, S.K. Aggregatibacter, A Low Abundance Pathobiont That Influences Biogeography, Microbial Dysbiosis, and Host Defense Capabilities in Periodontitis: The History of A Bug, And Localization of Disease. *Pathogens* **2020**, *9*, 179. [CrossRef]
8. Planet, P.J.; Kachlany, S.C.; Fine, D.H.; DeSalle, R.; Figurski, D.H. The widespread colonization island of *Actinobacillus actinomycetemcomitans*. *Nat. Genet.* **2003**, *34*, 193–198. [CrossRef]
9. Kachlany, S.C.; Fine, D.H.; Figurski, D.H. Secretion of RTX leukotoxin by *Actinobacillus actinomycetemcomitans*. *Infect. Immun.* **2000**, *68*, 6094–6100. [CrossRef]
10. Schreiner, H.; Li, Y.; Cline, J.; Tsiagbe, V.K.; Fine, D.H. A comparison of *Aggregatibacter actinomycetemcomitans* (Aa) virulence traits in a rat model for periodontal disease. *PLoS ONE* **2013**, *8*, e69382. [CrossRef]
11. Kaplan, J.B.; Meyenhofer, M.F.; Fine, D.H. Biofilm growth and detachment of *Actinobacillus actinomycetemcomitans*. *J. Bacteriol.* **2003**, *185*, 1399–1404. [CrossRef] [PubMed]
12. Kaplan, J.B. Biofilm dispersal: Mechanisms, clinical implications and potential therapeutic uses. *J. Dent. Res.* **2010**, *89*, 205–218. [CrossRef] [PubMed]
13. Shanmugam, M.; Gopal, P.; El Abbar, F.; Schreiner, H.C.; Kaplan, J.B.; Fine, D.H.; Ramasubbu, N. Role of exopolysaccharide in *Aggregatibacter actinomycetemcomitans*-induced bone resorption in a rat model for periodontal disease. *PLoS ONE* **2015**, *10*, e0117487. [CrossRef] [PubMed]
14. Fine, D.H.; Velliyagounder, K.; Furgang, D.; Kaplan, J.B. The *Actinobacillus actinomycetemcomitans* autotransporter adhesin Aae exhibits specificity for buccal epithelial cells from humans and old world primates. *Infect. Immun.* **2005**, *73*, 1947–1953. [CrossRef] [PubMed]
15. Yue, G.; Kaplan, J.B.; Furgang, D.; Mansfield, K.G.; Fine, D.H. A second *Aggregatbacter actinomycetemcomitans* autotransporter adhesin that exhibits specificity for buccal epithelial cells of humans and Old World Primates. *Infect. Immun.* **2007**, *75*, 4440–4448. [CrossRef]
16. Cugini, C.; Mei, Y.; Furgang, D.; George, N.; Ramasubbu, N.; Fine, D.H. Utilization of Variant and Fusion Proteins To Functionally Map the *Aggregatibacter actinomycetemcomitans* Trimeric Autotransporter Protein ApiA. *Infect. Immun.* **2018**, *86*, e00697-17. [CrossRef]
17. Lindholm, M.; Min Aung, K.; Nyunt Wai, S.; Oscarsson, J. Role of OmpA1 and OmpA2 in *Aggregatibacter actinomycetemcomitans* and Aggregatibacter aphrophilus serum resistance. *J. Oral. Microbiol.* **2019**, *11*, 1536192. [CrossRef]
18. Fine, D.H.; Patil, A.G.; Velusamy, S.K. *Aggregatibacter actinomycetemcomitans* (Aa) Under the Radar: Myths and Misunderstandings of Aa and Its Role in Aggressive Periodontitis. *Front. Immunol.* **2019**, *10*, 728. [CrossRef]
19. Loesche, W.J.; Gusberti, F.; Mettraux, G.; Higgins, T.; Syed, S. Relationship between oxygen tension and subgingival bacterial flora in untreated human periodontal pockets. *Infect. Immun.* **1983**, *42*, 659–667. [CrossRef]
20. Ebersole, J.L.; Cappelli, D.; Sandoval, M.N. Subgingival distribution of A. actinomycetemcomitans in periodontitis. *J. Clin. Periodontol.* **1994**, *21*, 65–75. [CrossRef]
21. Kononen, E.; Muller, H.P. Microbiology of aggressive periodontitis. *Periodontol. 2000* **2014**, *65*, 46–78. [CrossRef] [PubMed]
22. Aberg, C.H.; Kelk, P.; Johansson, A. *Aggregatibacter actinomycetemcomitans*: Virulence of its leukotoxin and association with aggressive periodontitis. *Virulence* **2015**, *6*, 188–195. [CrossRef] [PubMed]
23. Shillitoe, E.J.; Lehner, T. Immunoglobulins and complement in crevicular fluid, serum and saliva in man. *Arch. Oral. Biol.* **1972**, *17*, 241–247. [CrossRef] [PubMed]
24. Lambris, J.D.; Ricklin, D.; Geisbrecht, B.V. Complement evasion by human pathogens. *Nat. Rev. Microbiol.* **2008**, *6*, 132–142. [CrossRef] [PubMed]
25. Potempa, J.; Pike, R.N. Corruption of innate immunity by bacterial proteases. *J. Innate Immun.* **2009**, *1*, 70–87. [CrossRef]
26. Blom, A.M.; Hallstrom, T.; Riesbeck, K. Complement evasion strategies of pathogens-acquisition of inhibitors and beyond. *Mol. Immunol.* **2009**, *46*, 2808–2817. [CrossRef]
27. Hovingh, E.S.; van den Broek, B.; Jongerius, I. Hijacking Complement Regulatory Proteins for Bacterial Immune Evasion. *Front. Microbiol.* **2016**, *7*, 2004. [CrossRef]
28. Zipfel, P.F.; Hallstrom, T.; Riesbeck, K. Human complement control and complement evasion by pathogenic microbes--tipping the balance. *Mol. Immunol.* **2013**, *56*, 152–160. [CrossRef]
29. Asakawa, R.; Komatsuzawa, H.; Goncalves, R.B.; Izumi, S.; Fujiwara, T.; Nakano, Y.; Suzuki, N.; Uchida, Y.; Ouhara, K.; Shiba, H.; et al. Outer membrane protein 100, a versatile virulence factor of *Actinobacillus actinomycetemcomitans*. *Mol. Microbiol.* **2003**, *50*, 1125–1139. [CrossRef]
30. Walport, M.J. Complement. Second of two parts. *N. Engl. J. Med.* **2001**, *344*, 1140–1144. [CrossRef]
31. Janeway, C.J.; Travers, P.; Walport, M.; Shlomchik, M. *The Immune System in Healthb and Disease*, 5th ed.; Garland Science: New York, NY, USA, 2001.
32. Ripoche, J.; Day, A.J.; Harris, T.J.; Sim, R.B. The complete amino acid sequence of human complement factor H. *Biochem. J.* **1988**, *249*, 593–602. [CrossRef] [PubMed]
33. Kopp, A.; Hebecker, M.; Svobodova, E.; Jozsi, M. Factor h: A complement regulator in health and disease, and a mediator of cellular interactions. *Biomolecules* **2012**, *2*, 46–75. [CrossRef] [PubMed]
34. Schenkein, H.A. The role of complement in periodontal diseases. *Crit. Rev. Oral. Biol. Med.* **1991**, *2*, 65–81. [CrossRef] [PubMed]

35. Mei, Y. Functional Mapping of Aggregatibacter Actinomycetcomitans Autotransporter Adhesin Protein, ApiA. Ph.D. Thesis, Rutgers School of Dental Medicine, Newark, NJ, USA, 2014.
36. Komatsuzawa, H.; Kawai, T.; Wilson, M.E.; Taubman, M.A.; Sugai, M.; Suginaka, H. Cloning of the gene encoding the *Actinobacillus actinomycetemcomitans* serotype b OmpA-like outer membrane protein. *Infect. Immun.* 1999, *67*, 942–945. [CrossRef] [PubMed]
37. Cugini, C.; Ramasubbu, N.; Tsiagbe, V.K.; Fine, D.H. Dysbiosis From a Microbial and Host Perspective Relative to Oral Health and Disease. *Front. Microbiol.* 2021, *12*, 617485. [CrossRef]
38. Oscarsson, J.; Claesson, R.; Lindholm, M.; Hoglund Aberg, C.; Johansson, A. Tools of *Aggregatibacter actinomycetemcomitans* to Evade the Host Response. *J. Clin. Med.* 2019, *8*, 1079. [CrossRef]
39. Ouhara, K.; Komatsuzawa, H.; Shiba, H.; Uchida, Y.; Kawai, T.; Sayama, K.; Hashimoto, K.; Taubman, M.A.; Kurihara, H.; Sugai, M. *Actinobacillus actinomycetemcomitans* outer membrane protein 100 triggers innate immunity and production of beta-defensin and the 18-kilodalton cationic antimicrobial protein through the fibronectin-integrin pathway in human gingival epithelial cells. *Infect. Immun.* 2006, *74*, 5211–5220. [CrossRef]
40. Olsen, I.; Lambris, J.D.; Hajishengallis, G. *Porphyromonas gingivalis* disturbs host-commensal homeostasis by changing complement function. *J. Oral. Microbiol.* 2017, *9*, 1340085. [CrossRef]
41. McDowell, J.V.; Frederick, J.; Miller, D.P.; Goetting-Minesky, M.P.; Goodman, H.; Fenno, J.C.; Marconi, R.T. Identification of the primary mechanism of complement evasion by the periodontal pathogen, *Treponema denticola*. *Mol. Oral. Microbiol.* 2011, *26*, 140–149. [CrossRef]
42. Miller, D.P.; McDowell, J.V.; Rhodes, D.V.; Allard, A.; Caimano, M.; Bell, J.K.; Marconi, R.T. Sequence divergence in the *Treponema denticola* FhbB protein and its impact on factor H binding. *Mol. Oral. Microbiol.* 2013, *28*, 316–330. [CrossRef]
43. Miller, D.P.; McDowell, J.V.; Bell, J.K.; Goetting-Minesky, M.P.; Fenno, J.C.; Marconi, R.T. Analysis of the complement sensitivity of oral treponemes and the potential influence of FH binding, FH cleavage and dentilisin activity on the pathogenesis of periodontal disease. *Mol. Oral. Microbiol.* 2014, *29*, 194–207. [CrossRef] [PubMed]
44. Amano, A.; Chen, C.; Honma, K.; Li, C.; Settem, R.P.; Sharma, A. Genetic characteristics and pathogenic mechanisms of periodontal pathogens. *Adv. Dent. Res.* 2014, *26*, 15–22. [CrossRef] [PubMed]
45. Courts, F.J.; Boackle, R.J.; Fudenberg, H.H.; Silverman, M.S. Detection of functional complement components in gingival crevicular fluid from humans with periodontal diseases. *J. Dent. Res.* 1977, *56*, 327–331. [CrossRef] [PubMed]
46. Komatsuzawa, H.; Asakawa, R.; Kawai, T.; Ochiai, K.; Fujiwara, T.; Taubman, M.A.; Ohara, M.; Kurihara, H.; Sugai, M. Identification of six major outer membrane proteins from *Actinobacillus actinomycetemcomitans*. *Gene* 2002, *288*, 195–201. [CrossRef] [PubMed]
47. May, A.C.; Ehrlich, R.L.; Balashov, S.; Ehrlich, G.D.; Shanmugam, M.; Fine, D.H.; Ramasubbu, N.; Mell, J.C.; Cugini, C. Complete Genome Sequence of *Aggregatibacter actinomycetemcomitans* Strain IDH781. *Genome Announc.* 2016, *4*, e01285-16. [CrossRef]
48. Juarez-Rodriguez, M.D.; Torres-Escobar, A.; Demuth, D.R. Construction of new cloning, lacZ reporter and scarless-markerless suicide vectors for genetic studies in *Aggregatibacter actinomycetemcomitans*. *Plasmid* 2013, *69*, 211–222. [CrossRef]
49. Velusamy, S.K.; Sampathkumar, V.; Godboley, D.; Fine, D.H. Profound Effects of *Aggregatibacter actinomycetemcomitans* Leukotoxin Mutation on Adherence Properties Are Clarified in in vitro Experiments. *PLoS ONE* 2016, *11*, e0151361. [CrossRef]
50. Shanmugam, M.; El Abbar, F.; Ramasubbu, N. Transcriptome Profiling of Wild-Type and pga-Knockout Mutant Strains Reveal the Role of Exopolysaccharide in *Aggregatibacter actinomycetemcomitans*. *PLoS ONE* 2015, *10*, e0134285. [CrossRef]
51. Belibasakis, G.N.; Maula, T.; Bao, K.; Lindholm, M.; Bostanci, N.; Oscarsson, J.; Ihalin, R.; Johansson, A. Virulence and Pathogenicity of *Aggregatibacter actinomycetemcomitans*. *Pathogens* 2019, *8*, 222. [CrossRef]
52. Fives-Taylor, P.M.; Meyer, D.H.; Mintz, K.P.; Brissette, C. Virulence factors of *Actinobacillus actinomycetemcomitans*. *Periodontol. 2000* 1999, *20*, 136–167. [CrossRef]
53. Fine, D.H.; Kaplan, J.B.; Kachlany, S.C.; Schreiner, H.C. How we got attached to *Actinobacillus actinomycetemcomitans*: A model for infectious diseases. *Periodontol. 2000* 2006, *42*, 114–157. [CrossRef] [PubMed]
54. Rose, J.E.; Meyer, D.H.; Fives-Taylor, P.M. Aae, an autotransporter involved in adhesion of *Actinobaciillus actinomyctemcomitans* to epithelial cells. *Infect. Immun.* 2003, *71*, 2384–2393. [CrossRef] [PubMed]
55. Casadevall, A.; Pirofski, L.A. Host-pathogen interactions: Redefining the basic concepts of virulence and pathogenicity. *Infect. Immun.* 1999, *67*, 3703–3713. [CrossRef] [PubMed]
56. Casadevall, A.; Pirofski, L.A. Microbiology: Ditch the term pathogen. *Nature* 2014, *516*, 165–166. [CrossRef]
57. Shenker, B.J.; Walker, L.P.; Zekavat, A.; Korostoff, J.; Boesze-Battaglia, K. *Aggregatibacter actinomycetemcomitans* Cytolethal Distending Toxin-Induces Cell Cycle Arrest in a Glycogen Synthase Kinase (GSK)-3-Dependent Manner in Oral Keratinocytes. *Int. J. Mol. Sci.* 2022, *23*, 11831. [CrossRef]
58. Lally, E.T.; Golub, E.E.; Kieba, I.R.; Taichman, N.S.; Rosenblum, J.; Rosenblum, J.C.; Gibson, C.W.; Demuth, D.R. Analysis of the *Actinobacillus actinomycetemcomitans* leukotoxin gene. *J. Biol. Chem.* 1989, *264*, 15451–15456. [CrossRef]
59. Kachlany, S.C. *Aggregatibacter actinomycetemcomitans* leukotoxin from threat to therapy. *J. Dent. Res.* 2010, *89*, 561–570. [CrossRef]
60. Hajishengallis, G.; Lamont, R.J. Beyond the red complex and into more complexity: The polymicrobial synergy and dysbiosis (PSD) model of periodontal disease etiology. *Mol. Oral. Microbiol.* 2012, *27*, 409–419. [CrossRef]
61. Hallstrom, T.; Zipfel, P.F.; Blom, A.M.; Lauer, N.; Forsgren, A.; Riesbeck, K. Haemophilus influenzae interacts with the human complement inhibitor factor H. *J. Immunol.* 2008, *181*, 537–545. [CrossRef]

62. Taylor, P.W. Bactericidal and bacteriolytic activity of serum against gram-negative bacteria. *Microbiol. Rev.* **1983**, *47*, 46–83. [CrossRef]
63. Meri, T.; Amdahl, H.; Lehtinen, M.J.; Hyvarinen, S.; McDowell, J.V.; Bhattacharjee, A.; Meri, S.; Marconi, R.; Goldman, A.; Jokiranta, T.S. Microbes bind complement inhibitor factor H via a common site. *PLoS Pathog.* **2013**, *9*, e1003308. [CrossRef]
64. Galindo, C.L.; Rosenzweig, J.A.; Kirtley, M.L.; Chopra, A.K. Pathogenesis of *Y. enterocolitica* and *Y. pseudotuberculosis* in Human Yersiniosis. *J. Pathog.* **2011**, *2011*, 182051. [CrossRef] [PubMed]
65. McNeil, L.K.; Zagursky, R.J.; Lin, S.L.; Murphy, E.; Zlotnick, G.W.; Hoiseth, S.K.; Jansen, K.U.; Anderson, A.S. Role of factor H binding protein in *Neisseria meningitidis* virulence and its potential as a vaccine candidate to broadly protect against meningococcal disease. *Microbiol. Mol. Biol. Rev.* **2013**, *77*, 234–252. [CrossRef] [PubMed]
66. McDowell, J.V.; Lankford, J.; Stamm, L.; Sadlon, T.; Gordon, D.L.; Marconi, R.T. Demonstration of factor H-like protein 1 binding to *Treponema denticola*, a pathogen associated with periodontal disease in humans. *Infect. Immun.* **2005**, *73*, 7126–7132. [CrossRef] [PubMed]
67. Haubek, D.; Ennibi, O.K.; Poulsen, K.; Vaeth, M.; Poulsen, S.; Kilian, M. Risk of aggressive periodontitis in adolescent carriers of the JP2 clone of *Aggregatibacter* (*Actinobacillus*) *actinomycetemcomitans* in Morocco: A prospective longitudinal cohort study. *Lancet* **2008**, *371*, 237–242. [CrossRef] [PubMed]
68. Haubek, D.; Poulsen, K.; Kilian, M. Microevolution and patterns of dissemination of the JP2 clone of *Aggregatibacter* (*Actinobacillus*) *actinomycetemcomitans*. *Infect. Immun.* **2007**, *75*, 3080–3088. [CrossRef]
69. Schindler, M.K.; Schutz, M.S.; Muhlenkamp, M.C.; Rooijakkers, S.H.; Hallstrom, T.; Zipfel, P.F.; Autenrieth, I.B. Yersinia enterocolitica YadA mediates complement evasion by recruitment and inactivation of C3 products. *J. Immunol.* **2012**, *189*, 4900–4908. [CrossRef]

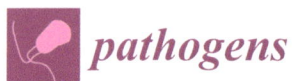

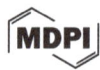

Review

Aggregatibacter actinomycetemcomitans Dispersin B: The Quintessential Antibiofilm Enzyme

Jeffrey B. Kaplan [1,*], Svetlana A. Sukhishvili [2], Miloslav Sailer [3], Khalaf Kridin [1,4] and Narayanan Ramasubbu [5]

[1] Laboratory for Skin Research, Institute for Medical Research, Galilee Medical Center, Nahariya 2210001, Israel; dr_kridin@hotmail.com
[2] Department of Materials Science and Engineering, Texas A&M University, College Station, TX 77843, USA; svetlana@tamu.edu
[3] Kane Biotech Inc., Winnipeg, MB R3T 6G2, Canada; msailer@kanebiotech.com
[4] The Azrieli Faculty of Medicine, Bar-Ilan University, Safed 1311502, Israel
[5] Department of Oral Biology, Rutgers School of Dental Medicine, Newark, NJ 07103, USA; ramasun1@sdm.rutgers.edu
* Correspondence: kaplanjb@american.edu

Abstract: The extracellular matrix of most bacterial biofilms contains polysaccharides, proteins, and nucleic acids. These biopolymers have been shown to mediate fundamental biofilm-related phenotypes including surface attachment, intercellular adhesion, and biocide resistance. Enzymes that degrade polymeric biofilm matrix components, including glycoside hydrolases, proteases, and nucleases, are useful tools for studying the structure and function of biofilm matrix components and are also being investigated as potential antibiofilm agents for clinical use. Dispersin B is a well-studied, broad-spectrum antibiofilm glycoside hydrolase produced by *Aggregatibacter actinomycetemcomitans*. Dispersin B degrades poly-*N*-acetylglucosamine, a biofilm matrix polysaccharide that mediates biofilm formation, stress tolerance, and biocide resistance in numerous Gram-negative and Gram-positive pathogens. Dispersin B has been shown to inhibit biofilm and pellicle formation; detach preformed biofilms; disaggregate bacterial flocs; sensitize preformed biofilms to detachment by enzymes, detergents, and metal chelators; and sensitize preformed biofilms to killing by antiseptics, antibiotics, bacteriophages, macrophages, and predatory bacteria. This review summarizes the results of nearly 100 in vitro and in vivo studies that have been carried out on dispersin B since its discovery 20 years ago. These include investigations into the biological function of the enzyme, its structure and mechanism of action, and its in vitro and in vivo antibiofilm activities against numerous bacterial species. Also discussed are potential clinical applications of dispersin B.

Keywords: biofilm matrix; biomaterial coating; DspB; EPS; exopolysaccharide; extracellular DNA; eDNA; matrix-degrading enzyme; PIA; PNAG; *Staphylococcus aureus*; *Staphylococcus epidermidis*

Citation: Kaplan, J.B.; Sukhishvili, S.A.; Sailer, M.; Kridin, K.; Ramasubbu, N. *Aggregatibacter actinomycetemcomitans* Dispersin B: The Quintessential Antibiofilm Enzyme. *Pathogens* **2024**, *13*, 668. https://doi.org/10.3390/pathogens13080668

Academic Editor: Vivi Miriagou

Received: 19 July 2024
Revised: 30 July 2024
Accepted: 6 August 2024
Published: 7 August 2024

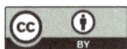

1. Introduction

Biofilms are densely packed communities of microorganisms, enclosed in a self-synthesized extracellular polymeric matrix, growing attached to a tissue or surface [1]. Biofilm is the primary mode of growth for microbes in most natural, industrial, and clinical environments. Biofilms exhibit a high tolerance to exogenous stress, and treatment of biofilms with biocides is usually ineffective at eradicating them [2]. Biofilms create many problems, ranging from industrial corrosion and biofouling to chronic and nosocomial infections.

Various antibiofilm strategies are currently being investigated. These include biomaterial surface modifications, quorum-sensing inhibitors, quorum-quenching enzymes, bacteriophages and phage-derived enzymes, and biofilm-matrix-degrading enzymes [3]. The biofilm matrix is a good target for antibiofilm agents because, unlike cells buried deep within the biofilm colony, the biofilm matrix is highly accessible to the outside environment and is inherently porous [4]. Agents that degrade or destabilize the biofilm matrix can inhibit biofilm formation or promote the detachment of established biofilm colonies [3]. Once the biofilm colony is dispersed, the cells exhibit increased sensitivity to killing by biocides and host defenses [2].

Numerous biofilm-matrix-degrading enzymes have been described [5–7]. These include various glycoside hydrolases, proteases, and nucleases, which degrade the polysaccharide, protein, and nucleic acid components of the biofilm matrix, respectively. These biopolymers have been shown to mediate fundamental biofilm-related phenotypes including surface attachment, intercellular adhesion, and biocide resistance [4]. The advantages of biofilm-matrix-degrading enzymes are that they exhibit broad-spectrum activity and they exert little or no selection pressure because they generally do not kill bacteria or inhibit their growth. The disadvantage of these enzymes is that they release microbial cells from the biofilm that can spread and cause infections at distant sites or elicit a hyper-inflammatory or hyper-immunogenic response [6]. Therefore, biofilm-matrix-degrading enzymes may be more useful for biofilm prevention rather than for the treatment of established biofilms, or they may need to be used in combination with antimicrobial agents to minimize these risks.

The glycoside hydrolase dispersin B is one of the best-studied biofilm-matrix-degrading enzymes. Dispersin B hydrolyzes poly-β(1,6)-*N*-acetylglucosamine (PNAG), a biofilm matrix polysaccharide that plays a role in surface attachment, biofilm formation, and biocide resistance in a wide range of Gram-negative and Gram-positive pathogens [8]. This review describes the initial discovery and characterization of dispersin B from *Aggregatibacter actinomycetemcomitans*, as well as subsequent studies on its structure and mechanism of action. Also highlighted are numerous studies demonstrating that dispersin B exhibits broad-spectrum antibiofilm activity against more than 25 phylogenetically diverse bacterial species in vitro and in vivo. Some potential clinical applications of dispersin B, such as medical device coatings, topical wound gels, and combination products, will also be discussed.

Discovery of dispersin B: The Gram-negative, non-motile periodontopathogen *A. actinomycetemcomitans* forms extremely tenacious biofilms on abiotic surfaces such as plastic and glass in vitro [9]. Its adherence is so strong that the broth shows no turbidity, removal of cells from the culture vessel surface by vortex agitation is negligible, and aliquots of medium taken from the culture are often sterile upon subculture. This remarkable phenotype makes *A. actinomycetemcomitans* a useful model for studying the process of biofilm dispersal, because cells that detach from mature biofilm colonies adhere tightly to the surface of the culture vessel and form independent daughter biofilm colonies that can be visualized and enumerated (Figure 1, left panel). Screening a transposon mutant library of *A. actinomycetemcomitans* strain CU1000 identified five mutant strains that were defective in biofilm dispersal (Figure 1, right panel). The transposons in three mutant strains inserted into genes required for lipopolysaccharide O-side-chain biosynthesis [10]; the transposon in one mutant strain inserted into *ptsI*, which encodes a regulator of sugar uptake and catabolite repression (J.B. Kaplan, unpublished results); and the transposon in one mutant strain (designated JK1023) inserted into a novel gene encoding a putative β-hexosaminidase enzyme [11]. The gene disrupted in the mutant strain JK1023 was named *dspB*, and the protein that it encodes was named dispersin B. A plasmid carrying a wild-type *dspB* gene restored the ability of JK1023 biofilm colonies to disperse [11].

Wild-type strain CU1000   ΔdspB mutant strain JK1023

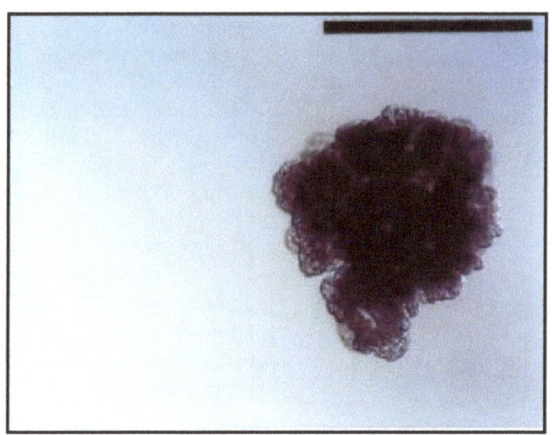

Figure 1. Dispersal of isolated *Aggregatibacter actinomycetemcomitans* biofilm colonies growing on the surface of polystyrene Petri dishes: (**left panel**) wild-type strain CU1000; (**right panel**) Δ*dspB* mutant strain JK1023. Satellite colonies surrounding the dispersed CU1000 biofilm colony were absent in the JK1023 culture. Photos were taken 3 d after inoculation. Scale bar = 1 mm. Image from [12].

Biological functions of dispersin B: Although the *A. actinomycetemcomitans dspB* mutant strain JK1023 exhibited a severe biofilm dispersal defect in broth, it exhibited wild-type surface attachment and biofilm formation phenotypes (Figure 1). Strain JK1023 also produced colonies on agar that had a hard texture and were extremely difficult to remove from the agar surface. In test tubes, JK1023 cells aggregated and settled to the bottom of the tube much more rapidly than cells of the wild-type strain CU1000 [11]. These phenotypes demonstrate that dispersin B decreases the intercellular adhesion of *A. actinomycetemcomitans* in vitro. Stacy et al. [13] constructed a Δ*dspB* mutation in a different *A. actinomycetemcomitans* parental strain (strain 624). They confirmed that dispersin B promotes biofilm dispersal in vitro and further demonstrated that dispersin-B-mediated biofilm dispersal is triggered by oxygen and H_2O_2. In a murine abscess model, the *A. actinomycetemcomitans* 624 Δ*dspB* mutant strain established similar single-species infections compared to the wild-type strain, but upon co-infection with *Streptococcus gordonii* the 624 Δ*dspB* mutant strain formed larger cell aggregates than those formed by the wild-type strain, and these aggregates were located closer to *S. gordonii* aggregates than those of the wild-type strain. These findings suggest that dispersin B can modulate the spatial organization of cells within multi-species biofilms in vivo.

Zhang et al. [14] constructed a Δ*dspB* mutation in *Actinobacillus pleuropneumoniae* strain 4074, a swine pathogen that produces an orthologue of *A. actinomycetemcomitans* dispersin B [15]. The *A. pleuropneumoniae* Δ*dspB* mutant strain exhibited increased autoaggregation and biofilm formation in vitro, phenotypes that were not evident when a wild-type *dspB* gene was supplied on a plasmid. These findings confirm that dispersin B modulates bacterial intercellular adhesion and biofilm formation in different species in vitro.

The *dspB* gene: The *A. actinomycetemcomitans dspB* gene encodes a protein of 381 amino acids that includes a 20-amino-acid N-terminal signal sequence that is cleaved upon secretion outside the cell. The genomes of at least 32 different bacterial species contain genes that exhibit >50% identity to *A. actinomycetemcomitans dspB* at the amino acid level (Table 1 and Figure 2) These include 16 species of *Pasteurellaceae*, 15 species of *Neisseriaceae*, and *Cardiobacterium hominis* (family *Cardiobacteriaceae*). *Pasteurellaceae* and *Neisseriaceae* have been found on the mucosal surfaces of the upper respiratory tracts of vertebrates and are often opportunistic pathogens [16]. *C. hominis* is a normal human oral and upper respiratory commensal that is rarely a cause of endocarditis [17]. The phylogeny of *dspB* homologues was congruent with the phylogenetic tree at the species level (Figure 2), suggesting that *dspB* emerged in an ancestor of these three bacterial families. All of the amino acid residues that play a critical role in *A. actinomycetemcomitans* dispersin B substrate hydrolysis (Arg27, Asp183, Glu184, Glu332; see below), as well as the three tryptophan residues at positions 216, 237, and 330 that line part of the substrate-binding pocket, were conserved in 31 of the 32 *dspB* homologues analyzed. Only the *Kingella oralis* homologue has substitutions at these critical positions (Arg27His, Glu184Ala, Trp237His, Trp330Glu, Glu332Asp). This suggests that most *dspB* homologues have the potential to encode functional dispersin B enzymes. Differences in the lengths of the predicted proteins result from N- or C-terminal extensions in the sequences of some species. Only small insertions/deletions of 1-4 amino acids are present within the core region of the protein.

Table 1. Orthologues of *A. actinomycetemcomitans dspB* in bacteria. Sequences were identified with a protein BLAST search using *A. actinomycetemcomitans* dispersin B (GenBank accession number WP_005566076) as a query sequence.

Species	Family	GenBank Accession No.	Amino Acids
Actinobacillus capsulatus	*Pasteurellaceae*	WP_018652103.1	378
Actinobacillus equuli	*Pasteurellaceae*	WP_039197353.1	378
Actinobacillus lignieresii	*Pasteurellaceae*	WP_126375001.1	377
Actinobacillus pleuropneumoniae	*Pasteurellaceae*	WP_005617581.1	377
Actinobacillus succinogenes	*Pasteurellaceae*	WP_012072607	508
Actinobacillus suis	*Pasteurellaceae*	WP_014991875.1	378
Actinobacillus ureae	*Pasteurellaceae*	WP_115607612.1	378
Actinobacillus vicugnae	*Pasteurellaceae*	WP_150540037.1	378
Aggregatibacter actinomycetemcomitans	*Pasteurellaceae*	WP_005566076	361
Aggregatibacter aphrophilus	*Pasteurellaceae*	OBY54997.1	403
Aggregatibacter kilianii	*Pasteurellaceae*	WP_275425143.1	339
Basfia succiniciproducens	*Pasteurellaceae*	WP_305367133	480
Cardiobacterium hominis	*Cardiobacteriaceae*	WP_281839854.1	528
Exercitatus varius	*Pasteurellaceae*	WP_317543108.1	508
Haemophilus pittmaniae	*Pasteurellaceae*	WP_269457014	381
Kingella oralis	*Neisseriaceae*	WP_315367803.1	405
Lonepinella koalarum	*Pasteurellaceae*	WP_228777406.1	363
Mannheimia succiniciproducens	*Pasteurellaceae*	AAU37718.1	501
Neisseria animaloris	*Neisseriaceae*	WP_199901419.1	517
Neisseria brasiliensis	*Neisseriaceae*	MRN37458.1	340
Neisseria canis	*Neisseriaceae*	WP_085415444.1	508
Neisseria chenwenguii	*Neisseriaceae*	WP_199720929.1	421
Neisseria dentiae	*Neisseriaceae*	WP_211276428.1	400
Neisseria dumasiana	*Neisseriaceae*	WP_085417823.1	395
Neisseria montereyensis	*Neisseriaceae*	WP_289623084.1	398
Neisseria musculi	*Neisseriaceae*	WP_187000616.1	388
Neisseria oralis	*Neisseriaceae*	WP_308022698.1	410

Table 1. *Cont.*

Species	Family	GenBank Accession No.	Amino Acids
Neisseria shayeganii	*Neisseriaceae*	WP_220457298.1	770
Neisseria wadsworthii	*Neisseriaceae*	WP_009115775.1	468
Neisseria weixii	*Neisseriaceae*	WP_096294699.1	392
Neisseria zalophi	*Neisseriaceae*	WP_318527728.1	398
Neisseria zoodegmatis	*Neisseriaceae*	WP_085364538.1	395

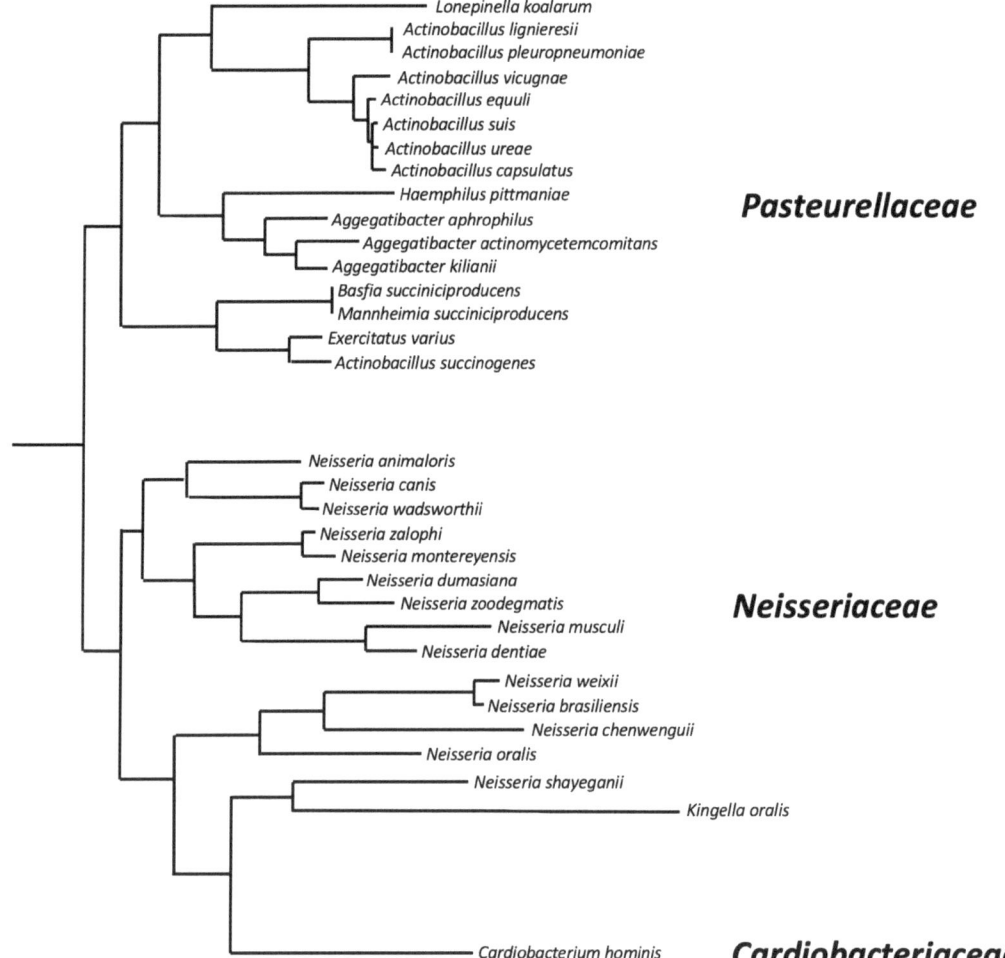

Figure 2. Phylogenetic relatedness of dispersin B homologues based on pairwise alignments of the amino acid sequences listed in Table 1. The alignment was generated using ClustalW, and the phylogenetic tree was generated using FastTree software. Lacto-*N*-biosidase from *Lactococcus lactis* (GenBank accession number AGY45663.1) was used as an outgroup to locate the root of the tree. Horizontal branch lengths are proportional to the number of amino acid differences in the pairwise alignments. Bacterial families are indicated on the right.

Several studies have investigated the transcriptional regulation of *A. actinomycetemcomitans dspB*, which is flanked by an upstream promoter sequence and a downstream rho-independent transcription terminator sequence and does not appear to be part of an operon. Stacy et al. [18] analyzed the transcriptome of *A. actinomycetemcomitans* strain VT1169 during oxic and anoxic growth using DNA microarrays. They found that *dspB* transcription was induced by oxygen. They also cloned the *dspB* promoter upstream of a *lacZ* reporter gene and then introduced the *dspB-lacZ* reporter gene into *A. actinomycetemcomitans* strains 624 and VT1169. When grown as colony biofilms, both reporter strains exhibited significant β-galactosidase activity under oxic conditions but little activity under anoxic conditions. Interestingly, *dspB* induction in both strains could be mitigated by exogenously added catalase or a mutation in *oxyR* which encodes a transcriptional regulator. These findings indicate that *dspB* transcription is activated during growth with oxygen in an OxyR-dependent manner, and that the activating factor is likely H_2O_2. Using these same two *dspB-lacZ* reporter strains, Stacy et al. [18] showed that transcription of *dspB* was increased >5-fold upon iron restriction. This induction was abolished when $FeSO_4$ was added to the medium. Furthermore, *dspB* transcription was increased >30-fold in a Δ*fur* mutant under the same conditions, confirming that the *dspB* promoter is regulated by iron and Fur. Other studies [19,20] showed that postbiotic compounds produced by lactic acid bacteria can modulate *dspB* expression and biofilm formation in *A. actinomycetemcomitans*, although more studies are needed to determine the mechanism of action and clinical utility of such compounds.

2. Production of Recombinant Dispersin B

Production of recombinant dispersin B in *Escherichia coli*: Kaplan et al. [11] constructed a plasmid (pRC1) that carries a gene encoding amino acids 21-381 of *A. actinomycetemcomitans* CU1000 dispersin B, fused to a 32-amino-acid C-terminal tail containing a hexahistidine metal-binding site and a thrombin protease cleavage site that can be used to cleave the C-terminal tail from the hybrid protein. This gene was located downstream from an IPTG-inducible *tac* promoter. *E. coli* strain BL21(DE3) was transformed with pRC1, induced with IPTG, and the protein was purified using Ni^{2+}-affinity chromatography. After cleavage with thrombin, the purified protein migrated with the expected molecular mass of 41.5 kDa. The yield of purified dispersin B was 10 mg/L of culture. Ramasubbu et al. [21] constructed a similar plasmid (pRC3) that encodes amino acids 21-381 of CU1000 *dspB*, fused directly to a hexahistidine metal-binding C-terminal tail to facilitate crystallization. When expressed from an IPTG-inducible *tac* promoter on a plasmid and purified by Ni^{2+}-affinity chromatography, this construct yielded up to 60 mg/L of dispersin B. Yakamdawala et al. [22] engineered a *dspB* gene devoid of the trinucleotide ACA. This was accomplished by silently and consecutively mutating each of the 14 occurrences of ACA in the wild-type *dspB* gene using PCR. Previous studies showed that mRNA transcripts lacking ACA sequences are protected from degradation by MazF, a sequence-specific endoribonuclease produced by *E. coli*. Expression of ACA-less *dspB* in *E. coli* strain Tuner(DE3)pLacI generated 236 mg/L of dispersin B versus 133 mg/L for wild-type *dspB* when expressed from a T7 promoter. Gökçen et al. [23] reported a dispersin B yield of about 60 mg/L when a codon-optimized *dspB* gene was cloned downstream from a tetracycline promoter/operator, transformed into *E. coli*, induced with anhydrotetracycline, and purified by Ni^{2+}-affinity chromatography. In addition, Zeng et al. [24] reported that hexahistidine-tagged dispersin B purified on Ni^{2+} ion-chelated magnetic nanoparticles exhibited higher purity and activity than protein purified on conventional Ni^{2+}-affinity columns.

Production of recombinant dispersin B in tobacco: Tobacco expression systems offer several advantages over *E. coli*, including lower costs, higher yields, and simplified downstream processing. Opdensteinen [25] expressed a codon-optimized, hexahistidine-tagged *A. actinomycetemcomitans dspB* gene in *Nicotiana tabacum* BY2 cells and *N. benthamiana* plants. *N. benthamiana* is a close relative of *N. tabacum* that is commonly used for "pharming" of recombinant proteins for clinical use. The recovery of dispersin B in planta was 75%, its purity was 96%, and a yield of up to 164 mg/kg of plant tissue was reported. These values were equivalent to those achieved in *E. coli*, suggesting that scalable purification of dispersin B in tobacco is feasible.

3. Dispersin B's Structure and Mechanism of Action

A. actinomycetemcomitans dispersin B was crystalized using the hanging-drop vapor diffusion technique, and its 3D structure in complex with a glycerol molecule and an acetate ion at the active site was solved and refined to a resolution of 2.0 Å using the automated structure solution pipeline autoSHARP [21]. Dispersin B is a monomeric enzyme whose primary amino acid structure corresponds to that of the glycoside hydrolase family 20 group of enzymes (CAZY GH_20). This family comprises diverse β-hexosaminidases produced by both prokaryotes and eukaryotes, as well as lacto-*N*-biosidase (EC 3.2.1.14), an enzyme involved in the degradation of human milk oligosaccharides in the gut microbiota of breast-fed infants.

Like all glycoside hydrolase family 20 enzymes, dispersin B adopts a TIM barrel protein fold consisting of eight α-helices and eight parallel β-strands that alternate along the polypeptide backbone (Figure 3). The active site of the enzyme is a large central cavity at the center of the TIM barrel that exhibits a negative electrostatic potential due to the presence of a number of polar acidic residues that are also conserved in other β-hexosaminidases (Figure 4A). Trp216 and Trp330 form the floor of the 12 Å deep substrate-binding pocket where the hexose ring binds. Asp183 and Glu184 are the catalytic residues that are conserved in all glycoside hydrolase family 20 enzymes [26–28].

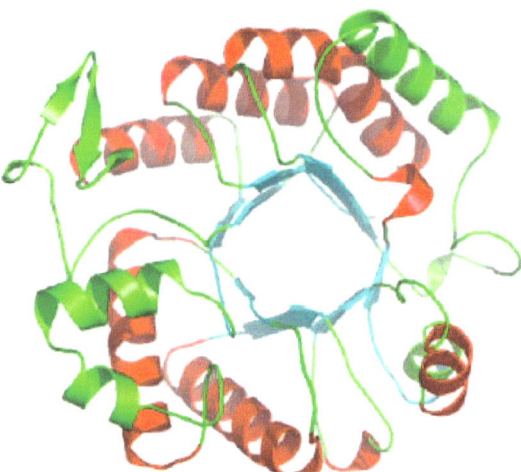

Figure 3. Ribbon diagram of *A. actinomycetemcomitans* dispersin B; α-helices are colored red and green; β-strands are colored blue. Image source: Wikimedia Commons.

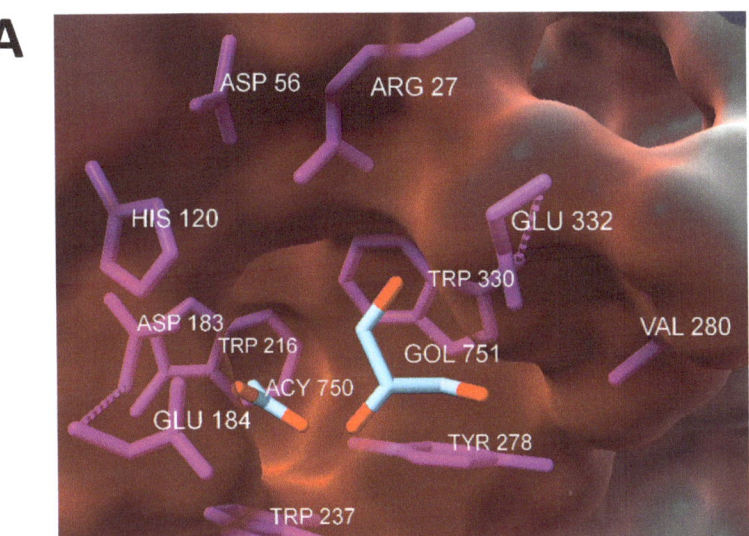

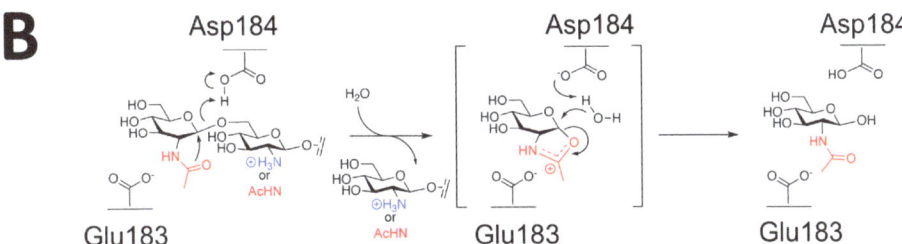

Figure 4. Dispersin B's active site and mechanism of action: (**A**) Electrostatic surface potential at the active site showing the negatively charged amino acids (Asp56, Asp183, Glu184, Glu332), which create a shallow anionic region in the catalytic pocket. The size of the pocket is approximately 12 Å. GOL, glycerol; ACY, acetate. Figure generated using ChimeraX [29]. (**B**) Substrate hydrolysis mechanism proposed for dispersin B and other glycoside hydrolase family 20 hexosaminidases. In this substrate-assisted mechanism, Glu184 acts as the acid/base. The nucleophile is the *N*-acetyl group of the substrate, which is assisted by Asp183. Both exo- (dPNAG) and endoglycosidic (PNAG) cleavage are shown, where the leaving group is either deacetylated or acetylated, respectively. A suitably positioned Asp183 helps stabilize the oxazolium ion in the transition state. Figure generated using ChemDraw (PerkinElmer).

Evidence suggests that dispersin B utilizes a substrate-assisted mechanism, commonly referred to as the double-displacement retaining mechanism, similar to other β-hexosaminidases (Figure 4B). A unique feature of this mechanism is the participation of the acetamido group of the substrate, which provides anchimeric assistance and acts as the nucleophile while a suitably juxtaposed amino acid residue acts the acid/base. This mechanism was confirmed using biochemical analyses of native dispersin B enzymes with different substrates, as well as mutational analyses [27,30–34]. In this mechanism, the active site residue Asp183 binds to the *N*-acetyl group of PNAG, and Glu184 serves as the catalytic acid/base (Figure 4B). Asp183 may also help stabilize the positive charge that develops in the oxazoline transition state (Figure 4B) or help distort the substrate to direct the 2-acetamido group toward the anomeric carbon [28]. Proteins with Asp183Asn and Glu184Gln mutations exhibited >10,000-fold and >70-fold decreased activity, respectively, compared to the wild-type enzyme, irrespective of the substrate used for hydrolysis. A mutation in another acidic residue located near the catalytic residues (Glu332) exhibited 2000-fold lower activity than the native enzyme. Glu332 may provide stabilization in the transition state while the terminal glucosamine is undergoing conformational changes [27]. Mutations in Asp147 and Asp245, which are also located in the anionic pocket near the active site, also exhibited decreased enzyme activity. These residues may play a role in recognition of the cationic PNAG substrate. Four aromatic amino acid residues (Tyr187, Tyr278, Trp237, Trp330) line the hydrophobic substrate-binding pocket, where they bind to and orient the PNAG substrate. As expected, mutations in these residues exhibited 5–2400-fold less activity that the wild-type enzyme. In addition to these acidic and aromatic amino acid residues, all β-hexosaminidases have a conserved arginine that is involved in substrate binding at the active site, equivalent to Arg27 of *A. actinomycetem-comitans* dispersin B. Enzymes with Arg27Lys and Arg27Ala mutations exhibited 2400-fold and >1700-fold reductions in activity, respectively. Overall, these mutational studies confirm that dispersin B utilizes the same substrate-assisted mechanism as that utilized by other glycoside hydrolase family 20 enzymes.

All PNAG exopolysaccharides have been shown to be post-translationally modified by partial deacetylation (ca. 15–20%), which is critical for PNAG-dependent biofilm formation [8]. Dispersin B exhibits both exo- and endoglycosidase activity against PNAG, depending on the nature of the substrate [27,31,32,35]. Dispersin B exhibits greater activity against fully deacetylated PNAG (dPNAG) than against fully acetylated PNAG. Thus, the mechanism of action of dispersin B evidently depends on different patterns of deacetylation [35,36]. Studies utilizing site-directed mutagenesis and synthetic PNAG oligosaccharides demonstrated that the increased rate of hydrolysis for dPNAG was mediated by interaction of the glucosamine residues of dPNAG with Asp147 and Asp242, which are located in a shallow anionic groove adjacent to the catalytic pocket [36,37]. Dispersin B containing an Asp242Asn mutation was highly deficient in endoglycosidase activity while maintaining exoglycosidase activity. These findings suggest that dispersin B exhibits endoglycosidic cleavage against dPNAG due to the absence of an acetamido group on dPNAG. The exhibition of both exo- and endoglycosidic activity by dispersin B might be critical during biofilm formation and dispersal, since this would catalyze the hydrolysis of both PNAG and dPNAG in an efficient manner.

4. Dispersin B as a Tool for Studying Biofilms

Dispersin B as a probe for PNAG production: PNAG has been identified as a highly conserved surface polysaccharide produced by diverse bacterial, fungal, and protozoal pathogens [38,39]. However, PNAG is difficult to isolate and purify because it is usually produced at low levels and is tightly bound to the cell surface. An alternative method for detecting PNAG is fluorescence confocal microscopy using the antigen-specific human IgG1 monoclonal antibody F598 [38]. Figure 5 shows that the immunoreactivity of *Yersinia pestis* cells with mAb F598 was lost after the cells were treated with dispersin B, but not with chitinase—a related glycoside hydrolase that degrades chitin, a polymer of β(1,4)-linked *N*-acetylglucosamine residues [40]. This same dispersin-B-induced loss of immunoreactivity with mAb F598 was observed in *Bacillus subtilis* [41] and several other prokaryotic and eukaryotic pathogens [38,42,43]. These findings demonstrate that dispersin B can function as a sensitive and specific probe for PNAG.

Dispersin B is often used along with proteinase K and DNase I to investigate the composition of the biofilm matrix. For example, dispersin B, but not proteinase K or DNase I, degraded insoluble extracellular matrix components of *S. aureus* strain SH1000 [44] and strain MR10 [45], confirming that the biofilm matrix of these strains primarily contains PNAG. This is consistent with the susceptibility of these strains to detachment by dispersin B.

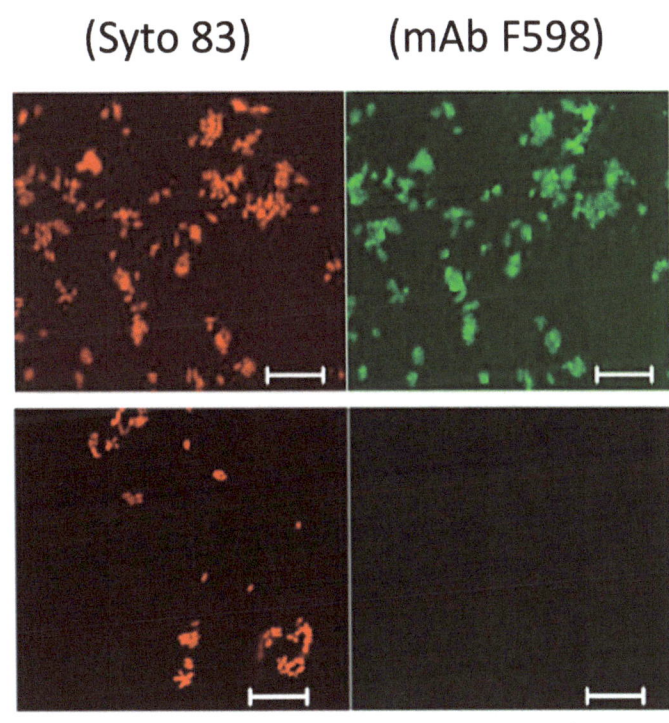

DNA stain
(Syto 83)

PNAG stain
(mAb F598)

Chitinase-
treated cells

Dispersin B-
treated cells

Figure 5. Confocal microscopic analysis of PNAG expression by *Y. pestis* strain KIM6+ grown at 28 °C overnight on Congo red agar. After treatment of bacterial cells with either chitinase (**top panels**) or dispersin B (**bottom panels**), cells were stained with Syto 83 to visualize DNA (red) and Alexa Fluor 488-conjugated mAb F598 to detect PNAG (green). Bars = 10 μm. Figure from Yoong et al. [40].

Eddenden et al. [46] and Eddenden and Nitz [47] leveraged the specificity of dispersin B to construct a probe (Dispersin B PNAG probe or DiPP) for monitoring and localizing PNAG production during biofilm formation. DiPP was created by mutating one amino acid in the dispersin B active site (E184), which rendered the enzyme catalytically inactive but still capable of binding to PNAG, and then fusing inactive dispersin B to green fluorescent protein (GFP-DiPP). Fluorescent imaging studies demonstrated that GFP-DiPP bound to PNAG-dependent cells and biofilms, but not to PNAG-independent cells and biofilms, thereby demonstrating the specificity of the probe for PNAG. DiPP binding experiments with the PNAG-producing *E. coli* strain MG1655 revealed a high concentration of PNAG at the bacterial cell surface, which was localized in discrete areas. These distinct areas appeared to slough from the cells and accumulate in interbacterial regions during the development of a PNAG-dependent biofilm. A helical distribution of staining was also observed, suggesting spatial organization of PNAG on the cell surface prior to biofilm formation These experiments demonstrate the potential value of a highly specific dispersin B probe for monitoring PNAG production.

Dispersin B as a probe for PNAG function: Several studies have used dispersin B to demonstrate that PNAG plays a role in bacterial intercellular adhesion, biofilm formation, biofilm porosity, and host cell binding. Al Laham et al. [48] found that *S. epidermidis* small-colony variants, which are sometimes associated with device infections, produced large cell aggregates when cultured under planktonic conditions. These cell aggregates were completely disintegrated by dispersin B, demonstrating that PNAG serves as an intercellular adhesin, a finding that was subsequently confirmed by indirect immunofluorescence assays with anti-PNAG antiserum. Similarly, Amini et al. [49] demonstrated that exogenously added PNAG enabled non-PNAG-producing strains of *E. coli* to form biofilms, a fact that was confirmed when dispersin B treatment abolished the activity. Ganeshnarayanan et al. [50] measured the transport of water and the cationic surfactant cetylpyridinium chloride (CPC) through *S. epidermidis* and *A. pleuropneumoniae* biofilms cultured in centrifugal filter devices. Significantly more water and CPC passed through the biofilms after treatment with dispersin B compared to the amount that passed through untreated biofilms. Similarly, significantly more water and CPC passed through *S. epidermidis* and *A. pleuropneumoniae* PNAG-mutant biofilms compared to wild-type biofilms. These findings suggest that PNAG impedes fluid convection and the transport of small molecules through biofilms. Similarly, Lin et al. [51] showed that pre-treating PNAG-expressing *S. carnosus* cells with dispersin B significantly decreased their ability to bind to human RPMI 2650 nasal epithelial cells.

Dispersin B as a tool for eDNA extraction: Extracellular DNA (eDNA) is an important matrix component of many bacterial biofilms, but it is sometimes difficult to isolate because it binds to other biofilm matrix components, including PNAG [52]. Wu and Xi [53] showed that when biofilms of *Acinetobacter* sp. grown in 6-well microtiter plates were pre-treated with dispersin B, they yielded more eDNA than untreated biofilms. Similarly, Wu and Xi [54] showed that dispersin B treatment significantly increased the yield of eDNA extracted from *Stenotrophomonas maltophilia* and *Acinetobacter baylyi* AC811 biofilms grown in 6-well plates. Thus, dispersin B may be a useful tool for eDNA extraction and analysis.

5. Modifications to Dispersin B

Chemical modification of dispersin B: Abdelkader et al. [55] covalently modified dispersin B with nine cyclodextrin molecules. Cyclodextrins are cone-shaped molecules that contain a hydrophobic central cavity that can bind to other hydrophobic molecules. The cyclodextrin modifications had no effect on the ability of dispersin B to detach preformed biofilms produced by four strains of *S. epidermidis*. The researchers then covalently linked ciprofloxacin to a hydrophobic adamantyl group and formed a complex between dispersin B/cyclodextrin and ciprofloxacin/adamantane to create an "all-in-one" drug delivery system that could destroy the biofilm matrix and simultaneously release the antibiotic. When tested against 24-hour-old biofilms produced by *S. epidermidis* strain 5 (a PNAG-overproducing strain) in 96-well microtiter plates, the enzyme/antibiotic complex exhibited a more than 2-log increase in biofilm eradication compared to dispersin B/cyclodextrin alone, thereby demonstrating the feasibility of this approach.

Dispersin-B-loaded nanoparticles: Various nanobiotechnology-based approaches for eradicating bacterial biofilms, including functionalized metallic nanoparticles, are being investigated. To this end, Liu et al. [56] created a fusion protein between dispersin B and MagR, a protein involved in responses to magnetism in *Drosophila melanogaster* that can be used as a fusion partner to functionally immobilize proteins on magnetic surfaces. MagR was fused to the C-terminus of dispersin B, expressed in *E. coli*, and purified by Ni^{2+}-affinity chromatography. The dispersin B-MagR fusion protein was immobilized on Fe_3O_4/SiO_2 magnetic nanoparticles and tested for its ability to detach preformed biofilms produced by *Bacillus cereus*, *Staphylococcus aureus*, and one additional staphylococcal strain in 24-well microtiter plates. The authors found that Fe_3O_4/SiO_2 nanoparticles loaded with the dispersin B-MagR fusion protein detached pre-biofilms more efficiently than Fe_3O_4/SiO_2 nanoparticles or the dispersin B-MagR fusion protein alone. In addition, immobilization of dispersin B-MagR on magnetic nanoparticles increased the stability of the enzyme and increased its optimal temperature from 30 °C to 37 °C. Theoretically, this system could be used to deliver dispersin B to specific sites under the function of a magnetic force. Similarly, Chen and Lee [57] fused a 12-amino-acid silver-binding peptide to the N-terminus of dispersin B in order to prepare Ag nanoparticles conjugated with dispersin B. The goal was to create an agent that could both disrupt biofilms and simultaneously kill planktonic cells released from the disrupted biofilms. Although Ag nanoparticles could not be conjugated with the dispersin B/Ag-binding peptide fusion protein because dispersin B precipitated in the presence of Ag ions, the fusion protein itself was found to detach preformed *S. epidermidis* biofilms grown on silicone sheets or glass coverslips twofold more efficiently than native dispersin B.

Dispersin B as a medical device coating: Implanted medical devices and wound dressings coated with dispersin B have the potential to reduce the incidence of device infections and promote wound healing. Strategies for grafting dispersin B onto solid surfaces rely on either non-covalent absorption/adsorption of the enzyme to the surface, or its covalent attachment to the surface. These strategies are designed to achieve a high local concentration of dispersin B in the vicinity of the biomaterial surface.

One example of non-covalent binding of dispersin B to biomaterials was reported by Hagan et al. [58], who adsorbed dispersin B and amikacin onto a commercially available, degradable hydrogel (VetriGel). Although these agents were successfully trapped within the hydrogel, the chemistry of the hydrogel did not support long-term retention of dispersin B, and the trapped molecules underwent rapid elution within the first 24 h. A similar approach was reported by Kaplan et al. [59], who adsorbed dispersin B onto unmodified polyurethane and Teflon catheters and showed that the coated catheters efficiently resisted biofilm formation by *S. epidermidis*. The amount of enzyme retained on the surface was not measured, although catheters that were pre-coated and dried retained their antibiofilm activity after one month of storage at 4 °C.

Additional studies quantified the adsorption of dispersin B on polyurethane disks, including those functionalized with acidic and basic groups [60]. These studies showed that coating polyurethane surfaces with dispersin B resulted in a >1 log unit reduction in *S. aureus* and *S. epidermidis* biofilms compared to the amount of biofilm formed on uncoated polyurethane. In addition, staphylococcal biofilms that were grown on dispersin-B-loaded polyurethane disks and rinsed exhibited increased sensitivity to killing by cefamandole nafate compared to biofilms grown on uncoated polyurethane disks. In a similar study, Darouiche et al. [61] showed that polyurethane central venous catheters coated with dispersin B and triclosan efficiently resisted colonization by *S. aureus*, *S. epidermidis*, *E. coli*, and *C. albicans*.

In other studies, dispersin B was trapped within a porous structure of biodegradable asymmetric membranes that were designed for wound dressing applications [62,63]. The efficiency of dispersin-B-loaded poly(3-hydroxybutyrate-co-4-hydroxybutyrate) membranes against *S. epidermidis* was modest (12% reduction) and occurred only in the case of preformed biofilms [62]. However, an improved membrane micro/nanostructure controlled by a polymeric porogen, as well as treatment of membrane surfaces with NaOH to create a surface charge, enhanced the antibiofilm activity of the membrane. Specifically, *S. epidermidis* biofilm formation was inhibited by 33%, while 26% of the preformed biofilm was destroyed [63]. By further improving the nanoporosity and efficiency of a poly(butylene-succinate-co-adipate)-based asymmetric membrane using a polymeric porogen, Bou Haidar et al. [64] showed that up to 80% of preformed *S. epidermidis* biofilms could be eradicated using this approach.

While a general feature of non-covalently adsorbed proteins is their tendency to desorb upon extensive dilution with a medium, controlling the nature and density of the adsorption sites can achieve strong binding of enzymes at surfaces. The latter scenario was realized by employing the layer-by-layer technique to construct surface hydrogels with a high density of basic groups, followed by trapping of dispersin B within the coatings [65]. Although dispersin B was retained within the coating only by electrostatic interactions, the coatings did not elute dispersin B in solution, were highly stable over a wide range of pH values, and maintained their antibiofilm function after a several-day-long pre-incubation in buffer solutions. These dispersin-B-loaded coatings inhibited biofilm formation by a clinical strain of *S. epidermidis* (Figure 6A). Importantly, this approach enables facile control of the amount of immobilized dispersin B by modulating the number of polymer layers in the surface hydrogels.

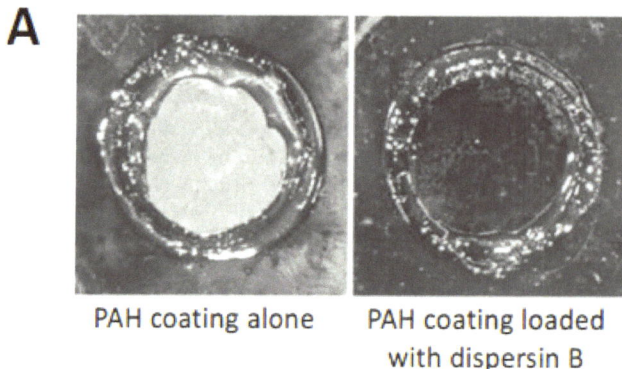

PAH coating alone | PAH coating loaded with dispersin B

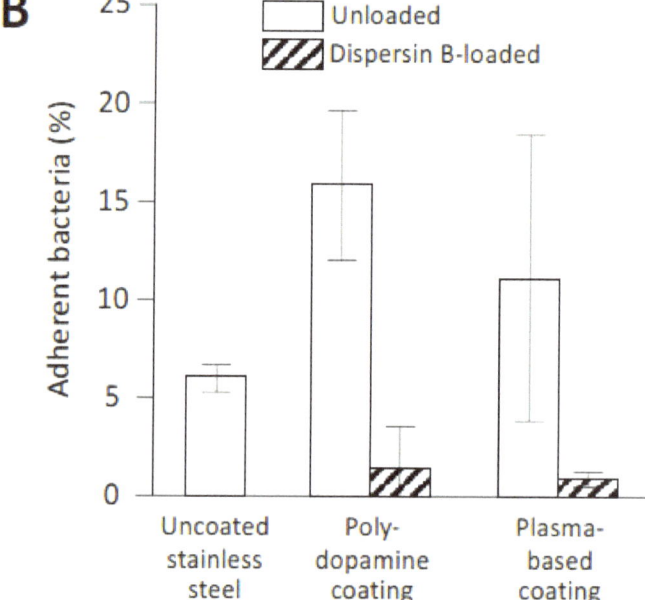

Figure 6. Abiotic surfaces coated with dispersin B resist *S. epidermidis* biofilm formation and surface attachment: (**A**) Biofilm formation by *S. epidermidis* strain NJ9709 on glass slides containing an ultrathin layered poly(allylamine hydrochloride) (PAH) hydrogel coating (**left panel**) or a PAH coating loaded with dispersin B (**right panel**). Bacteria were cultured inside plastic cloning cylinders (5 mm internal diameter) that were attached to the slide with high-vacuum grease. After 12 h, the biofilms were rinsed, the cloning cylinders were removed, and the slides were photographed. The rings correspond to the footprints of the cloning cylinders. The biofilm appeared as a white film on the unloaded PAH layer, which was absent on the dispersin-B-loaded PAH layer. (**B**) Attachment of *S. epidermidis* strain ATCC35984 to uncoated stainless steel disks, or to disks coated with polydopamine- or plasma-based coatings with or without grafted dispersin B. Source: (**A**) [65]; (**B**) redrawn from [66].

An alternative strategy for localized protection against biofilm growth is surface functionalization via covalent attachment of enzymes. For applications in regenerative medicine, biodegradable polyhydroxyalkanoate (PHA)-based fiber meshes were functionalized with dispersin B along with a synthetic antibacterial peptide by covalent conjugation, which was achieved by using reactive star-shaped macromolecules as an additive to a PHA solution [67]. Efficient prevention of bacterial adhesion (88%) and complete inhibition of *S. epidermidis* biofilm formation confirmed the successful presentation of the antibiofilm and antimicrobial agents at the fiber surface.

Covalent modification of solid surfaces, such as stainless steel mimicking the surfaces of biomedical implants, enables a convenient and rapid method for creating reactive surface groups using atmospheric plasma technology for the rapid modification of surfaces with protein-binding interlayers [66,68]. In one example, epoxy-rich films were created by introducing glycidyl methacrylate in the plasma, followed by covalent immobilization of dispersin B and a sulfomethoxazole-degrading enzyme (laccase). These coatings resulted in a 79–84% reduction in adherent *S. epidermidis* bacteria [68]. The atmospheric plasma technique was also used to deposit acrylic-based interlayers containing chemically reactive catechol/quinone groups on metallic surfaces for subsequent immobilization of dispersin B [66]. This biomimetic approach with both solution-adsorbed polydopamine (PDA) and plasma-based interlayers showed high antibiofilm activity against *S. epidermidis* (Figure 6B).

Faure et al. [69] used the redox and adhesive properties of 3,4-dihydroxy-L-phenylalanine (DOPA) to apply surface modifications on stainless steel surfaces for enzyme immobilization. While a cationic polyelectrolyte-bearing catechol unit that mimics the composition of adhesive proteins present in mussel feet was used to coat the surface, the capability of poly(methacrylamide)-bearing quinone groups for crosslinking with amine groups was used to prepare nanogels that could be easily deposited to stainless steel from aqueous solutions. Dispersin B containing thiol groups was then covalently anchored on the nanogels, resulting in coatings that provided long-term activity against *S. epidermidis* [69].

A different, potentially substrate-agnostic approach was recently developed that involves covalent conjugation of dispersin B to spider silk protein using the transpeptidase sortase A [70,71]. This approach is based on the ability of the silk protein to self-assemble via non-covalent interactions within a coating. The ability to use pre-assembly or post-assembly enzyme conjugation routes provides flexibility in optimizing the surface presentation of enzymes, because of the ease and efficiency of the conjugation procedure [70].

Despite the specific advantages and disadvantages of the above approaches, they all have the potential to create bioactive materials that allow local treatment of complex infections without the need for invasive procedures, and all deserve further development.

Dispersin-B-expressing bacteria as therapeutic agents: Several studies have investigated the use of genetically engineered bacterial strains expressing dispersin B as live therapeutics against biofilm-related infections. Garrido et al. [72] constructed an attenuated strain of *Mycoplasma pneumoniae* that secretes both dispersin B and lysostaphin, an endopeptidase that cleaves the pentaglycine crossbridge of the staphylococcal cell wall. This engineered strain significantly reduced *S. aureus* biofilm formation in polystyrene microtiter plates and on polyurethane catheters in vitro. In a murine *S. aureus* catheter infection model in vivo, mice treated with *M. pneumoniae* expressing both dispersin B and lysostaphin exhibited impaired biofilm formation compared to mice treated with *M. pneumoniae* expressing dispersin B alone. In addition, the engineered *M. pneumoniae* cells were significantly more efficient at inhibiting *S. aureus* biofilm formation than the purified dispersin B enzyme alone or supernatants from the engineered strain, suggesting that such strains have the potential to provide a continuous supply of dispersin B at infection sites. Since *M. pneumoniae* is a respiratory pathogen, these engineered strains may be useful for the treatment of biofilm-associated respiratory infections.

Ghalsasi and Sourjik [73] fused the secretion tag from *E. coli* OmpA to the N-terminus of dispersin B and transformed the hybrid gene into *E. coli* strain W3110, thereby creating a "disrupter" strain that secretes dispersin B into the surrounding medium. When tested against preformed biofilms produced by *E. coli* strain TRMG1655 in 96-well microtiter plates, the disrupter strain was found to detach 50% of the target biofilm in 12 h when induced with 100 mM IPTG. Similarly, Ragunath et al. [74] displayed dispersin B on the surface of *E. coli* by fusing dispersin B to a 290-amino-acid C-terminal region of *A. actinomycetemcomitans* Aae, an autotransporter protein involved in host cell binding. The C-terminal region of Aae inserts into the outer membrane and anchors the fusion partner in the membrane. *E. coli* cells that displayed dispersin B on their surface efficiently detached preformed *S. epidermidis* and *A. pleuropneumoniae* biofilms in a 96-well microtiter plate assay, further demonstrating the potential utility of this approach for biofilm control.

Enzymatic bacteriophages: Bacteriophages are being investigated as an alternative to antibiotics for the treatment of bacterial infections, including those caused by biofilms. Lu and Collins [75] engineered the lytic *E. coli*-specific phage T7 to express dispersin B intracellularly during infection so that dispersin B would be released into the extracellular environment upon cell lysis. When tested against preformed biofilms formed by *E. coli* strain TG1 on 96-peg lids, the engineered enzymatic phage reduced bacterial biofilm cell counts by ≈4.5 log units (≈99.997% removal), which was 2 log units greater than the reduction achieved with non-enzymatic phages. Schmerer et al. [76] confirmed that dispersin-B-expressing T7 phages were superior to non-enzymatic phages for eradicating *E. coli* biofilms grown for 12–16 h in 24-well microtiter plates, but they were only marginally better than non-enzymatic phages against *E. coli* biofilms grown for 7 d in silicone tubing. These studies demonstrate the feasibility of using engineered enzymatic bacteriophages as an antibiofilm strategy.

Enzyme cocktails: Wen et al. [77] tested different combinations of dispersin B, proteinase K, and DNase I against biofilms produced by 10 multidrug-resistant *Corynebacterium striatum* strains in 96-well microtiter plates. They found that the combination of 20 μg/mL dispersin B and 20 μg/mL proteinase K was most effective, dispersing at least 50% of the biofilm in 9/10 strains. Poilvache et al. [78] measured the ability of a tri-enzyme cocktail to detach biofilms produced by *S. aureus*, *S. epidermidis*, and *E. coli* on titanium surfaces. The enzymes were a nonspecific endonuclease from *Serratia marcescens*, an endoglucanase from *Aspergillus niger*, and dispersin B from *A. pleuropneumoniae*. The tri-enzyme combination exhibited greater biofilm-detaching activity than any of the individual enzymes against *S. epidermidis*, but the combination was not more effective than endonuclease alone against *S. aureus* or dispersin B alone against *E. coli*. Exposure of tri-enzyme-treated biofilms to antibiotics resulted in a 2–3 log unit reduction in the total CFUs compared to biofilms treated with antibiotics alone in all three species. In a similar study from the same laboratory, Ruiz-Sorribas et al. [79] measured the ability of the tri-enzyme cocktail to detach three-species biofilms formed by *S. aureus*, *E. coli*, and *Candida albicans* in 96-well microtiter plates and on glass coverslips. They found that the addition of *Bacillus subtilis* lyticase or *B. licheniformis* subtilisin A was necessary to achieve significant detachment of *C. albicans* biofilms. Pre-exposure of three-species biofilms to enzymes potentiated the activity of antimicrobials against the biofilms, including the activity of caspofungin against *C. albicans*. Waryah et al. [80] showed that despite the inferiority of dispersin B to DNase I in dispersing *S. aureus* biofilms in a 96-well microtiter plate assay, both enzymes were equally efficient in enhancing the antibacterial efficiency of tobramycin. However, a combination of these two enzymes was found to be significantly less effective in enhancing the antimicrobial efficacy of tobramycin than the individual enzymes alone. Finally, Chiba et al. [81] investigated the effects of combined RNase A and dispersin B treatment on *S. aureus* biofilm formation when grown in 96-well plates. When administered at low concentrations, neither enzyme alone dispersed the mature biofilms. However, efficient dispersal was achieved by incubation with both enzymes, even at low concentrations. Taken together, these findings suggest that combining dispersin B with other biofilm-matrix-degrading enzymes could increase their efficacy and spectrum of activity.

6. Antibiofilm Activities of Dispersin B against Bacteria

As outlined in Table 2, dispersin B exhibits various antibiofilm activities against more than 25 different species of Gram-negative and Gram-positive bacteria in vitro. These activities include (i) inhibition of biotic and abiotic surface attachment; (ii) inhibition of biofilm formation; (iii) detachment of preformed biofilms; (iv) inhibition of pellicle formation (biofilms at the air–liquid interface); (v) disaggregation of bacterial flocs (floating or suspended biofilms); (vi) sensitization of preformed biofilms to detachment by EDTA, SDS, proteinase K, DNase, and high-velocity water irrigation; (vii) sensitization of biofilms to killing by antibiotics (ampicillin, cefamandole nafate, ciprofloxacin, clindamycin, rifampicin, tetracycline, tobramycin, vancomycin), antiseptics (benzoyl peroxide, cetylpyridinium chloride, SDS, triclosan), antimicrobial peptides (KSL-W, LL-37, polymyxin B), bacteriophages, human macrophages, and predatory *Bdellovibrio* bacteria; and (viii) inhibition of hyphal aggregation and surface adhesion in *Streptomyces* spp. Taken together, these findings confirm that PNAG plays a role in diverse biofilm-related functions, and that dispersin B exhibits broad-spectrum antibiofilm activity.

Table 2. Antibiofilm activities of dispersin B against bacteria in vitro.

Species	Antibiofilm Activity	References
Achromobacter xylosoxidans	Inhibits biofilm formation; detaches preformed biofilms.	[82]
Acinetobacter baumannii	Inhibits "pellicle" formation at the air–liquid interface; inhibits biofilm formation; detaches preformed biofilms; sensitizes preformed biofilms to killing by antimicrobial peptide KSL-W.	[83,84]
Actinobacillus pleuropneumoniae	Inhibits biofilm formation; detaches preformed biofilms; sensitizes preformed biofilms to killing by ampicillin.	[14,15,50,85–90]
Aggregatibacter actinomycetemcomitans	Sensitizes planktonic cells to killing by human macrophages; sensitizes preformed biofilms to detachment by EDTA, SDS, proteinase K, and DNase; sensitizes preformed biofilms to killing by cetylpyridinium chloride and SDS; sensitizes preformed biofilms to killing by predatory *Bdellovibrio bacteriovorus* bacteria.	[91–94]
Bordetella pertussis, *B. parapertussis*	Inhibits biofilm formation; detaches preformed biofilms; sensitizes preformed biofilms to killing by antimicrobial peptides polymyxin B and LL-37.	[82,95–97]
Burkholderia cepacia complex	Inhibits biofilm formation; detaches preformed biofilms; sensitizes biofilms to killing by tobramycin.	[43,98]
Corynebacterium striatum	Detaches preformed biofilms.	[77]
Cutibacterium acnes	Inhibits surface attachment and biofilm formation; sensitizes biofilms to killing by benzoyl peroxide and tetracycline.	[99]
Escherichia coli	Inhibits biofilm formation; detaches preformed biofilms; sensitizes biofilms to killing by triclosan and bacteriophages.	[61,73,75,78,100,101]
Francisella novicida, *F. philomiragia*	Detaches preformed biofilms.	[102]
Klebsiella pneumoniae	Inhibits biofilm formation; sensitizes preformed biofilms to killing by antimicrobial peptide KSL-W.	[83,103]
Pectobacterium atrosepticum, *P. carotovorum*	Inhibits biofilm formation; detaches preformed biofilms.	[104,105]
Pseudomonas fluorescens	Inhibits biofilm formation; detaches preformed biofilms; inhibits attachment of planktonic cells to tomato roots.	[101]; J. B. Kaplan, unpublished data
Ralstonia solanacearum	Inhibits biofilm formation.	J. B. Kaplan, unpublished data
Solobacterium moorei	Inhibits biofilm formation.	[106]
Staphylococcus aureus	Inhibits biofilm formation; detaches preformed biofilms; sensitizes preformed biofilms to killing by triclosan, tobramycin, vancomycin, rifampicin, clindamycin, cefamandole nafate, and antimicrobial peptide KSL-W.	[60,61,83,103,107–111]
Staphylococcus capitis	Detaches preformed biofilms.	[112]

Table 2. *Cont.*

Species	Antibiofilm Activity	References
Staphylococcus epidermidis	Inhibits biofilm formation; detaches preformed biofilms; sensitizes preformed biofilms to killing by triclosan, cetylpyridinium chloride, ciprofloxacin, rifampicin, and antimicrobial peptide KSL-W.	[50,55,59,61,82,83,100, 103,108,109,112–118]
Staphylococcus pseudintermedius	Inhibits biofilm formation; detaches preformed biofilms.	[119]
Streptococcus mutans	Detaches preformed biofilms; sensitizes preformed biofilms to detachment by oral irrigation.	[120]
Streptomyces coelicolor, S. lividans	Inhibits surface attachment and hyphal aggregation.	[121]
Xanthomonas citri	Disaggregates bacterial flocs (floating or suspended biofilms).	J. B. Kaplan, unpublished data
Yersinia pestis	Inhibits biofilm formation.	[101]

Some studies have shown that the ability of dispersin B to inhibit biofilm formation and detach preformed biofilms depends on the shape, size, and composition of the culture vessel. For example, biofilm formation by *Cutibacterium acnes* was inhibited by dispersin B when biofilms were cultured in glass tubes, but not when cultured in 96-well polystyrene microtiter plates [99]. Similarly, dispersin B efficiently detached *A. actinomycetemcomitans* biofilms cultured in polystyrene tubes, but not in polystyrene microtiter plate wells [91]. These results may reflect differences in biofilm architecture or biofilm matrix composition resulting from differences in the culture vessel shape, culture volume, surface-to-volume ratio, or substrate material. In addition, some studies have found that dispersin B treatment appears to increase biofilm formation when the biofilm's biomass is measured using a crystal violet binding assay. For example, Izano et al. [91] found that treatment of preformed *A. actinomycetemcomitans* biofilms cultured in 96-well polystyrene microtiter plates with dispersin B resulted in a significant increase in crystal violet binding compared to mock-treated biofilms. Similarly, Atwood et al. [122] found that biofilms formed by *S. aureus rsbU* and *sigB* mutant strains in microtiter plates bound significantly more crystal violet dye when they were cultured in dispersin-B-supplemented broth compared to the amount of bound dye in unsupplemented broth. One possible explanation for these results is that dispersin B increases the volume and porosity of the biofilm matrix, thereby allowing more crystal violet dye molecules to enter the biofilm.

Numerous studies have reported that dispersin B exhibits no bacteriostatic or bactericidal activity against a wide range of Gram-positive and Gram-negative bacteria. These results are most often reported as "data not shown". However, LeBel et al. [106] found that dispersin B exhibited dose-dependent growth inhibition of *Solobacterium moorei* in microtiter plate wells, with approximately 50% growth inhibition at 5–50 µg/mL dispersin B. Other studies showed that dispersin B was not cytotoxic against human HEp-2 larynx carcinoma cells, human HaCaT keratinocytes, human THP-1 monocytes, human MG-63 osteoblasts, murine J774 macrophages, murine L929 fibroblasts, or sheep erythrocytes [60,64,79].

Antibiofilm activities of dispersin B against staphylococci: *S. aureus* has received considerable attention because it causes many serious biofilm-related infections and also forms PNAG-dependent biofilms. Nearly all *S. aureus* strains carry the *icaADBC* operon, which encodes the enzymes required for PNAG biosynthesis [8]. However, only some strains appear to rely on PNAG expression for biofilm formation in vitro and in vivo. This fact is reflected in the varied responses of *S. aureus* biofilms to dispersin B treatment. For example, Hogan et al. [107] measured the ability of dispersin B to detach 24-hour-old *S. aureus* biofilms grown in plasma-coated microtiter plate wells. They found that dispersin B at 0.125–4 µg/mL effectively detached biofilms formed by *S. aureus* strain SH1000, a methicillin-sensitive *S. aureus* (MSSA) strain, but not those formed by *S. aureus* strain JE2, a methicillin-resistant *S. aureus* (MRSA) strain. However, dispersin B at 1 μg/mL was able to sensitize both SH1000 and JE2 biofilms to killing by a combination of rifampicin and vancomycin, although the sensitization effect was significantly greater for strain SH1000 (6–7 log units) than for strain USA300 JE2 (1–2 log units). Similarly, Izano et al. [108] found that dispersin B efficiently detached preformed biofilms produced by MSSA strain SH1000 in 96-well microtiter plates, but not those produced by MRSA strain 252. However, dispersin B did not inhibit biofilm formation by either strain, and it did not sensitize MSSA strain SH1000 biofilms to killing by cetylpyridinium chloride. Asai et al. [109] found that only one of twelve *S. aureus* strains isolated from patients with catheter-related bloodstream infections was susceptible to detachment by dispersin B when cultured in 96-well microtiter plates. Instead, most strains were sensitive to detachment by proteinase K. Similarly, Sugimoto et al. [110] found that dispersin B exhibited very limited biofilm inhibition and detachment activities against a panel of 17 *S. aureus* strains (10 MSSA, 7 MRSA) isolated from hospital patients when tested in 96-well microtiter plates. In contrast, Rohde et al. [111] found that 18 out of 18 *S. aureus* strains isolated from prosthetic joint infections were efficiently detached from 96-well plates by dispersin B. These differences may reflect differences in the media, culture conditions, bacterial strains, or methods used.

Several studies have shown that dispersin B sensitizes *S. aureus* biofilms to killing by a variety of antimicrobial agents, including triclosan [59], cefamandole nafate [60], silver [103], the antimicrobial peptide KSL-W [83], and a combination of rifampicin and clindamycin [123]. In general, dispersin B appears to sensitize both MSSA and MRSA biofilms to antibiotic killing.

S. epidermidis is of interest because of its ability to cause biofilm-related implant infections and its high susceptibility to biofilm inhibition and detachment by dispersin B [59,113]. Unlike *S. aureus*, only some *S. epidermidis* strains carry the *icaADBC* operon. It is still unclear whether the presence of *icaADBC* in *S. epidermidis* is correlated with an increased risk of device infection. Numerous studies have shown that even low concentrations of dispersin B efficiently inhibit and detach PNAG-dependent *S. epidermidis* biofilms in vitro [61,67,82,100,109,111,112,114–117,124] and sensitize *S. epidermidis* biofilms to killing by antimicrobial agents such as cetylpyridinium chloride [50,108], silver [103], and rifampicin [118].

Antibiofilm activities of dispersin B against plant pathogens: Dispersin B exhibits antibiofilm activity against several PNAG-producing plant pathogens, including members of the genera *Ralstonia*, *Xanthomonas*, and *Pectobacterium*, as well as the plant biocontrol bacterium *Pseudomonas fluorescens* (Figure 7). *X. citri* subsp. *citri*, the causative agent of citrus canker, forms aggregates when cultured in broth (Figure 7A). These aggregates are readily dissolved by dispersin B, suggesting that PNAG mediates intercellular adhesion in this species. Dispersin B also inhibited biofilm formation by *R. solanacearum* in polystyrene microtiter plates (Figure 7B). *R. solanacearum* is a causative agent of bacterial wilt in wide range of host plants. Dispersin B also inhibited biofilm formation by *Pseudomonas fluorescens* [101], as well as the binding of *P. fluorescens* planktonic cells to tomato roots (Figure 7C). Dispersin B also blocked biofilm formation by *P. carotovorum* in 96-well plates in vitro [104], as well as *P. carotovorum* infection of tobacco leaves in planta when *dspB* was expressed as a transgene (Figure 7D). Taken together, these findings suggest that plant-associated bacteria produce PNAG, and that PNAG contributes to intercellular adhesion, biofilm formation, plant colonization, and phytopathogenicity in vivo.

In vivo studies: Four different studies have demonstrated that dispersin B exhibits antibiofilm activity against staphylococci in vivo. Kaplan et al. [125] showed that dispersin B decreased the ability of *S. epidermidis* to colonize pig skin by 66–78% compared to a no-enzyme control. Gawande et al. [103] found that dispersin B combined with a silver wound dressing showed an 80% reduction in *S. aureus* MRSA bioburden in a chronic wound mouse model, compared to a 14% reduction when wounds were treated with a silver wound dressing alone. Darouiche et al. [61] tested dispersin B against *S. aureus* in a rabbit catheter infection model. Only 1 out of 30 catheters coated with dispersin B plus triclosan was colonized with *S. aureus*, compared to 29/30 uncoated control catheters. Finally, Serrera et al. [126] showed that dispersin B, when used in combination with teicoplanin as a catheter lock solution in a sheep model of port-related bloodstream infection, reduced the number of *S. aureus* infections from 100% to 50% (8/8 versus 4/8) and the number of deaths from 50% to 0% (4/8 versus 0/8), compared to a teicoplanin catheter lock solution alone.

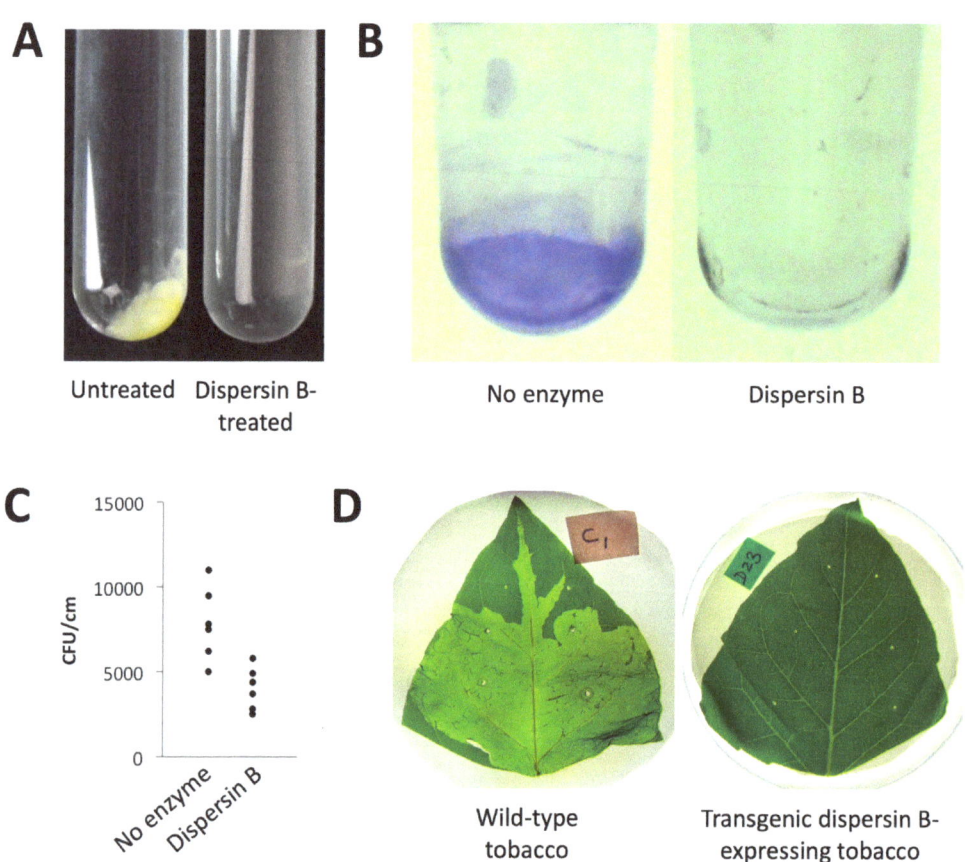

Figure 7. Effects of dispersin B on plant-associated bacteria: (**A**) *Xanthomonas citri* subsp. *citri* strain 306 forms aggregates when cultured in broth (**left panel**). These aggregates were rapidly dissolved upon dispersin B treatment (**right panel**). (**B**) Biofilm formation by *Ralstonia solanacearum* strain Molk2 in polystyrene microtiter plates in the absence or presence of 20 µg/mL dispersin B. Biofilms were stained with crystal violet. (**C**) Binding of *Pseudomonas fluorescens* strain WCS365 to tomato roots in the absence or presence of 20 µg/mL dispersin B. Bacteria were mixed with 6-day-old tomato roots for 90 min. The roots were then crushed, mixed by vortex agitation, diluted, and plated on agar for CFU enumeration. Each data point represents one individual root. (**D**) Tobacco leaves infected with *Pectobacterium carotovorum* subsp. *carotovorum* strain ATCC 15713. Leaves were photographed 24 h after inoculation: (**left**) wild-type tobacco leaf; (**right**) leaf from a transgenic tobacco plant expressing dispersin B. Source: (**A–C**) J.B. Kaplan, unpublished data; (**D**) Ragunath et al. [104], N. Ramasubbu, unpublished data.

7. Concluding Remarks

Dispersin B was licensed to the Canadian company Kane Biotech Inc. (Winnipeg, MB, Canada) in 2004, initially for the development of medical device coatings and cosmetics. Pharmaceutical-grade dispersin B (also known as DispersinB®) has been purified from a recombinant strain of *E. coli*, and the enzyme has undergone extensive biocompatibility testing. Recombinant dispersin B exhibited no cytotoxicity against L-929 cells in vitro and no mutagenicity or genotoxicity in the Ames test, in an in vitro human peripheral blood lymphocytes micronuclei assay, and in an in vivo rat blood reticulocyte assay that monitors chromosomal damage. Additional in vitro and in vivo biocompatibility testing showed that dispersin B was non-pyrogenic, non-sensitizing, and non-irritating, exhibited no acute or sub-chronic systemic toxicity, and was not detectable in blood when applied to full-thickness dermal wounds in pigs. These results suggest that dispersin B is biocompatible and safe for use on human skin. Dispersin B is also compatible with many antimicrobials, salts, preservatives, and excipients such as polyols, enabling it to be formulated into a plurality of products. For commercialization, dispersin B has been formulated into a gel containing poloxamer 407, glycerol, preservatives, and buffered phosphate. This formulation exhibits thermosensitive viscosity properties that enable it to form a gel on the skin. This dispersin B gel formulation has undergone stability and biocompatibility testing in accordance with ISO 10993 standards for prolonged exposure to breached/compromised skin, with positive results. Kane Biotech has also obtained promising results with dispersin B gel in a pig wound-healing study. The product has been designated as a biologic/device combination product, with the primary mode of action being the device. Dispersin B gel is currently undergoing the Investigational Device Exemption (IDE) review process with the FDA Center for Devices and Radiological Health (CDRH), with a plan to commence clinical trials for chronic wounds and acne vulgaris in 2025.

Dispersin B is a well-characterized PNAG-degrading enzyme that is both a useful tool for biofilm research and a potential therapeutic agent for the treatment and prevention of biofilm-related infections in plants and animals. Anti-PNAG antibodies have been shown to protect mice against local and/or systemic infections by various microbial pathogens, including *Streptococcus pyogenes*, *S. pneumoniae*, *Listeria monocytogenes*, *Neisseria meningitidis* serogroup B, *C. albicans*, and *Plasmodium berghei* ANKA, as well as against colonic pathology in a model of infectious colitis [38]. In addition, PNAG-based vaccines have been shown to be protective against a variety of PNAG-producing pathogens in animal models [39]. These findings validate PNAG as an antimicrobial target. Because of the large numbers of bacteria, fungi, and protozoa that produce PNAG [38,39], dispersin B may have applicability as a broad-spectrum antibiofilm agent. The most practical applications will be those where dispersin B can be used as a topical agent in the form of a gel, ointment, or spray in combination with an antimicrobial. These may include agents for the treatment of wounds, such as surgical site wounds, traumatic wounds, burns, and chronic wounds, including diabetic foot ulcers; for the treatment and prevention of dermatoses, such as atopic dermatitis and acne vulgaris; for the treatment of ocular infections, such as blepharitis and corneal ulcers; for the treatment of aural infections, such as otitis media; and as a pre-surgical skin antiseptic. Other potential applications include catheter lock solutions and irrigation solutions or coatings for implanted medical devices.

Author Contributions: J.B.K., S.A.S., M.S. and N.R. wrote the original draft of the manuscript. J.B.K., S.A.S., M.S., K.K. and N.R. reviewed and edited the manuscript. All authors have read and agreed to the published version of the manuscript.

Funding: This preparation and publication of this article was funded in part by the Health Corporation of the Galilee Medical Center (Nahariya, Israel) and Kane Biotech, Inc. (Winnipeg, MB, Canada).

Data Availability Statement: No new data were created or analyzed in this study. Data sharing is not applicable to this article.

Acknowledgments: Molecular graphics and analyses were performed with UCSF ChimeraX, developed by the Resource for Biocomputing, Visualization, and Informatics at the University of California, San Francisco, with support from National Institutes of Health grant R01-GM129325 and the Office of Cyber Infrastructure and Computational Biology, National Institute of Allergy and Infectious Diseases.

Conflicts of Interest: J.B.K. serves as an advisor for, owns equity in, and receives royalties from Kane Biotech Inc., Winnipeg, MB, Canada. This company is developing antibiofilm applications related to dispersin B. M.S. is an employee of Kane Biotech Inc., manufacturer of dispersin B (DispersinB®), and owns company stocks and stock options.

References

1. Penesyan, A.; Paulsen, I.T.; Kjelleberg, S.; Gillings, M.R. Three faces of biofilms: A microbial lifestyle, a nascent multicellular organism, and an incubator for diversity. *NPJ Biofilms Microbiomes* **2021**, *7*, 80. [CrossRef] [PubMed]
2. Penesyan, A.; Gillings, M.; Paulsen, I.T. Antibiotic discovery: Combatting bacterial resistance in cells and in biofilm communities. *Molecules* **2015**, *20*, 5286–5298. [CrossRef] [PubMed]
3. Abdelhamid, A.G.; Yousef, A.E. Combating bacterial biofilms: Current and emerging antibiofilm strategies for treating persistent infections. *Antibiotics* **2023**, *12*, 1005. [CrossRef] [PubMed]
4. Jiang, Y.; Geng, M.; Bai, L. Targeting biofilms therapy: Current research strategies and development hurdles. *Microorganisms* **2020**, *8*, 1222. [CrossRef] [PubMed]
5. Kaplan, J.B. Therapeutic potential of biofilm-dispersing enzymes. *Int. J. Artif. Organs* **2009**, *32*, 545–554. [CrossRef]
6. Ramakrishnan, R.; Singh, A.K.; Singh, S.; Chakravortty, D.; Das, D. Enzymatic dispersion of biofilms: An emerging biocatalytic avenue to combat biofilm-mediated microbial infections. *J. Biol. Chem.* **2022**, *298*, 102352. [CrossRef] [PubMed]
7. Wang, S.; Zhao, Y.; Breslawec, A.P.; Liang, T.; Deng, Z.; Kuperman, L.L.; Yu, Q. Strategy to combat biofilms: A focus on biofilm dispersal enzymes. *NPJ Biofilms Microbiomes* **2023**, *9*, 63. [CrossRef] [PubMed]
8. Nguyen, H.T.T.; Nguyen, T.H.; Otto, M. The staphylococcal exopolysaccharide PIA—Biosynthesis and role in biofilm formation, colonization, and infection. *Comput. Struct. Biotechnol. J.* **2020**, *18*, 3324–3334. [CrossRef] [PubMed]
9. Fine, D.H.; Furgang, D.; Kaplan, J.; Charlesworth, J.; Figurski, D.H. Tenacious adhesion of *Actinobacillus actinomycetemcomitans* strain CU1000 to salivary-coated hydroxyapatite. *Arch. Oral Biol.* **1999**, *44*, 1063–1076. [CrossRef]
10. Kaplan, J.B.; Meyenhofer, M.F.; Fine, D.H. Biofilm growth and detachment of *Actinobacillus actinomycetemcomitans*. *J. Bacteriol.* **2003**, *185*, 1399–1404. [CrossRef]
11. Kaplan, J.B.; Ragunath, C.; Ramasubbu, N.; Fine, D.H. Detachment of *Actinobacillus actinomycetemcomitans* biofilm cells by an endogenous beta-hexosaminidase activity. *J. Bacteriol.* **2003**, *185*, 4693–4698. [CrossRef] [PubMed]
12. Kaplan, J.B. Biofilm dispersal: Mechanisms, clinical implications, and potential therapeutic uses. *J. Dent. Res.* **2010**, *89*, 205–218. [CrossRef] [PubMed]
13. Stacy, A.; Everett, J.; Jorth, P.; Trivedi, U.; Rumbaugh, K.P.; Whiteley, M. Bacterial fight-and-flight responses enhance virulence in a polymicrobial infection. *Proc. Natl. Acad. Sci. USA* **2014**, *111*, 7819–7824. [CrossRef] [PubMed]
14. Zhang, Q.; Peng, L.; Han, W.; Chen, H.; Tang, H.; Chen, X.; Langford, P.R.; Huang, Q.; Zhou, R.; Li, L. The morphology and metabolic changes of *Actinobacillus pleuropneumoniae* during its growth as a biofilm. *Vet. Res.* **2023**, *54*, 42. [CrossRef] [PubMed]
15. Kaplan, J.B.; Velliyagounder, K.; Ragunath, C.; Rohde, H.; Mack, D.; Knobloch, J.K.; Ramasubbu, N. Genes involved in the synthesis and degradation of matrix polysaccharide in *Actinobacillus actinomycetemcomitans* and *Actinobacillus pleuropneumoniae* biofilms. *J. Bacteriol.* **2004**, *186*, 8213–8220. [CrossRef] [PubMed]
16. Michael, G.B.; Bossé, J.T.; Schwartz, S. Antimicrobial resistance in *Pasteurellaceae* of veterinary origin. *Microbiol. Spectr.* **2018**, *6*, ARBA-0022-2017. [CrossRef]
17. Ono, R.; Kitagawa, I.; Kobayashi, Y. *Cardiobacterium hominis* infective endocarditis: A literature review. *Am. Heart J. Plus* **2023**, *26*, 100248. [CrossRef]
18. Stacy, A.; Abraham, N.; Jorth, P.; Whiteley, M. Microbial community composition impacts pathogen iron availability during polymicrobial infection. *PLoS Pathog.* **2016**, *12*, e1006084. [CrossRef]
19. Ishikawa, K.H.; Bueno, M.R.; Kawamoto, D.; Simionato, M.R.L.; Mayer, M.P.A. Lactobacilli postbiotics reduce biofilm formation and alter transcription of virulence genes of *Aggregatibacter actinomycetemcomitans*. *Mol. Oral. Microbiol.* **2021**, *36*, 92–102. [CrossRef]
20. Shakya, S.; Danshiitsoodol, N.; Noda, M.; Inoue, Y.; Sugiyama, M. 3-Phenyllactic acid generated in medicinal plant extracts fermented with plant-derived lactic acid bacteria inhibits the biofilm synthesis of *Aggregatibacter actinomycetemcomitans*. *Front. Microbiol.* **2022**, *13*, 991144. [CrossRef]
21. Ramasubbu, N.; Thomas, L.M.; Ragunath, C.; Kaplan, J.B. Structural analysis of dispersin B, a biofilm-releasing glycoside hydrolase from the periodontopathogen *Actinobacillus actinomycetemcomitans*. *J. Mol. Biol.* **2005**, *349*, 475–486. [CrossRef] [PubMed]
22. Yakandawala, N.; Gawande, P.V.; LoVetri, K.; Romeo, T.; Kaplan, J.B.; Madhyastha, S. Enhanced expression of engineered ACA-less beta-1, 6-N-acetylglucosaminidase (dispersin B) in *Escherichia coli*. *J. Ind. Microbiol. Biotechnol.* **2009**, *36*, 1297–1305. [CrossRef] [PubMed]
23. Gökçen, A.; Vilcinskas, A.; Wiesner, J. Methods to identify enzymes that degrade the main extracellular polysaccharide component of *Staphylococcus epidermidis* biofilms. *Virulence* **2013**, *4*, 260–270. [CrossRef] [PubMed]
24. Zeng, K.; Sun, E.J.; Liu, Z.W.; Guo, J.; Yuan, C.; Yang, Y.; Xie, H. Synthesis of magnetic nanoparticles with an IDA or TED modified surface for purification and immobilization of poly-histidine tagged proteins. *RSC Adv.* **2020**, *10*, 11524–11534. [CrossRef] [PubMed]

25. Opdensteinen, P. Assessment of a Novel High-Throughput Process Development Platform for Biopharmaceutical Protein Production. Ph.D. Thesis, Aachen University, Aachen, Germany, 2023.
26. Prag, G.; Papanikolau, Y.; Tavlas, G.; Vorgias, C.E.; Petratos, K.; Oppenheim, A.B. Structures of chitobiase mutants complexed with the substrate di-*N*-acetyl-d-glucosamine: The catalytic role of the conserved acidic pair, aspartate 539 and glutamate 540. *J. Mol. Biol.* **2000**, *300*, 611–617. [CrossRef] [PubMed]
27. Manuel, S.G.; Ragunath, C.; Sait, H.B.; Izano, E.A.; Kaplan, J.B.; Ramasubbu, N. Role of active-site residues of Dispersin B, a biofilm-releasing beta-hexosaminidase from a periodontal pathogen, in substrate hydrolysis. *FEBS J.* **2007**, *274*, 5987–5999. [CrossRef] [PubMed]
28. Williams, S.J.; Mark, B.L.; Vocadlo, D.J.; James, M.N.; Withers, S.G. Aspartate 313 in the *Streptomyces plicatus* hexosaminidase plays a critical role in substrate-assisted catalysis by orienting the 2-acetamido group and stabilizing the transition state. *J. Biol. Chem.* **2002**, *277*, 40055–40065. [CrossRef] [PubMed]
29. Pettersen, E.F.; Goddard, T.D.; Huang, C.C.; Meng, E.C.; Couch, G.S.; Croll, T.I.; Morris, J.H.; Ferrin, T.E. UCSF ChimeraX: Structure visualization for researchers, educators, and developers. *Protein Sci.* **2021**, *30*, 70–82. [CrossRef]
30. Chibba, A.; Dasgupta, S.; Yakandawala, N.; Madhyastha, S.; Nitz, M. Chromogenic carbamate and acetal substrates for glycosaminidases. *J. Carbohydr. Chem.* **2011**, *30*, 549–558. [CrossRef]
31. Fazekas, E.; Kandra, L.; Gyemant, G. Model for beta-1,6-*N*-acetylglucosamine oligomer hydrolysis catalysed by DispersinB, a biofilm degrading enzyme. *Carbohydr. Res.* **2012**, *363*, 7–13. [CrossRef]
32. Fekete, A.; Borbas, A.; Gyemant, G.; Kandra, L.; Fazekas, E.; Ramasubbu, N.; Antus, S. Synthesis of beta-(1→6)-linked *N*-acetyl-D-glucosamine oligosaccharide substrates and their hydrolysis by Dispersin B. *Carbohydr. Res.* **2011**, *346*, 1445–1453. [CrossRef] [PubMed]
33. Kerrigan, J.E.; Ragunath, C.; Kandra, L.; Gyemant, G.; Liptak, A.; Janossy, L.; Kaplan, J.B.; Ramasubbu, N. Modeling and biochemical analysis of the activity of antibiofilm agent Dispersin B. *Acta Biol. Hung.* **2008**, *59*, 439–451. [CrossRef] [PubMed]
34. Wang, S.; Breslawec, A.P.; Poulin, M.B. Multifunctional fluorescent probes for high-throughput characterization of hexosaminidase enzyme activity. *Bioorg. Chem.* **2022**, *119*, 105532. [CrossRef]
35. Wang, S.; Breslawec, A.P.; Alvarez, E.; Tyrlik, M.; Li, C.; Poulin, M.B. Differential recognition of deacetylated PNAG oligosaccharides by a biofilm degrading glycosidase. *ACS Chem. Biol.* **2019**, *14*, 1998–2005. [CrossRef]
36. Breslawec, A.P.; Wang, S.; Monahan, K.N.; Barry, L.L.; Poulin, M.B. The endoglycosidase activity of Dispersin B is mediated through electrostatic interactions with cationic poly-beta-(1→6)-*N*-acetylglucosamine. *FEBS J.* **2023**, *290*, 1049–1059. [CrossRef] [PubMed]
37. Breslawec, A.P.; Wang, S.; Li, C.; Poulin, M.B. Anionic amino acids support hydrolysis of poly-beta-(1,6)-*N*-acetylglucosamine exopolysaccharides by the biofilm dispersing glycosidase Dispersin B. *J. Biol. Chem.* **2021**, *296*, 100203. [CrossRef]
38. Cywes-Bentley, C.; Skurnik, D.; Zaidi, T.; Roux, D.; Deoliveira, R.B.; Garrett, W.S.; Lu, X.; O'Malley, J.; Kinzel, K.; Zaidi, T.; et al. Antibody to a conserved antigenic target is protective against diverse prokaryotic and eukaryotic pathogens. *Proc. Natl. Acad. Sci. USA* **2013**, *110*, E2209–E2218. [CrossRef]
39. Gening, M.L.; Pier, G.B.; Nifantiev, N.E. Broadly protective semi-synthetic glycoconjugate vaccine against pathogens capable of producing poly-(1→6)-*N*-acetyl-D-glucosamine exopolysaccharide. *Drug Discov. Today Technol.* **2020**, *35–36*, 13–21. [CrossRef]
40. Yoong, P.; Cywes-Bentley, C.; Pier, G.B. Poly-N-acetylglucosamine expression by wild-type *Yersinia pestis* is maximal at mammalian, not flea, temperatures. *mBio* **2012**, *3*, e00217-12. [CrossRef]
41. Roux, D.; Cywes-Bentley, C.; Zhang, Y.F.; Pons, S.; Konkol, M.; Kearns, D.B.; Little, D.J.; Howell, P.L.; Skurnik, D.; Pier, G.B. Identification of poly-*N*-acetylglucosamine as a major polysaccharide component of the *Bacillus subtilis* biofilm matrix. *J. Biol. Chem.* **2015**, *290*, 19261–19272. [CrossRef] [PubMed]
42. Spiliopoulou, A.I.; Krevvata, M.I.; Kolonitsiou, F.; Harris, L.G.; Wilkinson, T.S.; Davies, A.P.; Dimitracopoulos, G.O.; Karamanos, N.K.; Mack, D.; Anastassiou, E.D. An extracellular *Staphylococcus epidermidis* polysaccharide: Relation to polysaccharide intercellular adhesin and its implication in phagocytosis. *BMC Microbiol.* **2012**, *12*, 76. [CrossRef] [PubMed]
43. Yakandawala, N.; Gawande, P.V.; LoVetri, K.; Cardona, S.T.; Romeo, T.; Nitz, M.; Madhyastha, S. Characterization of the poly-beta-1,6-*N*-acetylglucosamine polysaccharide component of *Burkholderia* biofilms. *Appl. Environ. Microbiol.* **2011**, *77*, 8303–8309. [CrossRef] [PubMed]
44. Sugimoto, S.; Iwamoto, T.; Takada, K.; Okuda, K.; Tajima, A.; Iwase, T.; Mizunoe, Y. *Staphylococcus epidermidis* Esp degrades specific proteins associated *with Staphylococcus aureus* biofilm formation and host-pathogen interaction. *J. Bacteriol.* **2013**, *195*, 1645–1655. [CrossRef] [PubMed]
45. Chiba, A.; Sugimoto, S.; Sato, F.; Hori, S.; Mizunoe, Y. A refined technique for extraction of extracellular matrices from bacterial biofilms and its applicability. *Microb. Biotechnol.* **2015**, *8*, 392–403. [CrossRef] [PubMed]
46. Eddenden, A.; Kitova, E.N.; Klassen, J.S.; Nitz, M. An Inactive dispersin B probe for monitoring PNAG production in biofilm formation. *ACS Chem. Biol.* **2020**, *15*, 1204–1211. [CrossRef] [PubMed]
47. Eddenden, A.; Nitz, M. Applications of an inactive dispersin B probe to monitor biofilm polysaccharide production. *Methods Enzymol.* **2022**, *665*, 209–231. [CrossRef] [PubMed]
48. Al Laham, N.; Rohde, H.; Sander, G.; Fischer, A.; Hussain, M.; Heilmann, C.; Mack, D.; Proctor, R.; Peters, G.; Becker, K.; et al. Augmented expression of polysaccharide intercellular adhesin in a defined *Staphylococcus epidermidis* mutant with the small-colony-variant phenotype. *J. Bacteriol.* **2007**, *189*, 4494–4501. [CrossRef] [PubMed]

49. Amini, S.; Goodarzi, H.; Tavazoie, S. Genetic dissection of an exogenously induced biofilm in laboratory and clinical isolates of *E. coli*. *PLoS Pathog.* **2009**, *5*, e1000432. [CrossRef]
50. Ganeshnarayan, K.; Shah, S.M.; Libera, M.R.; Santostefano, A.; Kaplan, J.B. Poly-*N*-acetylglucosamine matrix polysaccharide impedes fluid convection and transport of the cationic surfactant cetylpyridinium chloride through bacterial biofilms. *Appl. Environ. Microbiol.* **2009**, *75*, 1308–1314. [CrossRef]
51. Lin, M.H.; Shu, J.C.; Lin, L.P.; Chong, K.Y.; Cheng, Y.W.; Du, J.F.; Liu, S.-T. Elucidating the crucial role of poly *N*-acetylglucosamine from *Staphylococcus aureus* in cellular adhesion and pathogenesis. *PLoS ONE* **2015**, *10*, e0124216. [CrossRef]
52. Mlynek, K.D.; Bulock, L.L.; Stone, C.J.; Curran, L.J.; Sadykov, M.R.; Bayles, K.W.; Brinsmade, S.R. Genetic and biochemical Analysis of CodY-mediated cell aggregation in *Staphylococcus aureus* reveals an interaction between extracellular DNA and polysaccharide in the extracellular matrix. *J. Bacteriol.* **2020**, *202*, e00593-19. [CrossRef] [PubMed]
53. Wu, J.; Xi, C. Evaluation of different methods for extracting extracellular DNA from the biofilm matrix. *Appl. Environ. Microbiol.* **2009**, *75*, 5390–5395. [CrossRef] [PubMed]
54. Wu, J.; Xi, C. Enzymatic method for extracting extracellular DNA in biofilm matrix. *Cold Spring Harb. Protoc.* **2010**, *7*, pdb-prot5456. [CrossRef] [PubMed]
55. Abdelkader, J.; Alelyani, M.; Alashban, Y.; Alghamdi, S.A.; Bakkour, Y. Modification of dispersin B with cyclodextrin-ciprofloxacin derivatives for treating staphylococcal. *Molecules* **2023**, *28*, 5311. [CrossRef] [PubMed]
56. Liu, Z.; Zhao, Z.; Zeng, K.; Xia, Y.; Xu, W.; Wang, R.; Guo, J.; Xie, H. Functional immobilization of a biofilm-releasing glycoside hydrolase dispersin B on magnetic nanoparticles. *Appl. Biochem. Biotechnol.* **2022**, *194*, 737–747. [CrossRef] [PubMed]
57. Chen, K.J.; Lee, C.K. Twofold enhanced dispersin B activity by N-terminal fusion to silver-binding peptide for biofilm eradication. *Int. J. Biol. Macromol.* **2018**, *118*, 419–426. [CrossRef] [PubMed]
58. Hagen, C.R.M.; Singh, A.; Weese, J.S.; Marshall, Q.; Zur Linden, A.; Gibson, T.W.G. In vitro elution of amikacin and dispersin B from a polymer hydrogel. *Vet. Surg.* **2020**, *49*, 1035–1042. [CrossRef] [PubMed]
59. Kaplan, J.B.; Ragunath, C.; Velliyagounder, K.; Fine, D.H.; Ramasubbu, N. Enzymatic detachment of *Staphylococcus epidermidis* biofilms. *Antimicrob. Agents Chemother.* **2004**, *48*, 2633–2636. [CrossRef] [PubMed]
60. Donelli, G.; Francolini, I.; Romoli, D.; Guaglianone, E.; Piozzi, A.; Ragunath, C.; Kaplan, J.B. Synergistic activity of dispersin B and cefamandole nafate in inhibition of staphylococcal biofilm growth on polyurethanes. *Antimicrob. Agents Chemother.* **2007**, *51*, 2733–2740. [CrossRef]
61. Darouiche, R.O.; Mansouri, M.D.; Gawande, P.V.; Madhyastha, S. Antimicrobial and antibiofilm efficacy of triclosan and DispersinB combination. *J. Antimicrob. Chemother.* **2009**, *64*, 88–93. [CrossRef]
62. Marcano, A.; Ba, O.; Thebault, P.; Cretois, R.; Marais, S.; Duncan, A.C. Elucidation of innovative antibiofilm materials. *Colloids Surf. B Biointerfaces* **2015**, *136*, 56–63. [CrossRef]
63. Marcano, A.; Bou Haidar, N.; Marais, S.; Valleton, J.M.; Duncan, A.C. Designing biodegradable PHA-based 3D scaffolds with antibiofilm properties for wound dressings: Optimization of the microstructure/nanostructure. *ACS Biomater. Sci. Eng.* **2017**, *3*, 3654–3661. [CrossRef]
64. Bou Haidar, N.; Marais, S.; De, E.; Schaumann, A.; Barreau, M.; Feuilloley, M.G.J.; Duncan, A.C. Chronic wound healing: A specific antibiofilm protein-asymmetric release system. *Mater. Sci. Eng. C Mater. Biol. Appl.* **2020**, *106*, 110130. [CrossRef]
65. Pavlukhina, S.V.; Kaplan, J.B.; Xu, L.; Chang, W.; Yu, X.; Madhyastha, S.; Yakandawala, N.; Mentbayeva, A.; Khan, B.; Sukhishvili, S.A. Noneluting enzymatic antibiofilm coatings. *ACS Appl. Mater. Interfaces* **2012**, *4*, 4708–4716. [CrossRef] [PubMed]
66. Czuba, U.; Quintana, R.; De Pauw-Gillet, M.C.; Bourguignon, M.; Moreno-Couranjou, M.; Alexandre, M.; Detrembleur, C.; Choquet, P. Atmospheric plasma deposition of methacrylate layers containing catechol/quinone groups: An alternative to polydopamine bioconjugation for biomedical applications. *Adv. Healthc. Mater.* **2018**, *7*, e1701059. [CrossRef] [PubMed]
67. Piarali, S.; Marlinghaus, L.; Viebahn, R.; Lewis, H.; Ryadnov, M.G.; Groll, J.; Salber, J.; Roy, I. Activated polyhydroxyalkanoate meshes prevent bacterial adhesion and biofilm development in regenerative medicine applications. *Front. Bioeng. Biotechnol.* **2020**, *8*, 442. [CrossRef]
68. Camporeale, G.; Moreno-Couranjou, M.; Bonot, S.; Mauchauffé, R.; Boscher, N.D.; Bebrone, C.; Van de Weerdt, C.; Cauchie, H.-M.; Favia, P.; Choquet, P. Atmospheric-pressure plasma deposited epoxy-rich thin films as platforms for biomolecule immobilization—Application for anti-biofouling and xenobiotic-degrading surfaces. *Plasma Process. Polym.* **2015**, *12*, 1208–1219. [CrossRef]
69. Faure, E.; Falentin-Daudré, C.; Svaldo Lanero, T.; Vreuls, C.; Zocchi, G.; Van De Weerdt, C.; Martial, J.; Jérôme, C.; Duwez, A.-S.; Christophe Detrembleur, C. Functional nanogels as platforms for imparting antibacterial, antibiofilm, and antiadhesion activities to stainless steel. *Adv. Funct. Mater.* **2012**, *22*, 5271–5282. [CrossRef]
70. Nileback, L.; Widhe, M.; Seijsing, J.; Bysell, H.; Sharma, P.K.; Hedhammar, M. Bioactive silk coatings reduce the adhesion of *Staphylococcus aureus* while supporting growth of osteoblast-like cells. *ACS Appl. Mater. Interfaces* **2019**, *11*, 24999–25007. [CrossRef]
71. Seijsing, F.; Nileback, L.; Ohman, O.; Pasupuleti, R.; Stahl, C.; Seijsing, J.; Hedhammar, M. Recombinant spider silk coatings functionalized with enzymes targeting bacteria and biofilms. *Microbiologyopen* **2020**, *9*, e993. [CrossRef]
72. Garrido, V.; Pinero-Lambea, C.; Rodriguez-Arce, I.; Paetzold, B.; Ferrar, T.; Weber, M.; Garcia-Ramallo, E.; Gallo, C.; Collantes, M.; Penuelas, I.; et al. Engineering a genome-reduced bacterium to eliminate *Staphylococcus aureus* biofilms in vivo. *Mol. Syst. Biol.* **2021**, *17*, e10145. [CrossRef] [PubMed]

73. Ghalsasi, V.V.; Sourjik, V. Engineering *Escherichia coli* to disrupt poly-*N*-acetylglucosamine containing bacterial biofilms. *Curr. Synth. Syst. Biol.* **2016**, *4*, 1. [CrossRef]
74. Ragunath, C.; DiFranco, K.; Shanmugam, M.; Gopal, P.; Vyas, V.; Fine, D.H.; Cugini, C.; Ramasubbu, N. Surface display of *Aggregatibacter actinomycetemcomitans* autotransporter Aae and Dispersin B hybrid act as antibiofilm agents. *Mol. Oral Microbiol.* **2016**, *31*, 329–339. [CrossRef] [PubMed]
75. Lu, T.K.; Collins, J.J. Dispersing biofilms with engineered enzymatic bacteriophage. *Proc. Natl. Acad. Sci. USA* **2007**, *104*, 11197–11202. [CrossRef] [PubMed]
76. Schmerer, M.; Molineux, I.J.; Ally, D.; Tyerman, J.; Cecchini, N.; Bull, J.J. Challenges in predicting the evolutionary maintenance of a phage transgene. *J. Biol. Eng.* **2014**, *8*, 21. [CrossRef] [PubMed]
77. Wen, J.; Wang, Z.; Du, X.; Liu, R.; Wang, J. Antibioflm effects of extracellular matrix degradative agents on the biofilm of different strains of multi-drug resistant *Corynebacterium striatum*. *Ann. Clin. Microbiol. Antimicrob.* **2022**, *21*, 53. [CrossRef] [PubMed]
78. Poilvache, H.; Ruiz-Sorribas, A.; Cornu, O.; Van Bambeke, F. In vitro study of the synergistic effect of an enzyme cocktail and antibiotics against biofilms in a prosthetic joint infection model. *Antimicrob. Agents Chemother.* **2021**, *65*, e01699-20. [CrossRef] [PubMed]
79. Ruiz-Sorribas, A.; Poilvache, H.; Kamarudin, N.H.N.; Braem, A.; Van Bambeke, F. Hydrolytic enzymes as potentiators of antimicrobials against an inter-kingdom biofilm model. *Microbiol. Spectr.* **2022**, *10*, e0258921. [CrossRef] [PubMed]
80. Waryah, C.B.; Wells, K.; Ulluwishewa, D.; Chen-Tan, N.; Gogoi-Tiwari, J.; Ravensdale, J.; Costantino, P.; Gökçen, A.; Vilcinskas, A.; Wiesner, J.; et al. In vitro antimicrobial efficacy of tobramycin against *Staphylococcus aureus* biofilms in combination with or without DNase I and/or dispersin B: A preliminary investigation. *Microb. Drug Resist.* **2017**, *23*, 384–390. [CrossRef]
81. Chiba, A.; Seki, M.; Suzuki, Y.; Kinjo, Y.; Mizunoe, Y.; Sugimoto, S. *Staphylococcus aureus* utilizes environmental RNA as a building material in specific polysaccharide-dependent biofilms. *NPJ Biofilms Microbiomes* **2022**, *8*, 17. [CrossRef]
82. Dobrynina, O.Y.; Bolshakova, T.N.; Umyarov, A.M.; Boksha, I.S.; Lavrova, N.V.; Grishin, A.V.; Lyashchuk, A.M.; Galushkina, Z.M.; Avetisian, L.R.; Chernukha, M.Y.; et al. Disruption of bacterial biofilms using recombinant dispersin B. *Microbiology* **2015**, *84*, 498–501. [CrossRef]
83. Gawande, P.V.; Leung, K.P.; Madhyastha, S. Antibiofilm and antimicrobial efficacy of DispersinB®-KSL-W peptide-based wound gel against chronic wound infection associated bacteria. *Curr. Microbiol.* **2014**, *68*, 635–641. [CrossRef] [PubMed]
84. Nait Chabane, Y.; Marti, S.; Rihouey, C.; Alexandre, S.; Hardouin, J.; Lesouhaitier, O.; Vila, J.; Kaplan, J.B.; Jouenne, T.; De, E. Characterisation of pellicles formed by *Acinetobacter baumannii* at the air-liquid interface. *PLoS ONE* **2014**, *9*, e111660. [CrossRef] [PubMed]
85. Bossé, J.T.; Sinha, S.; Li, M.S.; O'Dwyer, C.A.; Nash, J.H.; Rycroft, A.N.; Kroll, J.S.; Langford, P.R. Regulation of *pga* operon expression and biofilm formation in *Actinobacillus pleuropneumoniae* by sigmaE and H-NS. *J. Bacteriol.* **2010**, *192*, 2414–2423. [CrossRef] [PubMed]
86. Grasteau, A.; Tremblay, Y.D.; Labrie, J.; Jacques, M. Novel genes associated with biofilm formation of *Actinobacillus pleuropneumoniae*. *Vet. Microbiol.* **2011**, *153*, 134–143. [CrossRef] [PubMed]
87. Izano, E.A.; Sadovskaya, I.; Vinogradov, E.; Mulks, M.H.; Velliyagounder, K.; Ragunath, C.; Kher, W.B.; Ramasubbu, N.; Jabbouri, S.; Perry, M.B.; et al. Poly-*N*-acetylglucosamine mediates biofilm formation and antibiotic resistance in *Actinobacillus pleuropneumoniae*. *Microb. Pathog.* **2007**, *43*, 1–9. [CrossRef] [PubMed]
88. Labrie, J.; Pelletier-Jacques, G.; Deslandes, V.; Ramjeet, M.; Auger, E.; Nash, J.H.; Jacques, M. Effects of growth conditions on biofilm formation by *Actinobacillus pleuropneumoniae*. *Vet. Res.* **2010**, *41*, 3. [CrossRef] [PubMed]
89. Li, Y.; Cao, S.; Zhang, L.; Yuan, J.; Lau, G.W.; Wen, Y.; Wu, R.; Zhao, Q.; Huang, X.; Yan, Q.; et al. Absence of TolC impairs biofilm formation in *Actinobacillus pleuropneumoniae* by reducing initial attachment. *PLoS ONE* **2016**, *11*, e0163364. [CrossRef]
90. Tremblay, Y.D.; Levesque, C.; Segers, R.P.; Jacques, M. Method to grow *Actinobacillus pleuropneumoniae* biofilm on a biotic surface. *BMC Vet. Res.* **2013**, *9*, 213. [CrossRef]
91. Izano, E.A.; Wang, H.; Ragunath, C.; Ramasubbu, N.; Kaplan, J.B. Detachment and killing of *Aggregatibacter actinomycetemcomitans* biofilms by Dispersin B and SDS. *J. Dent. Res.* **2007**, *86*, 618–622. [CrossRef]
92. Dashiff, A.; Kadouri, D.E. Predation of oral pathogens by *Bdellovibrio bacteriovorus* 109J. *Mol. Oral Microbiol.* **2011**, *26*, 19–34. [CrossRef] [PubMed]
93. Izano, E.A.; Sadovskaya, I.; Wang, H.; Vinogradov, E.; Ragunath, C.; Ramasubbu, N.; Jabbouri, S.; Perry, M.B.; Kaplan, J.B. Poly-*N*-acetylglucosamine mediates biofilm formation and detergent resistance in *Aggregatibacter actinomycetemcomitans*. *Microb. Pathog.* **2008**, *44*, 52–60. [CrossRef]
94. Venketaraman, V.; Lin, A.K.; Le, A.; Kachlany, S.C.; Connell, N.D.; Kaplan, J.B. Both leukotoxin and poly-*N*-acetylglucosamine surface polysaccharide protect *Aggregatibacter actinomycetemcomitans* cells from macrophage killing. *Microb. Pathog.* **2008**, *45*, 173–180. [CrossRef]
95. Fullen, A.R.; Gutierrez-Ferman, J.L.; Yount, K.S.; Love, C.F.; Choi, H.G.; Vargas, M.A.; Raju, D.; Corps, K.N.; Howell, P.L.; Dubey, P.; et al. Bps polysaccharide of *Bordetella pertussis* resists antimicrobial peptides by functioning as a dual surface shield and decoy and converts *Escherichia coli* into a respiratory pathogen. *PLoS Pathog.* **2022**, *18*, e1010764. [CrossRef] [PubMed]
96. Parise, G.; Mishra, M.; Itoh, Y.; Romeo, T.; Deora, R. Role of a putative polysaccharide locus in *Bordetella* biofilm development. *J. Bacteriol.* **2007**, *189*, 750–760. [CrossRef] [PubMed]

97. Irie, Y.; Preston, A.; Yuk, M.H. Expression of the primary carbohydrate component of the *Bordetella bronchiseptica* biofilm matrix is dependent on growth phase but independent of Bvg regulation. *J. Bacteriol.* **2006**, *188*, 6680–6687. [CrossRef]

98. Messiaen, A.S.; Nelis, H.; Coenye, T. Investigating the role of matrix components in protection of *Burkholderia cepacia* complex biofilms against tobramycin. *J. Cyst. Fibros.* **2014**, *13*, 56–62. [CrossRef] [PubMed]

99. Kaplan, J.B.; Cywes-Bentley, C.; Pier, G.B.; Yakandawala, N.; Sailer, M.; Edwards, M.S.; Kridin, K. Poly-beta-(1→6)-N-acetyl-D-glucosamine mediates surface attachment, biofilm formation, and biocide resistance in *Cutibacterium acnes. Front. Microbiol.* **2024**, *15*, 1386017. [CrossRef]

100. Burton, E.; Yakandawala, N.; LoVetri, K.; Madhyastha, M.S. A microplate spectrofluorometric assay for bacterial biofilms. *J. Ind. Microbiol. Biotechnol.* **2007**, *34*, 1–4. [CrossRef]

101. Itoh, Y.; Wang, X.; Hinnebusch, B.J.; Preston, J.F., 3rd; Romeo, T. Depolymerization of beta-1,6-N-acetyl-D-glucosamine disrupts the integrity of diverse bacterial biofilms. *J. Bacteriol.* **2005**, *187*, 382–387. [CrossRef]

102. Siebert, C.; Villers, C.; Pavlou, G.; Touquet, B.; Yakandawala, N.; Tardieux, I.; Renesto, P. *Francisella novicida* and *F. philomiragia* biofilm features conditionning fitness in spring water and in presence of antibiotics. *PLoS ONE* **2020**, *15*, e0228591. [CrossRef]

103. Gawande, P.V.; Clinton, A.P.; LoVetri, K.; Yakandawala, N.; Rumbaugh, K.P.; Madhyastha, S. Antibiofilm efficacy of DispersinB® wound spray used in combination with a silver wound dressing. *Microbiol. Insights* **2014**, *7*, 9–13. [CrossRef] [PubMed]

104. Ragunath, C.; Shanmugam, M.; Bendaoud, M.; Kaplan, J.B.; Ramasubbu, N. Effect of a biofilm-degrading enzyme from an oral pathogen in transgenic tobacco on the pathogenicity of *Pectobacterium carotovorum* subsp. *carotovorum. Plant Pathol.* **2012**, *61*, 346–354. [CrossRef]

105. Perez-Mendoza, D.; Coulthurst, S.J.; Sanjuan, J.; Salmond, G.P.C. N-Acetylglucosamine-dependent biofilm formation in *Pectobacterium atrosepticum* is cryptic and activated by elevated c-di-GMP levels. *Microbiology* **2011**, *157*, 3340–3348. [CrossRef]

106. LeBel, G.; Haas, B.; Adam, A.-A.; Veilleux, M.-P.; Ben Lagha, A.; Grenier, D. Effect of cinnamon (*Cinnamomum verum*) bark essential oil on the halitosis-associated bacterium *Solobacterium moorei* and in vitro cytotoxicity. *Arch. Oral Biol.* **2017**, *83*, 97–104. [CrossRef]

107. Hogan, S.; Zapotoczna, M.; Stevens, N.T.; Humphreys, H.; O'Gara, J.P.; O'Neill, E. Potential use of targeted enzymatic agents in the treatment of *Staphylococcus aureus* biofilm-related infections. *J. Hosp. Infect.* **2017**, *96*, 177–182. [CrossRef] [PubMed]

108. Izano, E.A.; Amarante, M.A.; Kher, W.B.; Kaplan, J.B. Differential roles of poly-N-acetylglucosamine surface polysaccharide and extracellular DNA in *Staphylococcus aureus* and *Staphylococcus epidermidis* biofilms. *Appl. Environ. Microbiol.* **2008**, *74*, 470–476. [CrossRef] [PubMed]

109. Asai, K.; Yamada, K.; Yagi, T.; Baba, H.; Kawamura, I.; Ohta, M. Effect of incubation atmosphere on the production and composition of staphylococcal biofilms. *J. Infect. Chemother.* **2015**, *21*, 55–61. [CrossRef]

110. Sugimoto, S.; Sato, F.; Miyakawa, R.; Chiba, A.; Onodera, S.; Hori, S.; Mizunoe, Y. Broad impact of extracellular DNA on biofilm formation by clinically isolated methicillin-resistant and -sensitive strains of *Staphylococcus aureus. Sci. Rep.* **2018**, *8*, 2254. [CrossRef]

111. Rohde, H.; Burandt, E.C.; Siemssen, N.; Frommelt, L.; Burdelski, C.; Wurster, S.; Scherpe, S.; Davies, A.P.; Harris, L.G.; Horstkotte, M.A.; et al. Polysaccharide intercellular adhesin or protein factors in biofilm accumulation of *Staphylococcus epidermidis* and *Staphylococcus aureus* isolated from prosthetic hip and knee joint infections. *Biomaterials* **2007**, *28*, 1711–1720. [CrossRef]

112. Fagerlund, A.; Langsrud, S.; Heir, E.; Mikkelsen, M.I.; Moretro, T. Biofilm matrix composition affects the susceptibility of food associated staphylococci to cleaning and disinfection agents. *Front. Microbiol.* **2016**, *7*, 856. [CrossRef]

113. Brindle, E.R.; Miller, D.A.; Stewart, P.S. Hydrodynamic deformation and removal of *Staphylococcus epidermidis* biofilms treated with urea, chlorhexidine, iron chloride, or DispersinB. *Biotechnol. Bioeng.* **2011**, *108*, 2968–2977. [CrossRef]

114. Chaignon, P.; Sadovskaya, I.; Ragunah, C.; Ramasubbu, N.; Kaplan, J.B.; Jabbouri, S. Susceptibility of staphylococcal biofilms to enzymatic treatments depends on their chemical composition. *Appl. Microbiol. Biotechnol.* **2007**, *75*, 125–132. [CrossRef] [PubMed]

115. Frank, K.L.; Patel, R. Poly-N-acetylglucosamine is not a major component of the extracellular matrix in biofilms formed by *icaADBC*-positive *Staphylococcus lugdunensis* isolates. *Infect. Immun.* **2007**, *75*, 4728–4742. [CrossRef] [PubMed]

116. Kaplan, J.B.; Jabbouri, S.; Sadovskaya, I. Extracellular DNA-dependent biofilm formation by *Staphylococcus epidermidis* RP62A in response to subminimal inhibitory concentrations of antibiotics. *Res. Microbiol.* **2011**, *162*, 535–541. [CrossRef] [PubMed]

117. Loughran, A.J.; Atwood, D.N.; Anthony, A.C.; Harik, N.S.; Spencer, H.J.; Beenken, K.E.; Smeltzer, M.S. Impact of individual extracellular proteases on *Staphylococcus aureus* biofilm formation in diverse clinical isolates and their isogenic *sarA* mutants. *Microbiologyopen* **2014**, *3*, 897–909. [CrossRef]

118. Lee, J.H.; Kaplan, J.B.; Lee, W.Y. Microfluidic devices for studying growth and detachment of *Staphylococcus epidermidis* biofilms. *Biomed. Microdevices* **2008**, *10*, 489–498. [CrossRef]

119. Turk, R.; Singh, A.; Rousseau, J.; Weese, J.S. In vitro evaluation of DispersinB on methicillin-resistant *Staphylococcus pseudintermedius* biofilm. *Vet. Microbiol.* **2013**, *166*, 576–579. [CrossRef]

120. Rmaile, A.; Ward, M.T.; Aspiras, M.; Stoodley, P. Disruption of dental biofilms by matrix-degrading enzymes. In Proceedings of the British Sociey for Oral and Dental Research BSODR, Conference Paper, Bath, UK, 10 September 2013.

121. van Dissel, D.; Willemse, J.; Zacchetti, B.; Claessen, D.; Pier, G.B.; van Wezel, G.P. Production of poly-beta-1,6-N-acetylglucosamine by MatAB is required for hyphal aggregation and hydrophilic surface adhesion by *Streptomyces. Microb. Cell* **2018**, *5*, 269–279. [CrossRef]

122. Atwood, D.N.; Loughran, A.J.; Courtney, A.P.; Anthony, A.C.; Meeker, D.G.; Spencer, H.J.; Gupta, R.K.; Lee, C.Y.; Beenken, K.E.; Smeltzer, M.S. Comparative impact of diverse regulatory loci on *Staphylococcus aureus* biofilm formation. *Microbiologyopen* **2015**, *4*, 436–451. [CrossRef]
123. Belfield, K.; Bayston, R.; Hajduk, N.; Levell, G.; Birchall, J.P.; Daniel, M. Evaluation of combinations of putative anti-biofilm agents and antibiotics to eradicate biofilms of *Staphylococcus aureus* and *Pseudomonas aeruginosa*. *J. Antimicrob. Chemother.* **2017**, *72*, 2531–2538. [CrossRef] [PubMed]
124. Sadovskaya, I.; Chaignon, P.; Kogan, G.; Chokr, A.; Vinogradov, E.; Jabbouri, S. Carbohydrate-containing components of biofilms produced in vitro by some staphylococcal strains related to orthopaedic prosthesis infections. *FEMS Immunol. Med. Microbiol.* **2006**, *47*, 75–82. [CrossRef] [PubMed]
125. Kaplan, J.B.; Mlynek, K.D.; Hettiarachchi, H.; Alamneh, Y.A.; Biggemann, L.; Zurawski, D.V.; Black, C.C.; Bane, C.E.; Kim, R.K.; Granick, M.S. Extracellular polymeric substance (EPS)-degrading enzymes reduce staphylococcal surface attachment and biocide resistance on pig skin in vivo. *PLoS ONE* **2018**, *13*, e0205526. [CrossRef] [PubMed]
126. Serrera, A.; del Pozo, J.L.; Martinez, A.; Alonso, M.; Gonzalez, R.; Leiva, J.; Vergara, M.; Lasa, I. Dispersin B therapy of *Staphylococcus aureus* experimental port-related bloodstream infection. In Proceedings of the 17th European Congress of Clinical Microbiology and Infectious Disease, Munich, Germany, 31 March–3 April 2007; Poster P1786.

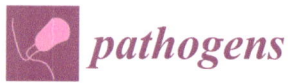

Review

Therapeutic Applications of *Aggregatibacter actinomycetemcomitans* Leukotoxin

Scott C. Kachlany * and Brian A. Vega †

Department of Oral Biology, Rutgers School of Dental Medicine, Newark, NJ 07103, USA
* Correspondence: kachlasc@rutgers.edu
† Current address: Nonclinical Drug Safety, Merck & Co., Inc., West Point, PA 19486, USA.

Abstract: *Aggregatibacter actinomycetemcomitans* is a Gram-negative oral bacterium that has been primarily studied for its role in causing periodontal disease. The bacterium has also been implicated in several systemic diseases such as endocarditis and soft tissue abscesses. Leukotoxin (LtxA) is perhaps the best studied protein virulence factor from *A. actinomycetemcomitans*. The protein can rapidly destroy white blood cells (WBCs), helping the bacterium to subvert the host immune system. The functional receptor for LtxA is lymphocyte function associated antigen-1 (LFA-1), which is expressed exclusively on the surfaces of WBCs. Bacterial expression and secretion of the protein are highly regulated and controlled by a number of genetic and environmental factors. The mechanism of LtxA action on WBCs varies depending on the type of cell that is being killed, and the protein has been shown to activate numerous cell death pathways in susceptible cells. In addition to serving as an important virulence factor for the bacterium, because of its exquisite specificity and rapid activity, LtxA is also being investigated as a therapeutic agent that may be used to treat diseases such as hematological malignancies and autoimmune/inflammatory diseases. It is our hope that this review will inspire an increased intensity of research related to LtxA and its effect on Aggressive Periodontitis, the disease that led to its initial discovery.

Keywords: LFA-1; inflammation; leukemia; lymphoma; autoimmune disease; translational research; drug development; protein drug; allergic asthma; inflammatory bowel disease; Crohn's disease; ulcerative colitis

Citation: Kachlany, S.C.; Vega, B.A. Therapeutic Applications of *Aggregatibacter actinomycetemcomitans* Leukotoxin. *Pathogens* **2024**, *13*, 354. https://doi.org/10.3390/pathogens13050354

Academic Editor: Anders Johansson

Received: 1 April 2024
Revised: 22 April 2024
Accepted: 23 April 2024
Published: 25 April 2024

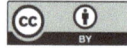
1. Introduction

Aggregatibacter actinomycetemcomitans produces numerous well-studied virulence factors including cytolethal distending toxin, tight adherence pili, cell-specific adhesins, and leukotoxin (LtxA). Leukotoxin from *A. actinomycetemcomitans* has been studied primarily as a bacterial virulence factor that contributes to the disease process. The protein is thought to help the bacterium to evade the host immune response during infection by eliminating certain white blood cells. The clinical relevance of LtxA is supported by the fact that patients who harbor the highly leukotoxic JP2 strain have an increased risk of developing aggressive periodontal disease [1]. Because of its numerous unique properties, our laboratory has also been studying how the protein can serve as a potent and safe therapeutic agent. Much like other bacterial proteins, such as botulinum toxin and *E. coli* asparaginase, which have been used as effective FDA-approved drugs, leukotoxin (LtxA) has significant potential to treat patients with various white blood cell (WBC) disorders, such as hematologic malignancies and autoimmune/inflammatory diseases.

The seminal discovery by Lally et al. [2,3] that LtxA binds specifically to lymphocyte function associated antigen-1 (LFA-1) laid the foundation for understanding how the protein interacts with host cells and, subsequently, how LtxA can be used to treat patients with disease. LFA-1 is a beta-2 integrin that is a dimer between CD11a and CD18 [4–6]. LFA-1 is surface localized and found exclusively on WBCs, which explains the target specificity of the protein. LFA-1 is highly conserved across species and considered essential for maintenance of a functional immune system. Initially, there was a controversy as to how LtxA was delivered [7–10]. Research suggested that LtxA was delivered in extracellular blebs and not secreted; however, it was subsequently discovered that LtxA was found in both secreted [11,12] and extracellular blebs [13–15], providing the toxin with both a direct attack on cell membranes (in the secreted form) and an intracellular attack mode (by blebs fusing with outer cell membranes).

The physiological role of LFA-1 in mammals is to interact with intercellular adhesion molecule-1 (ICAM-1) on vascular endothelial cells and mediate the proliferation and migration of the WBC from the blood stream into the surrounding tissue [6,16,17]. This migration occurs when WBCs are needed at certain locations in the body due to infection or injury. Inflammatory cytokines, such as IL-6 and IL-8, serve as signals to mediate the interaction between LFA-1 and ICAM-1 and subsequent trans-endothelial transmigration. However, not all WBCs in the body interact with ICAM-1 constantly. In fact, most WBCs exist in a resting state, whereby they are merely surveying the environment, waiting to be called upon by the immune system. The interaction between LFA-1 and ICAM-1 is controlled by the activation state of LFA-1. LFA-1 can exist in three different conformations: a low-, intermediate-, and high-affinity state [18–21]. In the low-affinity conformation, the CD11a and CD18 molecules are closed in a tucked-in structure that makes them unavailable to bind to ICAM-1. This is the resting state that the majority of circulating and tissue-resident WBCs exhibit. In the intermediate state, LFA-1 is extended and can interact with ICAM-1, albeit in a low-affinity capacity. In the high-affinity conformation, LFA-1 is extended and its ligand-binding site is fully available, allowing maximal interaction with ICAM-1. The activation state of LFA-1 is regulated by chemicals (such as PMA), metals (such as Mn^+, Mg^{2+}, and Ca^{2+}), and cytokines.

While interaction between LFA-1 and ICAM-1 under physiological conditions mediates the proliferation and migration of WBCs, contact between LFA-1 and LtxA results in very rapid cell death. Interestingly, it was discovered that LtxA preferentially kills activated WBCs that express the high-affinity LFA-1 conformation [22,23]. Physiologically, this preference makes the most sense since activated, proinflammatory WBCs pose the greatest threat to the bacterium. Hence, LtxA naturally targets the most active components of the immune system.

Studies on the WBC killing mechanisms by LtxA have revealed numerous fascinating and novel discoveries. There are significant differences in how LtxA kills macrophages and monocytes compared to lymphocytes. While these mechanisms have been described extensively elsewhere [24–29], a brief summary is described below. For macrophages and monocytes, LtxA interaction with active LFA-1 results in at least two downstream events: the activation of a caspase apoptotic pathway and endocytosis of the LtxA-LFA-1 complex and delivery to the lysosome. LtxA appears to cause significant disruption and damage to the lysosomal membrane, which seals the fate of the cell. Thus, it appears that LtxA activates at least two non-redundant killing pathways to ensure death of the cell.

For T-lymphocytes, LtxA initially contacts LFA-1 on the surface and then also appears to recruit FAS (CD95) death receptor to the complex to activate the FAS death receptor pathway. Normally, FAS death receptor requires contact with FAS ligand (FASL) for the activation and initiation of cell death. However, LtxA bypasses the requirement for FASL and is able to directly activate caspase-8 and the induction of cell death. It is interesting to note that macrophages and monocytes express very little FAS receptor on their surface, while lymphocytes are known to express abundant levels. Furthermore, macrophages and monocytes have a high lysosomal content, while lymphocytic cells contain a relatively small number of lysosomes. Hence, LtxA may have evolved numerous mechanisms to kill cells based on the death pathways available in each cell type.

While LtxA targets specifically cells that express LFA-1, not all cell types are equally sensitive to the bacterial protein. Both the surface levels of LFA-1 and activation state of the molecule affect sensitivity to LtxA. In general, neutrophils and monocytes have the highest expression levels of LFA-1, followed by T cells and then B cells. Indeed, the sensitivity of these cell types is roughly proportional to the levels of LFA-1, with monocytes and neutrophils being killed most efficiently by LtxA. In vitro and ex vivo studies have also shown that WBCs that are activated with molecules such as phorbol esters or certain activating antibodies exhibit 10–100 times greater sensitivity to LtxA than non-activated cells [22–24]. Furthermore, in vivo studies in rats and dogs have demonstrated that intravenously administered LtxA preferentially targets cells with the highest levels of active LFA-1.

A large number of white blood cell diseases are characterized by the overexpression and activation of LFA-1 such as certain hematologic malignancies and autoimmune/inflammatory diseases, including inflammatory bowel disease (Crohn's disease and ulcerative colitis), rheumatoid arthritis, psoriasis, multiple sclerosis, type I diabetes, allergic asthma, and dry-eye disease [30–37]. Given LtxA's preferential killing of cells expressing high levels of active LFA-1, we postulated that LtxA may serve as an ideal therapeutic agent for specifically and safely targeting diseased WBCs. This preferential attack on distinct cell populations is in need of further exploration in periodontal diseases. Below is a description of the multitudinous ways in which LtxA can be used for treating diseases other than periodontitis. This broad spectrum of effects supports the concept that LtxA can effect host immune regulation in several divergent ways.

2. Hematologic Malignancies

Leukemia and lymphoma are cancers of the immune system that are often difficult to treat [38–41]. The 5-year survival rate for patients with acute myeloid leukemia (AML) is 30%, which decreases with increasing age. Furthermore, nearly 50% of AML patients relapse after successful treatment. B cells and T cells can also become malignant and may circulate throughout the body or grow within lymph nodes. Because LtxA is able to potentially kill different subsets of WBCs selectively, we initially proposed that LtxA may be an ideal (effective and targeted) therapeutic agent to treat patients with leukemia and lymphoma. In these cases, the goal is merely to wipe out the cancerous WBCs.

We have evaluated LtxA in numerous animal models for leukemia and lymphoma [23,27]. In each study, just a few doses of LtxA were sufficient to eliminate the cancer, and the cancer never returned, suggesting that cells did not develop resistance to the protein. Interestingly, we never observed resistance to LtxA in any of the animal studies or in vitro studies using cancer cell lines derived from leukemia and lymphoma patients. Because LtxA employs numerous mechanisms to kill a cell, we believe that it would be difficult for a cell to develop resistance to the protein. This property could make LtxA a very effective therapy with a high unmet need.

We have also evaluated the levels of LFA-1 on WBCs from patients with various hematologic malignancies, including AML (Figure 1). We found that the levels of LFA-1 varied from low to very high levels on both newly diagnosed and relapsed AML patient samples. Furthermore, regardless of the levels of LFA-1, LtxA had a significant effect on the cells, suggesting that even low levels of LFA-1 are sufficient for activity (Figure 1). It may also be that these cells express the highly active conformation of LFA-1, making them even more sensitive to LtxA.

In 2021, a pharmaceutical company (Actinobac Biomed, Inc., manufactured in Baltimore, MD, USA) received IND approval from the FDA to evaluate intravenous LtxA in patients with relapsed/refractory leukemia and lymphoma, and these trials are pending.

LFA-1 plot	Disease	Percent killing with Leukothera
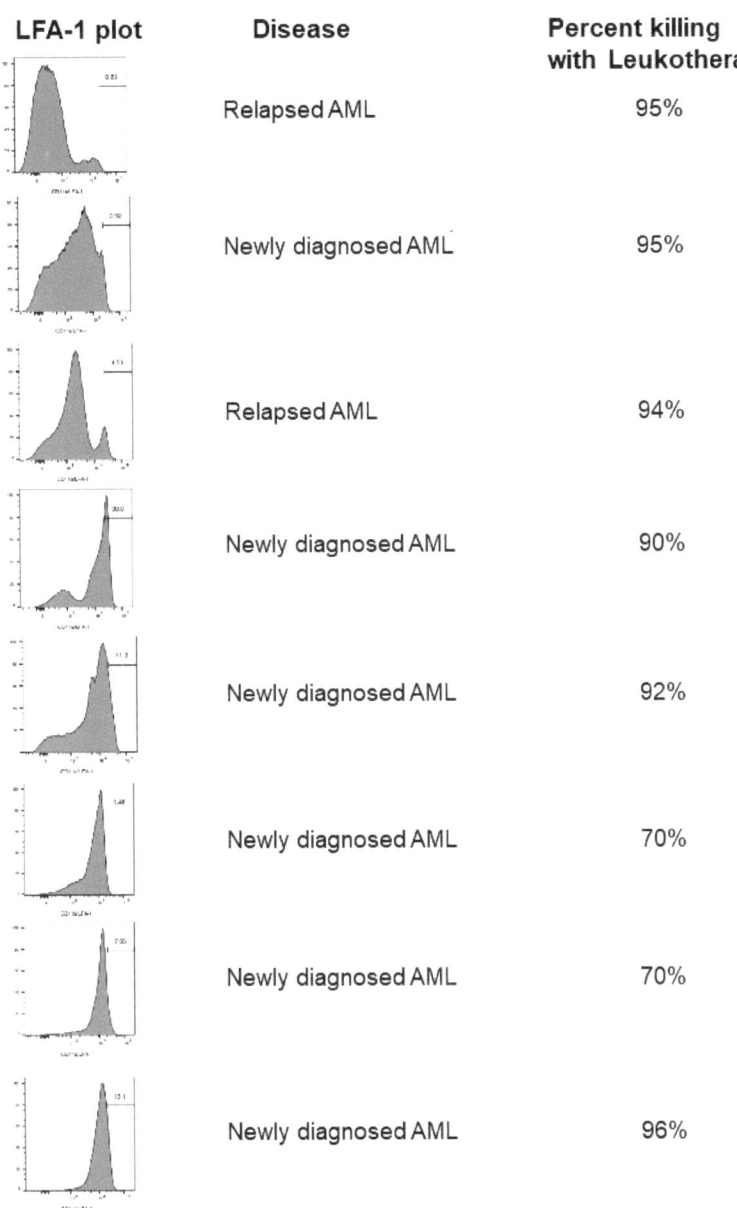	Relapsed AML	95%
	Newly diagnosed AML	95%
	Relapsed AML	94%
	Newly diagnosed AML	90%
	Newly diagnosed AML	92%
	Newly diagnosed AML	70%
	Newly diagnosed AML	70%
	Newly diagnosed AML	96%

Figure 1. LFA-1 on peripheral blood mononuclear cells (PBMCs) from AML patients. PBMC samples from patients with AML were stained with anti-CD11a antibodies and then analyzed via flow cytometry. The x-axis represents the levels of LFA-1, and the y-axis represents intensity of the peak. Cell viability was also measured in cells that had been separately treated with LtxA for 4 h. Viability was determined using the ATP-based Cell-Titer Glo Assay. Leukothera is a potential commercial name for LtxA.

3. Psoriasis

Psoriasis is the most common autoimmune disease, affecting about 2–3% of the population [42–45]. The disease presents in the form of dry, scaly skin that causes significant discomfort and itchiness for patients. The dry, patchy areas of skin, known as psoriatic plaques, are the result of keratinocytes proliferating and migrating to the surface of the skin much faster than normal, where they accumulate as a mass of cells. This enhanced proliferation and migration of skin cells is caused by proinflammatory cytokines that are secreted by over-reactive WBCs (predominantly T cells) in the underlying vasculature. Strategies to treat psoriasis include therapeutics directed against these cytokines, as well as drugs that suppress the immune system (such as steroids).

Given that LFA-1 plays a crucial role in the migration of T cells to the affected tissue in patients with psoriasis, we postulated that LtxA could be an effective strategy to eliminate the highly reactive immune cells without affecting the healthy, resting WBCs. We tested this hypothesis using a humanized mouse model for psoriasis [46]. In brief, human skin from patients with severe plaque psoriasis was grafted onto the backs of mice, and then the mice were treated with LtxA. In contrast to the vehicle control, LtxA treatment was able to essentially reverse the established disease and restore all parameters of healthy skin, including dermal and epidermal thickness, lymphocyte infiltration, and clinical psoriasis score (the visual appearance of the skin).

Further evidence that LtxA could be effective for treating inflammatory skin conditions was provided in a canine model for atopic dermatitis (AD), a common skin condition in dogs that results in extensive scratching and hair loss. Dogs with AD that were treated with a single dose of LtxA exhibited skin that was pathologically returned to health (unpublished results).

4. Allergic Asthma

Allergic asthma is a condition that is often activated by allergens such as house dust mite and pollen. The result is an accumulation of inflammatory WBCs, such as neutrophils and macrophages, in the lung tissue and the production of proinflammatory cytokines [47–51]. Since LFA-1 plays a significant role in the migration of WBCs to the lung tissue, we sought to determine if WBCs from patients with allergic asthma had higher levels of LFA-1 than those of healthy controls, as well as if LtxA could be effective in a mouse model for the disease [52].

Patients with allergic asthma exhibited WBCs that expressed significantly higher levels of LFA than those of controls. Most strikingly, these patients harbored a subpopulation of LFA-1-high, CD4-negative WBCs that was completely absent from healthy control subjects. It is possible that this unique subpopulation of cells is responsible for the over-reactive immune response in patients with allergic asthma. Furthermore, ex vivo treatment of WBCs from patients with LtxA revealed that LtxA preferentially eliminated the WBCs expressing the highest level of LFA-1, while not affecting the healthy, resting-state cells.

We evaluated LtxA in a mouse model for allergic asthma. Mice that are treated with house dust mite extract through inhalation develop pulmonary inflammation and a pathology that resembles the human condition. Most notably, a significant infiltrate of WBCs is detected in the lung sections of the mice. In the employed model, house dust mite extract treatment is administered for several weeks to allow the development of the disease. Systemic LtxA was then given to mice, and the treatment was compared to vehicle control. Mice that were treated with LtxA exhibited a significant reversal of disease based on WBC infiltrate levels in lung tissue and bronchoalveolar lavage (BAL) fluid and inflammatory cytokines in the BAL fluid. Interestingly, the WBCs in the BAL fluid expressed approximately 10-fold higher levels of LFA-1 than the WBCs in the peripheral blood, suggesting that cells migrating to the airways require LFA-1 to localize there.

5. Inflammatory Bowel Disease

Inflammatory bowel diseases (IBDs) such as Crohn's disease (CD) and ulcerative colitis are the result of an over-reactive immune system that targets the gastrointestinal tissue, resulting in inflammation and subsequent abdominal pain, bleeding, weight loss, and malnutrition [53–57]. Several studies have shown that LFA-1 plays a crucial role in the development of the disease.

Animal and human studies have shown that LFA-1 plays a critical role in the induction and progression of IBD. Multiple studies using the adoptive T-cell transfer model of chronic colitis indicated that the transfer of LFA-1 deficient T cells failed to induce chronic colitis in RAG-1$^{-/-}$ recipient mice, whereas the transfer of wild-type T cells induced severe colitis in the same immunodeficient recipients. Failure to induce colonic inflammation correlated with a significant reduction in CD3$^+$CD4$^+$ T cell numbers within the mesenteric lymph nodes (MLNs) and colonic interstitium. These data demonstrate that LFA-1 is critical for migration and/or priming within the MLN and the subsequent recruitment of these T cells into the colonic interstitium to initiate disease [58,59]. Additionally, in a dextran sodium sulfate (DSS)-induced model of colitis, the loss of LFA-1 significantly attenuated the development of disease by decreasing leukocyte infiltration and subsequent tissue damage in the intestine [60]. Furthermore, in a small open-label study with Efalizumab (anti-LFA-1 antibody), it was found that after 8 weeks of treatment, 67% of patients with moderate-to-severe refractory CD had a clinical response and 40% went into remission [61]. Collectively, these studies validate LFA-1 as a target in IBD.

We have conducted additional studies with the goal of assessing whether leukocytes derived from patients with IBD express a higher percentage of LFA-1 compared to healthy controls and whether these cells are sensitive to LtxA. We isolated PBMCs derived from healthy controls and IBD patients and assessed the percentage of PBMCs that express LFA-1 via flow cytometry (Figure 2). We found that PBMCs derived from IBD patients expressed significantly more LFA-1 compared to healthy controls (Figure 3). Furthermore, these highly expressing LFA-1 cells were sensitive to LtxA.

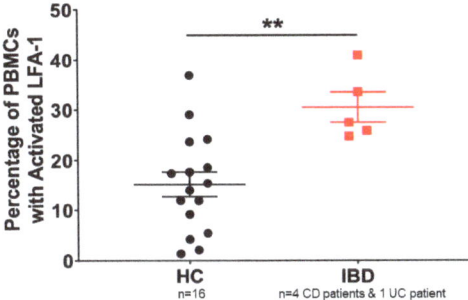

Figure 2. LFA-1 levels in PBMCs derived from healthy controls and patients with IBD. PBMCs were isolated and analyzed using anti-LFA-1 antibody and analyzed via flow cytometry. HC = healthy control; IBD = patients with Crohn's disease (CD) or ulcerative colitis (UC). ** indicates $p \leq 0.05$.

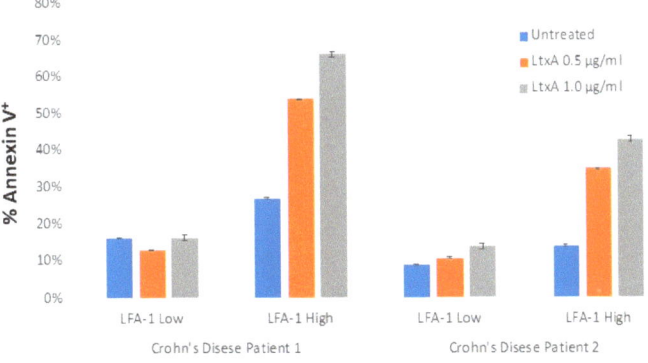

Figure 3. Sensitivity of PBMCs derived from CD patients to LtxA. PBMCs from two CD patients were treated with LtxA, and then cells were stained with anti-LFA-1 antibody (to separate high and low populations) and Annexin-V (to detect cell death).

We also carried out a study of intestinal tissue to determine if WBCs in the tissue sourced from Crohn's disease patients expressed higher levels of LFA-1 than those from non-CD patients. We found that LFA-1 staining in tissue from CD patients was significantly greater than similar tissue from non-CD patients (Figure 4). Thus, LtxA may be an effective approach to eliminate highly reactive immune cells in the GI tracts of patients suffering from IBD.

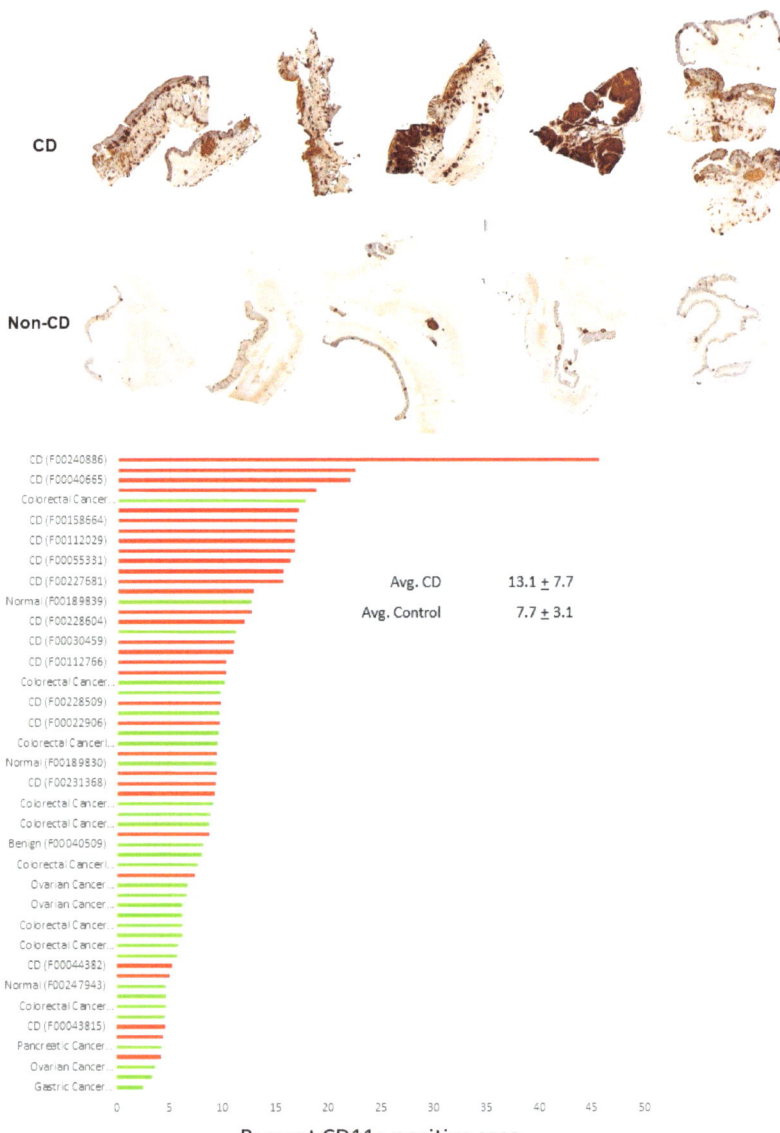

Figure 4. Immunohistochemical staining of LFA-1 on GI tissue. (**Top**) Intestinal tissue from CD patients or non-CD individuals were stained with anti-CD11a antibody and processed using immunohistochemistry. Shown are representative histological samples. (**Bottom**) The intensity of LFA-1 staining in the tissue samples was quantified as the percentage positive staining area compared to the total tissue area. Red bars represent CD samples, while green bars represent non-CD samples.

6. Conclusions

It is clear from the above review that LtxA has many ways of influencing the host response and affecting disease outcomes. In this review, we have highlighted the utility of LtxA as a therapeutic agent by modulating host immune responsiveness in a broad spectrum of immune cell diseases. It is our hope that showing this diverse efficacy can reinforce the idea that LtxA plays an important role in the disease of interest in this volume, namely periodontal disease.

Author Contributions: B.A.V. carried out studies, analyzed data, and assisted with the writing of the manuscript. S.C.K. analyzed data and wrote the manuscript. All authors have read and agreed to the published version of the manuscript.

Funding: Research for the IBD studies was funded by The Leona M. and Harry B. Helmsley Charitable Trust, grant number 1912-03606. Funding sources for the other studies noted in this manuscript are indicated in the primary literature in which the data first appeared.

Acknowledgments: We acknowledge the numerous students and staff who have conducted the studies discussed in this review.

Conflicts of Interest: SCK owns stock in the company that has licensed the use of LtxA for therapeutic applications (Actinobac). The funders had no role in the design of the study; the collection, analyses, or interpretation of data; the writing of the manuscript; or the decision to publish the results.

References

1. Haubek, D.; Ennibi, O.K.; Poulsen, K.; Vaeth, M.; Poulsen, S.; Kilian, M. Risk of aggressive periodontitis in adolescent carriers of the JP2 clone of Aggregatibacter (Actinobacillus) actinomycetemcomitans in Morocco: A prospective longitudinal cohort study. *Lancet* **2008**, *371*, 237–242. [CrossRef]
2. Lally, E.T.; Kieba, I.R.; Demuth, D.R.; Rosenbloom, J.; Golub, E.E.; Taichman, N.S.; Gibson, C.W. Identification and expression of the Actinobacillus actinomycetemcomitans leukotoxin gene. *Biochem. Biophys. Res. Commun.* **1989**, *159*, 256–262. [CrossRef]
3. Lally, E.T.; Kieba, I.R.; Sato, A.; Green, C.L.; Rosenbloom, J.; Korostoff, J.; Wang, J.F.; Shenker, B.J.; Ortlepp, S.; Robinson, M.K.; et al. RTX toxins recognize a beta2 integrin on the surface of human target cells. *J. Biol. Chem.* **1997**, *272*, 30463–30469. [CrossRef]
4. Evans, R.; Patzak, I.; Svensson, L.; De Filippo, K.; Jones, K.; McDowall, A.; Hogg, N. Integrins in immunity. *J. Cell Sci.* **2009**, *122*, 215–225. [CrossRef]
5. Hogg, N.; Harvey, J.; Cabanas, C.; Landis, R.C. Control of leukocyte integrin activation. *Am. Rev. Respir. Dis.* **1993**, *148*, S55–S59. [CrossRef]
6. Smith, A.; Stanley, P.; Jones, K.; Svensson, L.; McDowall, A.; Hogg, N. The role of the integrin LFA-1 in T-lymphocyte migration. *Immunol. Rev.* **2007**, *218*, 135–146. [CrossRef]
7. Tsai, C.C.; McArthur, W.P.; Baehni, P.C.; Hammond, B.F.; Taichman, N.S. Extraction and partial characterization of a leukotoxin from a plaque-derived Gram-negative microorganism. *Infect. Immun.* **1979**, *25*, 427–439. [CrossRef]
8. Tsai, C.C.; Shenker, B.J.; DiRienzo, J.M.; Malamud, D.; Taichman, N.S. Extraction and isolation of a leukotoxin from Actinobacillus actinomycetemcomitans with polymyxin B. *Infect. Immun.* **1984**, *43*, 700–705. [CrossRef]
9. DiRienzo, J.M.; Tsai, C.C.; Shenker, B.J.; Taichman, N.S.; Lally, E.T. Monoclonal antibodies to leukotoxin of Actinobacillus actinomycetemcomitans. *Infect. Immun.* **1985**, *47*, 31–36. [CrossRef]
10. Lally, E.T.; Golub, E.E.; Kieba, I.R.; Taichman, N.S.; Decker, S.; Berthold, P.; Gibson, C.W.; Demuth, D.R.; Rosenbloom, J. Structure and function of the B and D genes of the Actinobacillus actinomycetemcomitans leukotoxin complex. *Microb. Pathog.* **1991**, *11*, 111–121. [CrossRef]
11. Kachlany, S.C.; Fine, D.H.; Figurski, D.H. Secretion of RTX leukotoxin by Actinobacillus actinomycetemcomitans. *Infect. Immun.* **2000**, *68*, 6094–6100. [CrossRef]
12. Kachlany, S.C.; Fine, D.H.; Figurski, D.H. Purification of secreted leukotoxin (LtxA) from Actinobacillus actinomycetemcomitans. *Protein Expr. Purif.* **2002**, *25*, 465–471. [CrossRef]
13. Berthold, P.; Forti, D.; Kieba, I.R.; Rosenbloom, J.; Taichman, N.S.; Lally, E.T. Electron immunocytochemical localization of Actinobacillus actinomycetemcomitans leukotoxin. *Oral Microbiol. Immunol.* **1992**, *7*, 24–27. [CrossRef]
14. Kato, S.; Kowashi, Y.; Demuth, D.R. Outer membrane-like vesicles secreted by Actinobacillus actinomycetemcomitans are enriched in leukotoxin. *Microb. Pathog.* **2002**, *32*, 1–13. [CrossRef]
15. Ohta, H.; Kato, K.; Kokeguchi, S.; Hara, H.; Fukui, K.; Murayama, Y. Nuclease-sensitive binding of an Actinobacillus actinomycetemcomitans leukotoxin to the bacterial cell surface. *Infect. Immun.* **1991**, *59*, 4599–4605. [CrossRef]
16. Hogg, N.; Smith, A.; McDowall, A.; Giles, K.; Stanley, P.; Laschinger, M.; Henderson, R. How T cells use LFA-1 to attach and migrate. *Immunol. Lett.* **2004**, *92*, 51–54. [CrossRef]

17. Giblin, P.A.; Lemieux, R.M. LFA-1 as a key regulator of immune function: Approaches toward the development of LFA-1-based therapeutics. *Curr. Pharm. Des.* **2006**, *12*, 2771–2795. [CrossRef]

18. Ma, Q.; Shimaoka, M.; Lu, C.; Jing, H.; Carman, C.V.; Springer, T.A. Activation-induced conformational changes in the I domain region of lymphocyte function-associated antigen 1. *J. Biol. Chem.* **2002**, *277*, 10638–10641. [CrossRef]

19. Dransfield, I.; Cabanas, C.; Barrett, J.; Hogg, N. Interaction of leukocyte integrins with ligand is necessary but not sufficient for function. *J. Cell Biol.* **1992**, *116*, 1527–1535. [CrossRef] [PubMed]

20. Dransfield, I.; Cabanas, C.; Craig, A.; Hogg, N. Divalent cation regulation of the function of the leukocyte integrin LFA-1. *J. Cell Biol.* **1992**, *116*, 219–226. [CrossRef] [PubMed]

21. Porter, J.C.; Bracke, M.; Smith, A.; Davies, D.; Hogg, N. Signaling through integrin LFA-1 leads to filamentous actin polymerization and remodeling, resulting in enhanced T cell adhesion. *J. Immunol.* **2002**, *168*, 6330–6335. [CrossRef] [PubMed]

22. Hioe, C.E.; Tuen, M.; Vasiliver-Shamis, G.; Alvarez, Y.; Prins, K.C.; Banerjee, S.; Nadas, A.; Cho, M.W.; Dustin, M.L.; Kachlany, S.C. HIV envelope gp120 activates LFA-1 on CD4 T-lymphocytes and increases cell susceptibility to LFA-1-targeting leukotoxin (LtxA). *PLoS ONE* **2011**, *6*, e23202. [CrossRef] [PubMed]

23. Kachlany, S.C.; Schwartz, A.B.; Balashova, N.V.; Hioe, C.E.; Tuen, M.; Le, A.; Kaur, M.; Mei, Y.; Rao, J. Anti-leukemia activity of a bacterial toxin with natural specificity for LFA-1 on white blood cells. *Leuk. Res.* **2010**, *34*, 777–785. [CrossRef] [PubMed]

24. DiFranco, K.M.; Gupta, A.; Galusha, L.E.; Perez, J.; Nguyen, T.V.; Fineza, C.D.; Kachlany, S.C. Leukotoxin (Leukothera(R)) targets active leukocyte function antigen-1 (LFA-1) protein and triggers a lysosomal mediated cell death pathway. *J. Biol. Chem.* **2012**, *287*, 17618–17627. [CrossRef] [PubMed]

25. DiFranco, K.M.; Kaswala, R.H.; Patel, C.; Kasinathan, C.; Kachlany, S.C. Leukotoxin kills rodent WBC by targeting leukocyte function associated antigen 1. *Comp. Med.* **2013**, *63*, 331–337. [PubMed]

26. Kaur, M.; Kachlany, S.C. Aggregatibacter actinomycetemcomitans leukotoxin (LtxA; Leukothera) induces cofilin dephosphorylation and actin depolymerization during killing of malignant monocytes. *Microbiology* **2014**, *160*, 2443–2452. [CrossRef] [PubMed]

27. DiFranco, K.M.; Johnson-Farley, N.; Bertino, J.R.; Elson, D.; Vega, B.A.; Belinka, B.A., Jr.; Kachlany, S.C. LFA-1-targeting Leukotoxin (LtxA; Leukothera(R)) causes lymphoma tumor regression in a humanized mouse model and requires caspase-8 and Fas to kill malignant lymphocytes. *Leuk. Res.* **2015**, *39*, 649–656. [CrossRef] [PubMed]

28. Vega, B.A.; Schober, L.T.; Kim, T.; Belinka, B.A., Jr.; Kachlany, S.C. Aggregatibacter actinomycetemcomitans leukotoxin (LtxA; Leukothera(R)) requires death receptor Fas, in addition to LFA-1, to trigger cell death in T lymphocytes. *Infect. Immun.* **2019**, *87*, 10–1128. [CrossRef] [PubMed]

29. Prince, D.J.; Patel, D.; Kachlany, S.C. Leukotoxin (LtxA/Leukothera) induces ATP expulsion via pannexin-1 channels and subsequent cell death in malignant lymphocytes. *Sci. Rep.* **2021**, *11*, 18086. [CrossRef]

30. Hasegawa, Y.; Yokono, K.; Taki, T.; Amano, K.; Tominaga, Y.; Yoneda, R.; Yagi, N.; Maeda, S.; Yagita, H.; Okumura, K.; et al. Prevention of autoimmune insulin-dependent diabetes in non-obese diabetic mice by anti-LFA-1 and anti-ICAM-1 mAb. *Int. Immunol.* **1994**, *6*, 831–838. [CrossRef]

31. McMurray, R.W. Adhesion molecules in autoimmune disease. *Semin. Arthritis Rheum.* **1996**, *25*, 215–233. [CrossRef] [PubMed]

32. Yokomori, H.; Oda, M.; Yoshimura, K.; Nomura, M.; Ogi, M.; Wakabayashi, G.; Kitajima, M.; Ishii, H. Expression of intercellular adhesion molecule-1 and lymphocyte function-associated antigen-1 protein and messenger RNA in primary biliary cirrhosis. *Intern. Med.* **2003**, *42*, 947–954. [CrossRef] [PubMed]

33. Connolly, M.K.; Kitchens, E.A.; Chan, B.; Jardieu, P.; Wofsy, D. Treatment of murine lupus with monoclonal antibodies to lymphocyte function-associated antigen-1: Dose-dependent inhibition of autoantibody production and blockade of the immune response to therapy. *Clin. Immunol. Immunopathol.* **1994**, *72*, 198–203. [CrossRef] [PubMed]

34. Elovaara, I.; Lalla, M.; Spare, E.; Lehtimaki, T.; Dastidar, P. Methylprednisolone reduces adhesion molecules in blood and cerebrospinal fluid in patients with MS. *Neurology* **1998**, *51*, 1703–1708. [CrossRef]

35. Engelhardt, B. Molecular mechanisms involved in T cell migration across the blood-brain barrier. *J. Neural Transm.* **2006**, *113*, 477–485. [CrossRef] [PubMed]

36. Thomson, A.W.; Satoh, S.; Nussler, A.K.; Tamura, K.; Woo, J.; Gavaler, J.; van Thiel, D.H. Circulating intercellular adhesion molecule-1 (ICAM-1) in autoimmune liver disease and evidence for the production of ICAM-1 by cytokine-stimulated human hepatocytes. *Clin. Exp. Immunol.* **1994**, *95*, 83–90. [CrossRef] [PubMed]

37. Yusuf-Makagiansar, H.; Anderson, M.E.; Yakovleva, T.V.; Murray, J.S.; Siahaan, T.J. Inhibition of LFA-1/ICAM-1 and VLA-4/VCAM-1 as a therapeutic approach to inflammation and autoimmune diseases. *Med. Res. Rev.* **2002**, *22*, 146–167. [CrossRef]

38. Aureli, A.; Marziani, B.; Venditti, A.; Sconocchia, T.; Sconocchia, G. Acute Lymphoblastic Leukemia Immunotherapy Treatment: Now, Next, and Beyond. *Cancers* **2023**, *15*, 3346. [CrossRef]

39. Eisfeld, A.K. Disparities in acute myeloid leukemia treatments and outcomes. *Curr. Opin. Hematol.* **2024**, *31*, 58–63. [CrossRef]

40. Mikhael, J.; Cichewicz, A.; Mearns, E.S.; Girvan, A.; Pierre, V.; Rawashdh, N.A.; Yellow-Duke, A.; Cornell, R.F.; Nixon, M. Overall Survival in Patients with Multiple Myeloma in the U.S.: A Systematic Literature Review of Racial Disparities. *Clin. Lymphoma Myeloma Leuk.* **2024**, *24*, e1–e12. [CrossRef]

41. Schimmoeller, C.J.; Bastian, C.; Fleming, J.; Morales, J. A Review of Hodgkin Lymphoma in the Era of Checkpoint Inhibitors. *Cureus* **2023**, *15*, e41660. [CrossRef] [PubMed]

42.	Afvari, S.; Beck, T.C.; Kazlouskaya, M.; Afrahim, R.; Valdebran, M. Diet, sleep, and exercise in inflammatory skin diseases. *Our Dermatol. Online* **2023**, *14*, 430–435. [CrossRef]
43.	Bhagwat, A.P.; Madke, B. The Current Advancement in Psoriasis. *Cureus* **2023**, *15*, e47006. [CrossRef]
44.	Lie, E.; Choi, M.; Wang, S.P.; Eichenfield, L.F. Topical Management of Pediatric Psoriasis: A Review of New Developments and Existing Therapies. *Paediatr. Drugs* **2024**, *26*, 9–18. [CrossRef] [PubMed]
45.	Reali, E.; Ferrari, D. From the Skin to Distant Sites: T Cells in Psoriatic Disease. *Int. J. Mol. Sci.* **2023**, *24*, 15707. [CrossRef]
46.	Stenderup, K.; Rosada, C.; Dam, T.N.; Salerno, E.; Belinka, B.A.; Kachlany, S.C. Resolution of psoriasis by a leukocyte-targeting bacterial protein in a humanized mouse model. *J. Investig. Dermatol.* **2011**, *131*, 2033–2039. [CrossRef] [PubMed]
47.	Dunn, J.L.M.; Rothenberg, M.E. 2021 year in review: Spotlight on eosinophils. *J. Allergy Clin. Immunol.* **2022**, *149*, 517–524. [CrossRef]
48.	Kim, Y.M.; Kim, Y.S.; Jeon, S.G.; Kim, Y.K. Immunopathogenesis of allergic asthma: More than the th2 hypothesis. *Allergy Asthma Immunol. Res.* **2013**, *5*, 189–196. [CrossRef]
49.	Matos-Semedo, F.; Cruz, C.; Inacio, F.; Gama, J.M.R.; Nwaru, B.I.; Taborda-Barata, L. House dust mite (HDM) and storage mite (SM) molecular sensitisation profiles and association with clinical outcomes in allergic asthma and rhinitis: Protocol for a systematic review. *BMJ Open* **2021**, *11*, e046519. [CrossRef]
50.	Medeleanu, M.V.; Qian, Y.C.; Moraes, T.J.; Subbarao, P. Early-immune development in asthma: A review of the literature. *Cell. Immunol.* **2023**, *393*, 104770. [CrossRef]
51.	Woloski, J.R.; Heston, S.; Escobedo Calderon, S.P. Respiratory Allergic Disorders. *Prim. Care* **2016**, *43*, 401–415. [CrossRef] [PubMed]
52.	Gupta, A.; Espinosa, V.; Galusha, L.E.; Rahimian, V.; Miro, K.L.; Rivera-Medina, A.; Kasinathan, C.; Capitle, E.; Aguila, H.A.; Kachlany, S.C. Expression and targeting of lymphocyte function-associated antigen 1 (LFA-1) on white blood cells for treatment of allergic asthma. *J. Leukoc. Biol.* **2015**, *97*, 439–446. [CrossRef]
53.	Abdulla, M.; Mohammed, N. A Review on Inflammatory Bowel Diseases: Recent Molecular Pathophysiology Advances. *Biol. Targets Ther.* **2022**, *16*, 129–140. [CrossRef]
54.	Imbrizi, M.; Magro, F.; Coy, C.S.R. Pharmacological Therapy in Inflammatory Bowel Diseases: A Narrative Review of the Past 90 Years. *Pharmaceuticals* **2023**, *16*, 1272. [CrossRef]
55.	Khan, S.; Sebastian, S.A.; Parmar, M.P.; Ghadge, N.; Padda, I.; Keshta, A.S.; Minhaz, N.; Patel, A. Factors influencing the quality of life in inflammatory bowel disease: A comprehensive review. *Dis. Mon.* **2023**, *70*, 101672. [CrossRef]
56.	Mihai, I.R.; Burlui, A.M.; Rezus, I.I.; Mihai, C.; Macovei, L.A.; Cardoneanu, A.; Gavrilescu, O.; Dranga, M.; Rezus, E. Inflammatory Bowel Disease as a Paradoxical Reaction to Anti-TNF-alpha Treatment-A Review. *Life* **2023**, *13*, 1779. [CrossRef]
57.	Sousa, P.; Bertani, L.; Rodrigues, C. Management of inflammatory bowel disease in the elderly: A review. *Dig. Liver Dis.* **2023**, *55*, 1001–1009. [CrossRef] [PubMed]
58.	Ostanin, D.V.; Furr, K.L.; Pavlick, K.P.; Gray, L.; Kevil, C.G.; Shukla, D.; D'Souza, D.; Hoffman, J.M.; Grisham, M.B. T cell-associated CD18 but not CD62L, ICAM-1, or PSGL-1 is required for the induction of chronic colitis. *Am. J. Physiol. Gastrointest. Liver Physiol.* **2007**, *292*, G1706–G1714. [CrossRef] [PubMed]
59.	Pavlick, K.P.; Ostanin, D.V.; Furr, K.L.; Laroux, F.S.; Brown, C.M.; Gray, L.; Kevil, C.G.; Grisham, M.B. Role of T-cell-associated lymphocyte function-associated antigen-1 in the pathogenesis of experimental colitis. *Int. Immunol.* **2006**, *18*, 389–398. [CrossRef]
60.	Abdelbaqi, M.; Chidlow, J.H.; Matthews, K.M.; Pavlick, K.P.; Barlow, S.C.; Linscott, A.J.; Grisham, M.B.; Fowler, M.R.; Kevil, C.G. Regulation of dextran sodium sulfate induced colitis by leukocyte beta 2 integrins. *Lab. Investig. A J. Tech. Methods Pathol.* **2006**, *86*, 380–390. [CrossRef]
61.	James, D.G.; Seo, D.H.; Chen, J.; Vemulapalli, C.; Stone, C.D. Efalizumab, a human monoclonal anti-CD11a antibody, in the treatment of moderate to severe Crohn's Disease: An open-label pilot study. *Dig. Dis. Sci.* **2011**, *56*, 1806–1810. [CrossRef] [PubMed]

MDPI AG
Grosspeteranlage 5
4052 Basel
Switzerland
Tel.: +41 61 683 77 34

Pathogens Editorial Office
E-mail: pathogens@mdpi.com
www.mdpi.com/journal/pathogens

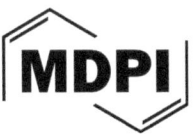

www.ingramcontent.com/pod-product-compliance
Lightning Source LLC
LaVergne TN
LVHW072341090526
838202LV00019B/2456